INTEGRATED CARE PATHWAYS
IN MENTAL HEALTH

Commissioning Editor: Steven Black
Development Editor: Catherine Jackson
Project Manager: Elouise Ball
Designer: George Ajayi
Illustration Manager: Bruce Hogarth

INTEGRATED CARE PATHWAYS IN MENTAL HEALTH

Editors

Julie Hall RMN BSc(Hons) MSc PGCAP MA

Head of Performance and Administration Forensic Services Directorate, Nottinghamshire Healthcare NHS Trust, Rampton Hospital, Retford, Nottinghamshire

David Howard MEd PhD RMN RGN CertEd DipN

Senior Mental Health Lecturer and Director MSc Organisational Leadership in Health and Social Care, The University of Nottingham, Nottingham

Foreword by

Antony Sheehan DSci MPhil BEd(Hons) RN DipHSM CertEd(FE) HMFPHM

Director of Care Services, Department of Health; Professor of Health and Social Care Strategy, University of Central Lancashire

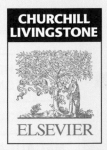

CHURCHILL LIVINGSTONE

ELSEVIER

Edinburgh London New York Oxford Philadelphia St Louis Sydney Toronto 2006

CHURCHILL
LIVINGSTONE
ELSEVIER

First published 2006

ISBN 0 443 10172 8
ISBN 13: 978 0443 101724

British Library Cataloguing in Publication Data
A catalogue record for this book is available from the British Library

Library of Congress Cataloging in Publication Data
A catalog record for this book is available from the Library of Congress

Notice
Knowledge and best practice in this field are constantly changing. As new research and experience broaden our knowledge, changes in practice, treatment and drug therapy may become necessary or appropriate. Readers are advised to check the most current information provided (i) on procedures featured or (ii) by the manufacturer of each product to be administered, to verify the recommended dose or formula, the method and duration of administration, and contraindications. It is the responsibility of the practitioner, relying on their own experience and knowledge of the patient, to make diagnoses, to determine dosages and the best treatment for each individual patient, and to take all appropriate safety precautions. To the fullest extent of the law, neither the publisher nor the editors assumes any liability for any injury and/or damage.

The Publisher

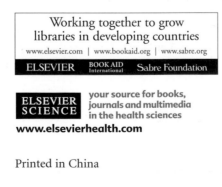

Working together to grow
libraries in developing countries
www.elsevier.com | www.bookaid.org | www.sabre.org

ELSEVIER   BOOK AID International   Sabre Foundation

ELSEVIER SCIENCE   your source for books, journals and multimedia in the health sciences
www.elsevierhealth.com

Printed in China

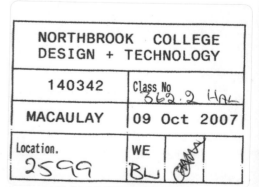

Contents

Contributors

Joanna Chave BA(Hons) RMN DipThorn
Nurse Manager, Rehabilitation Day Services, Rotherham, Yorkshire.

Jeannette Connolly BA(Hons) Adv Dip(PTSD) DipN RMN
Senior Crisis Resolution Worker, Crisis Resolution and Home Treatment Service, Sycamore Assessment Unit Grantham, Lincolnshire.

Mark Fleming BSc Dip RMN
Clinical Development Manager, NHS Ayrshire and Arran, Ayrshire Central Hospital, Irvine.

Angus Forsyth MSc BA RMN RGN PGCE ENB650
Nurse Consultant, Acute In-Patient Services, Newcastle North Tyneside & Northumberland NHS Trust, Newcastle-upon-Tyne.

Barrie Green MA(Crim) BA(Hons)(Forensic) DipMDO RMN
Forensic Nurse Consultant, Humber Centre for Forensic Psychiatry, Humber Mental Health Teaching NHS Trust, Hull.

Julie Hall RMN BSc(Hons) MSc PGCAP MA
Head of Performance and Administration Forensic Services Directorate, Nottinghamshire Healthcare NHS Trust, Rampton Hospital, Retford, Nottinghamshire

David Howard MEd PhD RMN RGN CertEd DipN
Director MSc Organisational Leadership in Health and Social Care, The University of Nottingham, Nottingham

Ashley Irons BA(Hons)
Mental Health Partner, Capsticks Solicitors, 77–83 Upper Richmond Street London SW15 2TT

Carol Jackson RN DipHE BSc(Hons) MSc
Integrated Care Pathway Co-ordinator, Cherry Valley Mental Health Services, Downshire Hospital, Downpatrick.

Karen J. Jenkins BSc(Hons) PhD CertMgmt(Open)
Clinical Effectiveness Integrated Care Pathway Coordinator, Greater Glasgow Primary Care Division, Gartnavel Royal Hospital, Glasgow, formerly Clinical Effectiveness Facilitator for Integrated Care Pathways, The State Hospital, Carstairs, Lanark.

Julie Lambert RMN Dip(Child and Adolescent Mental Health Nursing) Tier 1 Worker in Community
Primary Mental Health Nurse, Lincolnshire Partnership NHS Trust, Lincolnshire

Richard Oldham RN
Acting Clinical Team Leader, Lincolnshire Partnership NHS Trust, Lincolnshire

Ruth E. Page RMN BSc MSc
Product Manager, IDX Systems UK Ltd, London

Jon Painter BSc(Hons) RMN Thorn BMedSc(Hons)
Integrated Care Pathways Manager, Doncaster and South Humber Healthcare NHS Trust, Yorkshire

Malcolm Peet MBCHb FRCPsych
Consultant Psychiatrist, Doncaster and South Humber NHS Trust; Professor Associate, School of Health and Related Research, University of Sheffield, Sheffield.

Alan Pringle RGN RMN BSc(Hons)
Health Lecturer (Mental Health), University of Nottingham, Mansfield Education Centre, Nottinghamshire.

Marie Rawdon DipNursing(Mental Health)
Community Nurse Specialist/ Foster Carer Support Worker, Sleaford, Lincolnshire.

Adrian Roberts BA(Hons) PgDINF
National Pathways Coordinator, BUPA Hospitals Researcher, Clifford Price Associates

Rafael Sorribas DipHighEd
Health Informatics Development Manager, Buckinghamshire and Oxfordshire Mental Health NHS Trusts, Oxford.

Susan Wakefield MA ARQE PG Cert AdvDip(Counselling) RMN
Senior Lecturer in Mental Health Nursing, Faculty of Health and Well-Being, Sheffield Hallam University, Sheffield.

Simon Wood MB ChB MMedSc FRCPsych
Clinical Director, Humber Centre for Forensic Psychiatry, Humber Mental Health Teaching NHS Trust, Hull

Foreword

As health and social care organisations respond to the current mental health modernisation agenda, the use of integrated care pathways is growing rapidly. Care pathways, which detail the expected multidisciplinary interventions within a care experience and use variances to monitor care and quality, have been emerging throughout UK mental health services over the last few years. Although they are advocated within health policy, their introduction has been generally unco-ordinated. The idea of this book arose from the dearth of accessible information about integrated care pathways in mental health within the UK. This book is thus a timely gathering together of the recent developments in this field in which the authors combine discussion of relevant and developing theory with accounts of real-time developments in practice.

Integrated care pathways have strong relationships with many of the contemporary drivers that underpin the delivery of mental health services. They are advocated as a means of ensuring consistent, evidence-based, high-quality care and are integral to the modernisation process to ensure that care experiences are built around the needs of service users, their families and carers.

Providing the background of integrated care pathways in mental health, and of their implementation, the opening chapters of this book introduce the theories of integrated care pathways in order to give insight to readers who are new to the concept, and to develop more experienced users' understanding of the professional, legal and political issues that surround their development.

From this base, the second part of the book details the development of integrated care pathways in the major areas of mental health practice. It is intended for this book to be used as a resource by health and social care teams and to facilitate this, case studies of current mental health care pathways are included within each chapter. These focus on describing the process of developing the integrated care pathway, illustrating the main challenges and identifying the benefits of its implementation. These accounts 'bring alive' the process of developing and implementing an integrated care pathway and offer insights to others who are planning to undertake such an endeavour.

This combination of knowledgeable discussion and the credible experience of each author ensures this is an innovative text which will be of great value to those who are challenged with developing mental health care services within an inclusive environment. There is a wealth of evidence in this book to suggest that integrated care pathways are able to support philosophies that place service users and carers at the centre of the care process, yet define clearly the roles and responsibilities of the supporting services.

Securing high standards is a challenge faced by all healthcare providers. This book then is a valuable resource for managers and practitioners to develop and provide evidence of quality mental health services within their own areas of practice.

An introduction to mental health integrated care pathways

Julie Hall and David Howard

INTEGRATED CARE PATHWAYS – A DEFINITION

THE PROVENANCE OF INTEGRATED CARE
PATHWAYS

DEVELOPMENTS IN THE UNITED KINGDOM

QUALITY AND GOVERNANCE

THE CONCEPTUAL FRAMEWORK

BENEFITS AND LIMITATIONS

A MODEL OF ICP DEVELOPMENT

SERVICE USER AND CARER INVOLVEMENT
AND EXPERIENCE

INTEGRATED CARE PATHWAY CONTENT

WORKING ON AN INTEGRATED CARE PATHWAY
PROGRAMME

ICP PROGRAMME AIM

EVALUATION

REFERENCES

INTEGRATED CARE PATHWAYS – A DEFINITION

Over recent years the term 'care pathway' has been used in a variety of ways with various intentions. It has been used to describe various concepts from guidelines and protocols to general descriptions of a patient's journey or high-level process maps of services and processes of care. Consequently it has become difficult to interpret the expression 'integrated care pathway' in a consistent way. In response to this ambiguity, it is therefore important to define clearly what an integrated care pathway actually is, both within this text, and in relation to other literature.

Most definitions agree that an integrated care pathway is a multi-professional plan of care that provides detailed guidance for each stage in the care of a patient with a specific condition, over a given period of time (Riley 1998). The pathway exists as all or part of the clinical documentation, mapping what should be done, when, and by whom, and predicting the time and type of response. Any deviation from this plan is subsequently documented as a variance and forms the basis of the evaluation of effectiveness of the interventions made. In turn, this information forms the basis of both day-to-day monitoring and periodic analysis for quality improvement. A care pathway thus spans an episode of care for a defined patient group. It documents the anticipated evidence based on multi-professional care (including investigations, interventions, activities, assessments etc.) required to achieve agreed outcomes. This differentiates integrated care pathways from protocols, guidelines and process maps, particularly since the latter cases are rarely used as part of the patient record, to track the care given or to monitor variance on a concurrent basis.

While integrated care pathways were ideally suited to areas with clearly defined symptom management, the ambiguity of presentations within mental health made the application of pathway frameworks more obscure. To help to clarify definitions of integrated care pathways in mental health, a subgroup of the National Pathways Association (NPA) in 1999 established generic criteria for care pathways. This group collated a collection of care pathways that had been used in mental health to enable them to be available to others as reference material. A standard set of criteria was developed to ensure that the material intended for this library was indeed integrated care pathways and not something else and, following a period of consultation and refinement, this was developed into a composite model for care pathways (Box 1.1).

Although these criteria are several years old, they remain valid in their contribution to understanding the concept of integrated care pathways. Indeed, the clarity this framework provides will assist the reader to analyse the characteristics of integrated care pathways in the examples that are given in the chapters in the second part of this book.

THE PROVENANCE OF INTEGRATED CARE PATHWAYS

The origins of Integrated Care Pathways (ICPs) arise from the insurance-based United States (US) healthcare system. They were originally developed in an attempt to improve the effectiveness without compromising quality. Dykes (1998) describes how ICPs are part of the US managed mental healthcare system, focusing upon careful design of the care process and reducing costs whilst still achieving outcomes.

US mental healthcare teams began to experiment with ICPs in the early 1980s. One notable centre of this activity was the New England Medical Center in Boston headed by Karen Zander. At this time the US government was in the process of reducing state healthcare spending and had capped the revenues related to inpatient cases. This corresponded with the introduction of diagnosis-related reimbursement and the introduction of set rates for Medicare patients. Subsequently, all payers for health care became cost-conscious consumers.

Zander led a multi-professional team with a remit to develop mental health specific pathways. A major premise that underpinned the team's philosophy was that the misuse of nursing care and technology increased the cost of hospitalisation and technology. Following initial trials they believed that ICPs would focus activities on interventions that contributed most to the desired outcomes. In turn, this approach limited the costs of unnecessary technology and reduced the patient's length of stay, without compromising outcomes (Zander 1998).

Box 1.1 CRITERIA FOR CARE PATHWAYS (adapted from Mental Health Subgroup 1999)

A care pathway should meet the following criteria:

1. The pathway is for a specific condition, process or patient group (i.e. diagnosis, symptom or need) and includes the interventions detailing expected care.
2. The pathway has identified start and finish points.
3. Not all pathways have a physical matrix appearance but are structured on the concept of having two axes: one based on time or stages of care, and the other on interventions, goals or standards.
4. Outcomes, goals or aims are identified. Where appropriate, these should be agreed with the service users and their carers.
5. It is used as all or part of the clinical record, and in most cases includes multi-professional input.
6. The pathway is a tool for the clinician, and/or users/carers, in making decisions about the agreed care.
7. There is the ability to track actual care given against care that is planned.
8. The pathway records any variance from the pathway and the associated reasons for this.
9. The pathway document should comply with standards for record keeping. It must include the date that it was developed and the date of review.
10. There should be evidence of accountability for recorded clinical care.
11. Relevant guidelines and/or protocols are incorporated within the care pathway.
12. Outcomes, goals or aims can be for the patient to achieve, or for the staff to achieve on behalf of the patient, or may be process outcomes (i.e. administrative procedure).
13. The care pathway is a tool for identifying where decisions about care and treatment are being made, and when it is appropriate to include the patient and/or carer in that process.
14. The ability to track care given can be separate from the ability to track care that is planned. Tracking assists with the management of both the individual patient and groups of patients. It is also used for audit and review, and other analytical purposes.
15. Having a place to record variation on the care pathway meets the basic level of expectation. But a more detailed care pathway will provide specific information about the process, and identify why there is variance and/or action taken in response to this.

Unsurprisingly however, these changes were the target for several critics. Sack (1996) and Glazer (1997), both medical directors, asserted that there would be negative consequences for patient privacy, therapeutic relationships and care standards. It was claimed that a lack of agreed care guidelines, outcome measures and decision support tools would leave professional care at the mercy of administrators and profit makers. While the empirical basis for pathway development was to curtail unnecessary admission and reduce variation in treatment programmes, there were concerns over the reduction in length of stay, and the unpredictable course of mental health problems. Consequently, it was even argued that this managed care approach would be unsuitable for the philosophy of mental health care. Nevertheless, as organisations became focused upon outcomes, quality measurement and attempts to quantify care, ICPs increasingly became featured as the tool of choice. Use of ICPs (or critical pathways as they are often termed in the US) became more widespread and investigation of variations that related to patient outcomes and service providers' expectations became commonplace. Evidence began to emerge that using ICPs for inpatient mental health care meant lengths of stay were reduced significantly and that for the first time clinical outcomes were associated with diagnosis, outcome measures for each patient, and all underpinned by processes that included quality management reporting (Dykes 1998).

DEVELOPMENTS IN THE UNITED KINGDOM

During the 1990s the use of ICPs began to grow in the United Kingdom (UK), predominantly within the area of acute general medicine. However, UK mental health services became aware of the potential benefits of ICPs. A significant commentator on their adoption in the UK has been Adrian Jones, who has worked in developing and implementing an ICP for service users experiencing psychosis, and has published a series of papers examining the concept of ICPs and their application within UK mental health services (Jones 1996, 1997, 1999). There are significant social and political differences between health care in the US and UK, and in these papers Jones questioned whether the espoused benefits of ICPs could be transferred simply. He forecasted that because of these differences it was likely that even experienced teams in the UK would struggle with the task of developing ICPs. Nevertheless, he identified the benefits of ICPs as role clarification, improved decision-making and increased achievement of clinical outcomes. It became recognised that using ICPs meant that care processes could be easily audited, and variations could be identified and possibly rectified.

It is precisely their ability to standardise and monitor care that led to a considerable uptake of ICPs within contemporary practice in the NHS, a transformation that in a large part was led by the modernisation agenda and associated clinical governance targets. However, it was not until the late 1990s that ICP development in mental health gathered pace in the UK. Here, ICPs were developed both along process-orientated lines, based upon the systems that contribute to the patient journey, and for particular diagnostic groups (Browning & Hollingberry 2000, Hall 2004) and by the year 2000 several trusts were describing various care pathways in use for several mental health diagnostic groups. Due to the esoteric presentation of mental illnesses however, it was difficult to align the development of ICPs with the individualised nature of mental health experiences; therefore various strategies were adopted to ensure that individualisation could still be possible alongside managing care using an ICP.

In contrast to the fiscal-led US system, the drivers for the development in the UK were generally focused upon clinical governance and the implementation of evidence-based practice (Browning & Hollingberry 2000). Furthermore, it was noticeable that development in the UK included service user and carer involvement whilst trying to ensure that the aspirations of the organisation were also incorporated. The information from ICPs thus enabled service users and carers to understand more fully what would be made available to them, promoting more choice. This is a very different impression from earlier themes of restricted patient autonomy and choice (Bryant 1999).

The esoteric nature of mental illness presentations, however, has required a move away from specific illness-focused pathways. In their development of ICPs, Wakefield & Peet (2003) use a method that joins small, discrete processes together. For example, by combining a pre-admission ICP for psychosis with an admission ICP, a psychosis treatment ICP and a discharge ICP, an individualised package is formed to span the patient journey.

Wakefield & Peet (2003) used opportunities to develop ICPs in new services where the historical or cultural issues experienced by Jones were not so profound. It was believed that communicating with staff and their involvement in ICP development contributed to their support and engagement for implementation. Wakefield & Peet (2003) concluded that in their experience ICPs have been useful for focusing on technical procedures and activities. However, they caution that it is easy to overlook the human and interpersonal elements of mental health. It is therefore important, when developing ICPs, to incorporate mechanisms that ensure these more human processes are included.

QUALITY AND GOVERNANCE

As pathways involve some degree of standardisation, service users can expect at least equitable treatment and rising standards. It is important to realise though that a pathway only documents minimum standards. Even so, ensuring a minimum standard may indeed improve upon past experiences characterised by lack of contact and active intervention. Several authors also propose that an increase in multi-professional collaboration resulting from the care pathway approach to working leads to an increase in patient satisfaction (Mosher et al 1992, Petryshen & Petryshen 1992, Tucci & Bartels 1998). However, often studies do not adopt any formal methodology to measure correlation between pathway use and a subsequent increase in patient satisfaction. Many evaluative studies are retrospective in nature and therefore the administration of patient satisfaction surveys as a means of measuring improvement is impractical. A notable exception is Stead et al's (1995) study of a surgical pathway which showed a 12% increase in patient satisfaction over two clinical areas following implementation. Unfortunately the low response rate (33%) limits the impact of the study's findings. Examples of reviews of service users' satisfaction have been factored into the evaluation of some ICPs in this book – a specific example of this is described in Chapter 14. As yet, however, few studies have been carried out in the UK on the impact of mental health integrated care pathways upon service user satisfaction.

THE CONCEPTUAL FRAMEWORK

Considering these developments, it is possible to identify a clear conceptual framework underpinning the development and use of ICPs, and these common elements of integrated care pathways are summarised in Box 1.2. In mental health pathway development (Wakefield & Peet 2003), it is important to ensure that all stakeholders who have a vested interest in the care process are involved. Adrian Roberts demonstrates this in Chapter 13 where he describes the value of developing ICPs from pluralistic viewpoints to coordinate interventions in older people's mental health services. This helped organisations move from compart-mentalised working to cross-organisation agreements, improving the experience of receiving care. ICPs describe the anticipated care – an expected standard that is to be offered. Arguably, arranging care using a predetermined philosophy may seem illusive, impractical or inappropriate to some professionals. However, in services which have been sporadically characterised by portrayals of fragmented patient journeys, the alleged benefits of integrated care pathways warrant further consideration, especially by those charged with modernising services. Clearly, the ICP has to acknowledge the need for individualisation as well as the underpinning guidelines and content. That has been addressed in many ICPs through the use of cues for choice, service user and carer narratives and monitoring of variances

Box 1.2   ELEMENTS OF AN INTEGRATED CARE PATHWAY

- Developed by all stakeholders
- Plan of anticipated care
- Includes measurable outcomes
- Defines standards of care to promote consistency and equity
- Follows a timeline (days, hours, outcomes, stages)
- System of integrated recording
- Forms all or part of the clinical record (on paper or electronically)
- Designed to meet local needs and constraints
- Incorporates evidence-based guidelines
- Uses variance tracking for day-to-day monitoring and review of performance
- Crosses organisational and professional boundaries
- Is never finalised and is a continually evolving tool in response to variance analysis and research.

(described further in Chapter 2). All the example pathways in this book are incorporated into the patient record either electronically or on paper and serve as a record of the care given. The examples have been developed locally within organisations. They have often been specifically developed to target quality problems or the implementation of clinical guidelines. Review of the available literature supports the claim that the benefits of integrated care pathways relate to clinical effectiveness, evidence-based practice, risk management, inter-professional working and appropriate bed management. This corresponds with the rationale for their development as described in later chapters. Once a care pathway has been developed and is in use, it requires maintenance. ICP content has a limited lifespan as the evidence base continually changes and service provision is subject to review.

BENEFITS AND LIMITATIONS

Using ICPs in mental health is associated with improved use of clinical information, role clarification, implementation of guidelines, improved risk management, practitioner and user education, potential to reduce costs and continuous quality improvement. It is possible to consider these benefits using tailored evaluation strategies (as subsequent chapters describe) or through using benefits realisation.

Benefits realisation is a process adapted from Benefits Management (Office of Government Commerce 2004). Using this process, it is possible to map the care pathway objectives, organisational changes, change mechanisms, benefits and requirements in a benefits network for a specific ICP – as shown in Figure 1.1. Using this approach it is vital to consider and agree at the outset the proposed objectives and benefits of the ICP. All stakeholders need to be involved in this process and those responsible for implementation need to consider critically the organisational changes required to support the developments and the change mechanisms required to underpin the achievement of benefits. Using this benefits approach is useful for managing ICP development and ensuring that the necessary organisational changes and change mechanisms are planned for. By involving different stakeholders it is clear from the start what the anticipated benefits of the ICP can be, and the changes that will be needed to underpin the benefits. Of course, to simply espouse the benefits of any modernisation, change or ICP is not sufficient and it is crucial to provide evidence that they have (or have not) been achieved. Measurement of benefits is described in later chapters of this book, including the use of variance analysis, audit of health records, interviews with service users, questionnaires, focus groups and measurement of specific indicators pre and post pathway.

As well as specific benefits related to particular ICPs there are many generic and commonly claimed benefits such as:

- improved multi-professional communication and cooperation
- a reduction in the duplication of services

Figure 1.1
Acute inpatient
integrated care pathway
benefits network.
MDT-multidisciplinary
team, ICP-integrated
care pathway,
DoH-Department of
Health, CPA-Care
Programme Approach.

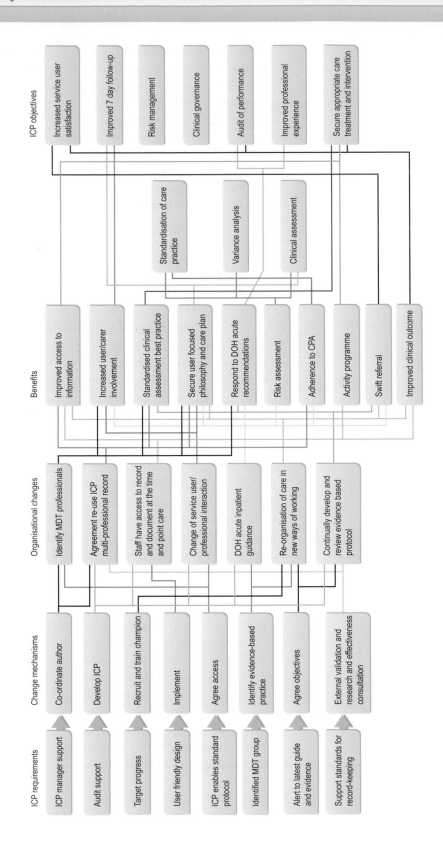

- a length of hospital stay which corresponds with need
- an increased service user satisfaction and a reduction in the number of complaints
- a reduction in the number of errors
- improved achievement of outcomes
- the development of practice based upon research, guidelines and national standards
- improved staff morale and job satisfaction
- less time spent on documentation
- development of multi-professional documentation
- consistent standards of care delivery through preferred specific goals, interventions, investigations and treatments
- early identification of variance i.e. complications/relapse
- improved risk management
- continual quality improvement.

As the mental health modernisation agenda pursues collaborative integrated systems, many current directives, initiatives and innovations have important associations with integrated care pathways. Care pathway development requires in-depth discussion and negotiation in order to develop a shared understanding of a patient journey. Developing and using a multi-professional integrated care pathway strengthens inter-professional accountability for patient outcomes which, in turn, is very much in tune with the clinical governance agenda. Describing a seamless pathway of care and articulating expected interventions bring increased pressure to ensure effective care delivery, and many organisations have used care pathways in developing the new services required to achieve modernisation targets. Pathway development is thus an apt opportunity to consider the anticipated elements of care for a particular journey through services.

A frequently claimed benefit is that ICPs enable organisations to target interventions to produce the greatest clinical effect. Clear care processes enable efficient checks to establish whether professionals are working towards quality standards as they identify clinical interventions, timescales and anticipated outcomes. Consequently, they offer a succinct framework to measure effectiveness. Analysis of the data generated by variation is used to refine practice, update the pathway and inform organisations about service needs. In turn, the regular review of pathway content and supporting evidence base informs training needs and ensures that high-quality patient care is maintained.

Organisations can also collect data to establish whether outcomes are achieved over defined periods. This enables several journeys of care to be measured in terms of length of stay and effect upon health outcomes. Not surprisingly, some stakeholders are suspicious of this viewpoint and perceive that their position and autonomy are threatened. It has also been suggested that there is a fear amongst healthcare professionals that pathways too easily indicate deficiencies in care. The concern is that this information may then be used against care providers as evidence of failures in duty or standards of care (this is discussed in greater depth in Chapter 5). However, as the structures and strategies to increase corporate responsibility grow, care pathways are a likely vehicle for refining clinical governance mechanisms.

Disadvantages of ICPs have been described as reduced professional autonomy, lack of individualised care, lack of commitment to development by professionals, poor availability of outcome measures and the view that mental health patient journeys are too complex to fit into a pre-formulated process. It is acknowledged that pathways are significantly easier to develop in cases where there is less variance in the clinical course of the condition between patients (Kitchener et al 1996), and issues such as those identified by Jones (1996) who demonstrated how the unpredictable nature of serious mental illness led to complex mental health pathway development and implementation. In particular, a predicted timeline that offers structure to the content of ICPs is often absent in mental disorders as the experience of mental health problems is unique and difficult to generalise in terms of duration. Indeed, many individuals experience complications or experience outcomes which do not correspond with the pre-planned nature of pathways. However, it is argued that in the current state of high demand and reduced resources, it is still necessary to use a process like ICPs to strive for efficiency and effectiveness.

Jones (1999) also found that professionals involved in ICP development expressed difficulty in articulating their interventions or desired outcomes. They believed that care processes needed to remain individualised and could not be pre-formulated in the way that ICPs require. It is this perception that the ICP is too simplistic to capture the essence of mental health care and stifles individualised care that remains a potential stumbling block. Roebuck (1998) identifies the time-consuming nature of ICP development as a disadvantage along with the commitment of resources required in the change process. This scenario is familiar to those charged with facilitating change in health and social care. A great deal of leadership, commitment and drive is required to ensure that changes in practice are embraced into day-to-day reality. Implementing change in mental health services has to contend with this context and its culture. The difficulties experienced in maintaining minimum staffing levels, lack of funding and competing priorities impact upon commitment. It is probable that levels of stress and morale can contribute to a climate that militates against improvements in services. Development processes must therefore be flexible and creative in an environment where meaningful change is difficult to sustain.

A MODEL OF ICP DEVELOPMENT

Over the last decade differing approaches to care pathway development have been developed. By comparing these, it has been possible to establish a composite model of ICP life cycle and development (Table 1.1). Drawing significantly on the works of Johnson (1997), Stephens (1997), Campbell et al (1998) and Ignatavicius &

Table 1.1
Development model

Conceptualisation phase

Specific steps	Involved activity
Select a case type or client group	Data are collected to determine the service user population. High-cost, high-volume, high-risk and difficult to manage case groups are prioritised, in addition to specific groups targeted by current policy initiatives. These are usually identified through diagnostic label, stage/phase of treatment, specific procedures, patient dependency data and risk assessments. Other sources may also be drawn upon such as a high level of interest among local staff, or where variations in practice occur resulting in inconsistent service delivery.
Establish, develop and educate the authoring team	To determine local stakeholders' interests and to secure support from the clinical setting, multi-professional team and service user/carer representatives.
Select the timeframe and parameters	This determines where the pathway begins and ends. The timeframe enables the care to be mapped in hours, days, weeks or in phases or stages of treatment/intervention.
Determine the goals and outcomes	Once established, the pathway team must determine the goals and outcomes of care within the chosen parameters of care. These can be identified in terms of service user and process outcomes.

Development phase

Specific steps	Involved activity
Process mapping	All stakeholders map the major steps and activities onto the timeframe. A review of related medical records provides the evidence for current patterns of practice. Identify the role of all stakeholders at each stage of the process, and identify possible problems and conflicts. The team also needs to attach time parameters for each stage, and identify whether it is likely that other pathways will be running in parallel and the influence that these may have on progress.
Search for evidence-based interventions	Review the literature, established guidelines and national recommendations which influence the expected integrated care pathway.
Analysis	Review critically the care process map and associated steps for appropriateness and timeliness. Determine any role conflicts, duplications, delays as well as identifying any added value. Compare with current practice and with established clinical guidelines. If possible, it is useful to benchmark the pathway across other organisations. Identify key areas for pathway/service development.

Continued

Table 1.1
(Continued)

Development phase—cont'd

Specific steps	Involved activity
Redesign	Redesign the process around the experience of receiving care. Revise processes in terms of coordination, preplanning, and removing steps with no added value. Incorporate evidence-based interventions, extend roles and match capacity to demand. Develop, consult and review a sustainable, feasible vision based upon best practice.
Map the anticipated care and write the pathway	Integrate the care process map into the corporate care pathway template, variance analysis system and prevailing clinical documentation.
Review, consult and revise	Initially review internally by the pathway development team. To increase the validity, and to ensure that local issues do not adversely influence the pathway, it is useful at this point to arrange for a critical review by an expert outside of the local organisation. Following this, the pathway can be presented confidently for organisational approval.

Implementation phase

Specific steps	Involved activity
Develop implementation plan	This involves disseminating the pathway information and consulting with local stakeholders. In particular, it is imperative that there are adequate resources, and some areas will probably need development. To this end 'champions' are appointed locally to lead the implementation and to identify areas of staff development/education. Initially, the pathway should be piloted over a period of 3-6 months during which the area is monitored to assess the level of completion. This is supplemented by variance analysis, which should occur after 30 cases.
Fully implement	Review the pilot, revise and fully implement. Monitor and evaluate usability, content and influence upon outcomes.
ICP in use	Variance analysis should occur every 3 months, with the findings presented to representatives of the multi-professional team and the organisation. These should be considered in the context of local clinical activity and care processes. Ensure that positive feedback is given to all stakeholders and develop action plans and the pathway to address any adverse variances.

Maintenance phase

Specific steps	Involved activity
Annual review	Revise and upgrade pathway content according to emerging evidence, variance analysis and organisational developments. Communicate findings and modifications to all stakeholders.

Hausman (1995), this model illustrates how the life of a pathway moves through four phases of conceptualisation, development, implementation and maintenance:

- Conceptualisation is very much involved with developing the focus and parameters of the ICP. If this is a first ICP within an organisation, much more needs to be agreed at the stage relating to the format the ICP will take and how it will be used as part of the health record.
- Development is the impetus for securing the process and content. Consideration is given to the evidence base, contemporary policy initiatives, and to the perspectives of all stakeholders.
- Implementation is the phase of getting the ICP into daily use – this generally involves piloting the ICP. Once this is satisfactory, it is followed by training and supporting all users of the ICP.
- Maintenance refers to the ongoing review to ensure the content remains contemporary and appropriate. This phase also identifies when the life of the ICP is at an end. Although this can occur for a number of reasons, most frequently it is due to changes in service provision.

Considered in more detail, care pathway development begins by selecting a case type or client group that will access the pathway. This is often determined by the local patient population, particularly those from high-cost, high-volume, high-risk or difficult to manage case groups. There are also occasions where pathways have been developed for certain patient groups because of a high level of interest and expertise among local professionals. Alternatively, organisations may discover considerable variations between their areas of practice, and which may have adversely affected patient outcomes. In this case a pathway may be developed in an attempt to improve practice by standardisation. Additionally, within the contemporary health and social care environment, organisations are constantly evolving. This may result in adjusting their provision of service, the geographical location and nature of practice, incorporating different grades of staff and re-quiring existing staff to change their roles. This requires radical consideration of how the service will be delivered and, in turn, this adds to the impetus driving care pathway development.

The process of developing the pathway begins by establishing a small authoring team who take responsibility for leading the pathway's progress. However, as has been emphasised, to develop a care pathway involves collaboration between all stakeholder groups. Consequently, these people need to be brought together to advise the authoring team in the form of an ICP development group. Once in place, this group begins by defining the parameters of the pathway timeframe i.e. where the pathway begins and ends. This in turn provides the framework which enables the care to be mapped in hours, days and weeks; or stages of treatment/intervention. It may well involve bridging the primary and secondary care inter-face, and it is very likely to cross traditional organisational boundaries, adding to the complexities of the task. Common sources of data are patient diaries, focus groups and review of medical records to establish practice patterns and it is the role of the authoring team to collate and summarise this information, returning to the development group to review the aims and outcomes (both service user and process focused) of the mapping process.

After the focus, timeframe, outcomes and mapping have been completed there will be sufficient information to identify keywords and terms to enable the authoring team to search for evidence-based interventions. These should include established guidelines, systematic reviews, meta-analyses and national recommendations which influence the expected integrated care pathway content. This is then returned to the pathway development group who examine the process map critically. Each step is scrutinised for appropriateness and timeliness, to clarify roles; and to identify duplications, delays and added value. Interventions are compared with established clinical guidelines and benchmarked across other organisations. This enables the process map to be reviewed to identify any areas for development.

Following this initial development, the map is considered from the perspective of a person receiving the care. Processes are considered specifically in terms of coordination and preplanning. Those steps with no added value are removed.

Once evidence-based interventions are incorporated, roles can be defined and the organisation's capacity reviewed to ensure it is able to match the demand. From this context, a sustainable, feasible vision of the pathway based upon best available evidence is developed and disseminated for consultation, following which final modifications are made and the final pathway is written within the corporate pathway template, variance analysis system and prevailing clinical documentation.

Every integrated care pathway will thus have its own implementation plan which considers dissemination/consultation, staff education, establishing champions in the clinical areas, pilot duration, monitoring and variance analysis. The pilot version of the ICP is used for a controlled period and then reviewed in respect of usability, content and influence upon outcomes. The pathway is then revised and fully implemented. Quarterly variance analysis is performed with data presented to specified members of the multi-professional team and organisation and, in light of this analysis, clinical activities and care processes are reviewed with action plans being developed to address adverse variances.

To ensure completeness, an annual review to revise and upgrade pathway content according to emerging evidence, variance analysis and organisational developments is also recommended. However, within the context of changes in contemporary health and social care, it is highly possible that these time periods may recur more frequently than those we suggest within this model.

SERVICE USER AND CARER INVOLVEMENT AND EXPERIENCE

Service users are the only stakeholders who experience the whole system of care, making their involvement fundamental throughout planning and evaluating pathways if user-focused services are to be sustained. Different stakeholder groups may prioritise efficiency, democracy, choice and respect differently, and services often fail to consider the views of all stakeholders (Berk & Rossi 1999, Rossi & Wright 1977). In addition, the views of professionals alone rarely reveal the limitations of services with the clarity and recognition offered by those who actually use them (Heyman 1995). To address this, a pathway approach should aim for service users and professionals to work collaboratively. By gathering a range of views into the process of care, areas of good practice will be identified as well as how and why limitations arise and can be addressed. Incorporating these contrasting views within care pathway planning enables service users to become central to pathway design, in turn, resulting in a powerful user-focused service.

There are a variety of ways to ensure that service user and carer involvement not only occurs during planning but follows through into the content of the ICP. Specifying interventions and processes ensures that all involved are aware of anticipated care, and the contributions they have to offer. Service user involvement in process mapping is fundamental here and some organisations have used process maps either written exclusively by service users, or based on service users' stories and diaries, to influence ICP content. An example of a service user process map is shown in Figure 1.2.

Although the process of care pathway development we advocate involves all stakeholders, the discourse about social control and medicalisation must be considered at this point. Service users in the care pathway development process may raise awareness about impressions of enforced care and powerlessness, particularly if the medical rationale for care dominates. To some extent, by ensuring that all stakeholders are represented in pathway development, the organisation has recognised that the medical solution may not be optimal in all instances. However, the location of mental health services within a medically led environment may well disadvantage other perspectives on care delivery, particularly if the majority of members of the remainder of the group derive their power from this situation, and it will take a very assertive individual to argue against quite powerful medically based arguments. This phenomenon was identified by Faulkner (2004) who suggests the use of advocates to support service users in such an environment.

When developing care pathways, therefore, it is important to recognise that some members of the group may feel intimidated (Read 1996). Consequently, it is essential that this is addressed effectively, to avoid tokenism. Respect, empathy, time, normalisation, inclusion and skilled interventions are the underpinning values of contemporary pathways themselves and should, in turn, underpin their development. This ideology ensures that care pathways do not impede individualised care or contribute to the social distance between heath and social care workers and service users.

INTEGRATED CARE PATHWAY CONTENT

Cues for ICP content generally come from two main sources – process mapping activities and systematic reviews of the literature. Developing the initial process

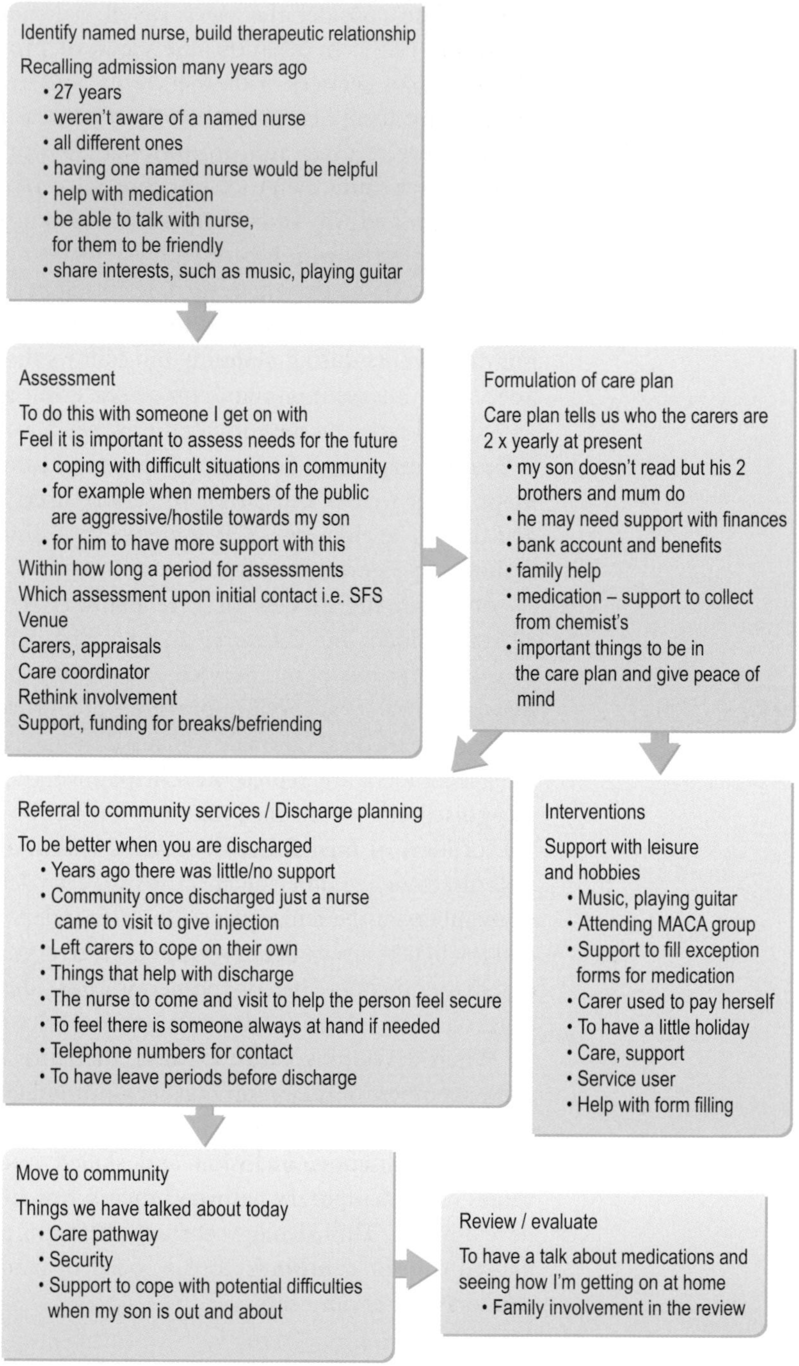

Figure 1.2
Example of mapping by
service users

Identify named nurse, build therapeutic relationship

Recalling admission many years ago
- 27 years
- weren't aware of a named nurse
- all different ones
- having one named nurse would be helpful
- help with medication
- be able to talk with nurse,
  for them to be friendly
- share interests, such as music, playing guitar

Assessment

To do this with someone I get on with
Feel it is important to assess needs for the future
- coping with difficult situations in community
- for example when members of the public
  are aggressive/hostile towards my son
- for him to have more support with this
Within how long a period for assessments
Which assessment upon initial contact i.e. SFS
Venue
Carers, appraisals
Care coordinator
Rethink involvement
Support, funding for breaks/befriending

Formulation of care plan

Care plan tells us who the carers are
2 x yearly at present
- my son doesn't read but his 2
  brothers and mum do
- he may need support with finances
- bank account and benefits
- family help
- medication – support to collect
  from chemist's
- important things to be in
  the care plan and give peace of
  mind

Referral to community services / Discharge planning

To be better when you are discharged
- Years ago there was little/no support
- Community once discharged just a nurse
  came to visit to give injection
- Left carers to cope on their own
- Things that help with discharge
- The nurse to come and visit to help the person feel secure
- To feel there is someone always at hand if needed
- Telephone numbers for contact
- To have leave periods before discharge

Interventions

Support with leisure
and hobbies
- Music, playing guitar
- Attending MACA group
- Support to fill exception
  forms for medication
- Carer used to pay herself
- To have a little holiday
- Care, support
- Service user
- Help with form filling

Move to community

Things we have talked about today
- Care pathway
- Security
- Support to cope with potential difficulties
  when my son is out and about

Review / evaluate

To have a talk about medications and
seeing how I'm getting on at home
- Family involvement in the review

mapping to define the interventions to be incorporated into the pathway inevitably involves asking clinical questions, then searching for and appraising the evidence. This undoubtedly is the most time-consuming activity in ensuring that the ICP content is underpinned by a rigorous evidence base. This involves completing a systematic literature review in regard to specific interventions, treatments and approaches to care using bibliographic databases such as MEDLINE, CINAHL and the Cochrane Library, in addition to reliable web-based resources such as the National Institute of Clinical Excellence (www.nice.org.uk), the National Electronic Library for Health (www.nelh.nhs.uk) and the National Institute for Mental Health in England (www.nimhe.org.uk). The aim is to have an ICP which encompasses the latest clinical evidence and that the evidence is made accessible to those who will use the ICP. In addition, it is essential that this evidence base and the ICP are kept up to date, requiring the ICP authoring team to develop strategies for regular review of the appropriateness of the pathway. The outcome of these processes then is ICP content that encompasses information from primary and secondary studies, published clinical guidelines, clinical expertise and the perspectives of service users and carers.

WORKING ON AN INTEGRATED CARE PATHWAY PROGRAMME

There are several ways in which organisations develop care pathways. Some organisations have accepted that care pathways are developed by one team and the use of that pathway is restricted to that locality. Such pathways rarely form part of an organisational strategy and are considered as isolated projects. In these cases ICP development is usually led by interested individuals who are motivated by improving care over that specific process. In this case then the 'vested interest' is high. ICPs of this nature are discussed by some contributors in this book and have been shown to have a high level of success. Other organisations have developed many ICPs for different services which, depending on the size or nature of the organisation, are often not replicated across several teams or locations. For example they have one assertive outreach team which uses an ICP, one day service clinic which uses an ICP and so forth. Where there are several ICPs within an organisation there are more likely to be specific resources dedicated to supporting ICPs. This may take the form of a dedicated ICP facilitator and perhaps audit support. There are examples of organisations that use several ICPs, which are themselves replicated over several different teams. Organisations that have several ICPs in use over different localities are generally supported by dedicated ICP resources and operate within an organisational framework for ICP development and use.

Where several ICPs are used over different locations there is a need for rigorous programme management. Before considering an organisational ICP programme, it is necessary to consider what has been done to date, in previous or parallel initiatives, and how to build on this. It is essential to consider the need for ICPs within the organisation, why they are important and what needs to be achieved by their use. ICP programme management involves programme governance (i.e. determining the lines of accountability and responsibility within ICP development and implementation). The Joint Information Systems Committee (2003) offers a suitable programme management process to follow. Typically, organisations have an ICP advisory board and an ICP facilitator who acts as a programme manager. The advisory board should represent all stakeholders and different levels of the organisation. These boards are responsible for helping executives to steer the ICP programme and sending regular reports, usually to trust boards. Members of the ICP advisory board play an important role in steering the ICP programme and are able to oversee activities like planning strategies for evaluation, dissemination and exit/sustainability, and may advise on areas like standards and best practice. They may also advise on relationships between the ICP programme and external organisations, and play a role in steering the projects in the ICP programme. The board help to ensure that ICP authoring teams and the facilitator work together on the implementation of ICP developments, and ensure that ICP outputs are sustainable, and taken up by the organisation and wider community if appropriate. ICP facilitators generally:

- manage ICPs from development to closedown
- provide a framework for evaluation, dissemination and sustainability at programme level
- guide and support authoring teams in the development of ICPs
- coordinate projects within the ICP programme often related to medical records, information technology, reporting and performance
- arrange meetings, training and other events
- arrange for the dissemination of ICPs and their related information
- monitor the performance of ICPs through progress reports, site visits, etc.
- ensure that ICP deliverables are submitted on time and are aligned with organisational developments
- support teams and individuals in the development of evidence-based ICP content
- lead implementation and support local ICP champions (identified individuals who lead implementation within teams)
- develop the variance reporting process which supports purchasing, governance and performance monitoring
- enable evaluation so that the progress and impact of ICPs can be monitored and 'steered' dynamically.

It is important that ICP developments are embraced within existing mechanisms for communication, be this board, governance and locality meetings or the organisation's websites and newsletters. An ICP strategy and programme should make clear the methods of communication and it is usual to follow a recognised project planning process giving the relevant background, aims and objectives (as shown below).

ICP PROGRAMME AIM

The aim of this strategy is to improve the experience of receiving services by using care pathways as a tool for monitoring, coordinating and improving standards of care. This approach will be used to help secure a culture of practice development and a pursuit of improvement in outcomes which places service users at the centre of care.

ICP programme objectives

All care pathways developed and implemented will:

1. Be a consequence of rigorous review of existing practices and involve all stakeholders in development.
2. Adopt an integrative philosophy and deliberately use teamworking and shared belief systems from the outset. Collaboration will be visible during development, within pathway content and in subsequent feedback of variance.
3. Form all or part of the patient record and describe a seamless pathway of care that articulates expected interventions. The document, in conjunction with others, will satisfy existing standards of record keeping and be multi-professional in nature.
4. Describe effective interventions targeted to effect the greatest clinical benefit. This will incorporate evidence-based practice and clear reference to available clinical guidelines, outcome measures, benchmarks, research and expert opinion.
5. Identify through variance analysis clinical deterioration, variation in care delivery and clinical outcomes. This specific information is used to facilitate clinical decision-making, risk management, individualised interventions and continuous quality improvement.
6. Focus upon benefits management – reviewing service availability, 'gate-keeping' arrangements and reducing delays, duplications, hold-ups and deficiencies.

It is common for ICP strategies to offer guidelines for choosing target processes for ICP development and a specific model of development that should be adopted. It may be possible as part of the strategy and programme to offer standards around ICP outputs. These may refer to a criterion around the ICPs to be developed, although experience has shown that ICP outputs can change, especially since, as ICPs move from paper to electronic versions, their format within health care changes as do the variance reporting strategies used. Organisations should consider the outcomes envisaged, the changes ICPs will stimulate or enable, and their likely impact on the experience of receiving care. A stakeholder analysis should consider who has a vested interest in the ICP programme or will be affected by its outcomes. It is appropriate to consider why they will be interested in or affected by ICPs, and what their stake is. There is a need to be creative and think of how each stakeholder could be affected, either positively or negatively, and this will help in deciding who needs to be on board to make ICPs a success. ICP programmes commonly follow a project plan approach which maps out the work and shows how an organisation intends to achieve its ICP objectives. As work progresses the plan can be updated and the ICP advisory board can take time out to think about how things are going, what is being learned, and adjust the plan. ICP programmes, as with any development, carry an element of risk. A risk analysis at the start of the ICP programme will help to predict the risks that could prevent ICPs from delivering on time or even failing. It will also help to manage the risks should they occur. A risk analysis addresses the following questions:

- what could possibly go wrong?
- what is the likelihood of it happening?
- how will it affect the project?
- what can be done about it?

Risks may relate to staffing, the organisation or technical issues. An analysis at the beginning of the programme will help minimise the risks that may occur. If a risk does occur, the ICP advisory board can consider how to minimise its impact in practice. During the ICP development the ICP facilitator can maintain an 'issues and risk' log for use at reviews by the advisory board.

EVALUATION

Like any other modernisation or development, integrated care pathways require considered evaluation. Evaluation should be considered as part of the development process and should consider the objectives of the pathway and/or the success (or not) of implementation. Evaluation could be considered at an individual ICP and ICP programme level. Evaluation can focus upon quality, e.g. whether the ICP is useful, meets the needs of service users and is implemented in the expected way. In the case of an ICP programme, evaluation focuses on whether the model used was effective, whether development achieved its objectives, and what was the impact upon the experience of receiving or giving the service. The aim is to undertake the evaluation in an objective way and this can be either formative or summative in nature. Formative evaluation can be routinely undertaken during ICP implementation perhaps after a pilot. Information gained can be used to improve the ICP, influence the outcomes of the ICP and the likelihood of it being successfully implemented. Summative evaluation of ICPs is typically completed when one or more ICPs have been in use for some time and provide evidence of achievement.

Evaluation methods vary in relation to specific ICPs (as illustrated in later chapters). Methods used vary depending on the objectives set and the outcomes envisaged. Measures of success vary by outcome or objectives. Questionnaires are frequently used in the evaluation of ICPs to gather opinions from service users, carers and health or social care professionals in a systematic way using closed and open-ended questions. They are a common and versatile way of collecting data, which is relatively cheap. Interviews are often used with the same stakeholders and are useful for exploring opinions and issues in more depth on a one-to-one basis. Focus groups have been used in informal evaluation of ICPs and have allowed evaluators to gather a range of views (not a consensus) about ICPs or their outcomes and explore how strongly views are held or change as the issue is discussed. Whatever methods are used, it is important to involve stakeholders, as this will increase their commitment to ICPs, their confidence in the results and the likelihood they will act on the findings. Organisations may choose to involve an outside evaluator, e.g. to help plan the studies or advise on analysing results. When planning evaluation, it is important to get independent views on the methods. Credible evaluation is fraught with methodological difficulty and rigorously conducted evaluations of integrated care pathways are rare. Measuring success even when specific objectives have been set is complicated by the perspective of success held by various stakeholders and the difficulty in attributing causality.

REFERENCES

Berk RA, Rossi PH 1999 Thinking about program evaluation 2. Sage, London

Browning R, Hollingberry T 2000 For good measure. Health Service Journal 5 October:34-35

Bryant L 1999 National Care Pathways Association Annual Conference 22 July 1999, York Racecourse

Campbell H, Hotchkiss R, Bradshaw N et al 1998 Integrated care pathways. British Medical Journal 10 January 316:113-137

Dykes PC 1998 Psychiatric clinical pathways. Aspen, New York

Faulkner A 2004 Strategies for surviving acute care. In: Harrison M, Howard D, Mitchell D (eds) Acute mental health nursing: from acute concerns to the capable practitioner. Sage, London

Glazer W M 1997 Managed care: nowhere to run. Psychiatric Times. Http://www.mhsource.com/edu/psytimes/p971221.html posted December 1997, accessed 12.05.1998

Hall J 2004 Mental health integrated care pathways in the UK: a review of their content. Journal of Integrated Care Pathways 8:14-18

Heyman B 1995 Utilitarian, historical and methodological issues. In: Heyman B (ed) Researching user perspectives on community healthcare. Chapman & Hall, London

Ignatavicius D, Hausman K 1995 Clinical pathways for collaborative practice. Saunders, London

Johnson S 1997 Pathways of care. Blackwell Science, London

Joint Information Systems Committee 2003 JISC project management framework http://www.jisc.ac.uk/index.cfm?name=proj_manguide developed: 22 December 2003, accessed: 21 December 2004

Jones A 1996 Managed care: length of stay as a measure of quality. Mental Health Nursing 16(6):12-13

Jones A 1997 Managed care strategy for mental health services. British Journal of Nursing 6(10):564-568

Jones A 1999 A modernized mental health service: the role of care pathways. Journal of Nursing Management 7:331-338

Kitchener D, Davidson C, Burnard P 1996 Integrated Care Pathways: effective tools for continuous evaluation of clinical practice. Journal of Evaluation of Clinical Practice 2(1):65-69

Mental Heath Subgroup 1999 National Pathways Association Mental Health Subgroup, meetings minutes. Meeting at the Kings Fund, London

Mosher C, Cronk P, Kidd A et al 1992 Upgrading practice with critical pathways. American Journal of Nursing Jan 41-44

Office of Government Commerce 2004 Benefits Management http://www.ogc.gov.uk/sdtoolkit/reference/deliverylifecycle/benefits_mgmt.html developed 09.04, accessed 28.01.05

Petryshen PR, Petryshen PM 1992 The case management model: an innovative approach to the delivery of patient care. Journal of Advanced Nursing 17:1188-1194

Read J 1996 What do we want from mental health services? In: Read J, Reynolds J Speaking our minds. Open University Press, Milton Keynes

Riley K 1998 Paving the way. Health Service Journal 108:30-31

Roebuck A 1998 Critical pathways: an aid to practice. Nursing Times 94 (26):50-51

Rossi PH, Wright SR 1977 Evaluation research – an assessment of theory, practice and politics. Evaluation Quarterly 1(1):5-53

Sack L 1996 What will managed care do to the profession of psychiatry. Psychiatric Times www.webmaster@mhsource.com posted August 1996, accessed 12.05.1998

Stead L, Arthur C, Cleary A et al 1995 Multidisciplinary pathways of care series – do multidisciplinary pathways affect patient satisfaction. Healthcare Risk Report November, p 13-14

Stephens R 1997 Setting up care pathways in mental health. In: Wilson J (ed) Integrated care management. Butterworth Heinemann, London p 151-171

Tucci RA, Bartels KL 1998 Ovarian cancer surgery: a clinical pathway. Clinical Journal of Oncology Nursing 2(2):65-66

Wakefield S, Peet M 2003 Developing integrated care pathways in mental health: critical success factors. Journal of Integrated Care Pathways 7:47-49

Zander K 1998 Psychiatric clinical pathways – an interdisciplinary approach. Aspen, New York

Variance reporting and quality improvement

Julie Hall

This chapter focuses upon how variance information is used as an approach to improve quality in mental health services. This information is used to examine practice critically, monitor the implementation of guidelines and in continuous evaluation of the service user's journey. Variance reporting has long been described as a central component of integrated care pathways but is often problematic to implement. This account describes a system that has been successful and consistent in using variance information to support governance and assurance. Initially, the theory underpinning variance information is outlined and its basis within quality improvement, clinical governance and performance management. This is illustrated with the use of a case study, which guides the reader through the process of identifying and recording variances.

WHAT IS A VARIANCE?

Care pathways detail the flow of care for a typical service user episode. These often relate to a specific diagnosis or need, specifying service user outcomes and interventions. Their primary aim is to ensure that, through process mapping, latest evidence and research is incorporated into day-to-day practice (Johnson 1994).

Most care pathways are developed upon the basis of meeting the needs of most people, most of the time. This raises immediate issues for implementation of integrated care pathways in mental health. What happens when a service user journey does not progress as expected and the course of illness changes or recovery is delayed? What about choice, negotiation or individualised care? Consequently, integrated care pathways in mental health must also acknowledge and respond to variation.

As integrated care pathways define expected interventions, a variance can be defined as when activities described on the pathway either do not happen or when interventions not described on the pathway are delivered (i.e. those you would not usually expect to offer). A variance is digression from the planned pathway. For example, in a care pathway for early intervention in psychosis, a service user should have their health and social needs assessed within 10 working days of referral to the early intervention team. If this did not occur, e.g. due to a waiting list, this would be a variance. Similarly, if an acute admission pathway required a service user to have a physical examination on admission to hospital and the service user refused, this too would be a variance from the anticipated care.

It is important to understand why variances occur. The variance from the early intervention in psychosis care pathway example above has a system type cause. In the second example, where the service user refused a physical examination, the cause could be a matter of individual choice or an exacerbation of illness.

Although variances sometimes indicate interventions which have not been delivered, or outcomes that have not been achieved, it is not always the case. Variance should therefore not always be viewed negatively, or as a failure, as many have their basis in individualised care (e.g. the service user declining the medical examination above). They may also indicate positive factors such as rapid clinical improvement and recovery. Consequently, variance information requires interpretation before assumptions can be made. Capturing where interventions are offered which are not within the pathway is also a valuable source of variance information and affords great benefits within governance and performance structures.

CLINICAL GOVERNANCE

From a governance perspective, care pathways enable organisations to target effective interventions to effect the greatest clinical benefit. As care pathways identify clinical interventions, timescales and anticipated outcomes they offer a succinct framework to measure effectiveness. Variance data are collected as an integral part of documenting care delivery, enabling each service user's journey to be measured in terms of interventions and effect upon health outcomes. Analysis of variation from the pathway is used to refine practice, update the pathway and inform service needs. Regular review of pathway content and the supporting evidence base informs training needs and ensures that quality is maintained.

Not surprisingly though, some stakeholders are suspicious of this viewpoint and perceive that their authority and autonomy are threatened by such structures. However, as the strategies to secure corporate responsibility grow, care pathways are a likely vehicle to refine assurance arrangements. Certainly one of the barriers to effective governance and assurance is inadequate identification of the processes of care to achieve outcomes. Care pathways therefore offer a process which is also advantageous to governance arrangements.

Many organisations have approached pathways as vehicles to incorporate clinical guidelines within practice. Edwards (1998) describes the implementation of clinical guidelines as sporadic and proposes care pathways as an aid to secure their implementation. He argues evidence for the content of pathways should be obtained from systematic literature reviews including evidence-based guidelines, technology appraisals, meta analyses, primary research and expert opinion. (The United Kingdom National Institute for Clinical Excellence guidelines are also a major source of effective treatments and care processes.) In turn, incorporation of this evidence within care pathways ensures that professionals have a framework for routinely applying research findings and that service users and carers have access to interventions that are current. Consequently, the integrated care pathway sees through the implementation of guidelines at practice level and allows variance from guidelines and protocols to be reviewed and examined.

Defining the interventions incorporated into a pathway thus involves asking clinical questions, searching for and appraising the evidence. This process enables all stakeholders to review critically what is offered in the context of local services and agreements and it is the integration of professional expertise, scientific inquiry and service user perspectives that forms the basis of pathway content. Care pathway development consequently enables change and helps to ensure that evidence-based practice becomes part of day-to-day care delivery.

Care pathways are also cited widely as a risk management tool. They can reduce risk by agreeing and controlling the parameters of care. Improved communication and the implementation of guidance promote consistency and reduce variation in outcomes. Using the pathway process to monitor needs provides benefits to service users and lowers the level of clinical risk by reducing errors.

Risk management is in turn associated with variance analysis (Kitchener & Wilson 1995). As care pathways specify outcomes, any failure, delay or omission can therefore be clearly identified. The emphasis is on securing the correct interventions at the right time in as many instances as possible. Care pathways do this by communicating effective interventions and preventing adverse incidents. Wilson (1995) describes opportunities to use the pathway to reduce uncertainty and delays, eliminate duplication and identify unexplained variation. Furthermore, it is possible that deviations from expected recovery identify clinical relapse and deterioration. This specific information is used to facilitate decision-making and shape individual interventions aimed at managing risk. In the longer term, systematically collecting variance data is credible and reliable for developing changes in practice that are clinically led (Kitchener & Wilson 1995). These data enable organisations to identify interventions that are ineffective, or have not been delivered. Both scenarios present significant risks and this information can be analysed to consider how omissions and errors can be minimised. The consequence is gaining a wider understanding of service user journeys and minimising exposure to risk.

PERFORMANCE MANAGEMENT AND ORGANISATIONAL LEARNING

Performance management and organisational learning in health and social care thrive upon critical examination of current practice. Implementation of clinical guidelines and continuous appraisal of outcomes are fundamental to a quality improvement approach to care. Recorded variances, as part of the pathway process, provide information for clinical audit. Issues of cost, activity and quality can all be scrutinised rigorously by different stakeholders. One of the common themes within contemporary health and social care practice is this requirement for organisations to use information for day-to-day decision-making and the achievement of strategy. Information from variance reports has the benefit of being meaningful and pluralistic in its contribution to assurance processes. Over a period of time, these data can be examined to establish trends, develop action plans and improve practice.

In the same way that variance information can be used for quality improvement, it can also be readily applied to performance measurement (Bridge et al 2002). Bridge et al (2002) link care pathways to an organisation's ability to improve services and success in accreditation schemes. Responding to complaints and claims from an assurance perspective involves identifying and controlling risks, a feature of the variance information process. Combining variance information with outcome measures thus allows the efficiency of a service user's episode to be identified. Outcomes, variance, cost and indicators, when used together, offer a powerful analysis and organisations that have used these methods have demonstrated significant improvements in performance characterised by reduced length of stay, reduction in costs and improved outcomes (Wood et al 1992).

Certain structural and cultural conditions within an organisation are required to enable the success of this approach, however:

- competence in care delivery
- interdisciplinary commitment and collaboration
- effective information systems
- structures which align information with day-to-day decision-making and the achievement of strategy.

Given these conditions, variance information enables different stakeholders and organisations to examine patterns and trends within service user episodes, thus forming the basis of learning, seeking solutions and modernisation, all aimed at improving the experience of receiving care. The association with performance management and aligning day-to-day activity with decision-making is obvious. Variance information has its basis within the service user journey and offers information about systems, the environment and outcomes. This is used to manage change and strengthen processes, all aligned to improving performance. Targets and performance indicators are discernible in many examples of care pathway content in the UK. The information produced from variance reports therefore supplements existing sources of performance information. The data can show how the achievement of targets varies according to the team or locality. The information can drill down to timeframes, settings, choice, clinical circumstances and variations in systems. Traditional sources of performance information do not reveal situations in the direct and rich way that variance information does.

RECORDING VARIANCES

The remainder of this chapter focuses on developing a successful variance information system. Variances relate to an activity that did not occur or is supplementary to the expected process of care. They are recorded contemporaneously and the first step is to identify the activity in question. For example, in the early intervention in psychosis pathway stated previously, the activity was that a service user should have their health and social needs assessed within 10 working days of referral to the service. This would be written into the care pathway, usually with an accompanying activity code which corresponds to each activity (Figure 2.1).

At points within the pathway there will be prompts to record variances within the different timeframes, enabling easy identification of variances within the care pathway. This is particularly useful where professionals use the care pathway to manage care step by step.

It is also important to record why the variance occurred. In this example of why a service user did not have their health and social needs assessed within 10 working days of referral there could be several reasons. For the purpose of this example though, we could say that there were 'no staff available'. In most reporting systems the reason or cause of the variance is aligned to a choice of codes known as variance codes. The choice of the variance codes is shown at the foot of Figure 2.2. Altogether, this information (on paper-based pathways) is recorded on a register of variances usually found at the end of the document.

The activity code on the variance register in Figure 2.2 is 1.1. Alongside this is the variance code selected from the list at the base of the register. In this case, the variance code 2.3 has been chosen suggesting that the activity has not been completed as the staff or service is not available. The variance source codes offer a choice of situations explaining why an activity has not been completed. Alternative models of variance codes can be found internationally although clear patterns can be seen in that variance source codes represent service users and their carers, systems or services, care givers and health themes. The model of variance codes shown (in Figure 2.2) has user/carer codes, system codes and other agencies and is used by several National Health Service (NHS) trusts in the United Kingdom.

Figure 2.1
Care pathway extract
showing activity codes

Code	Activity completed within 10 working days by an Early Intervention in Psychosis Specialist
1.1	A specialist assessment of health and social needs is completed

Figure 2.2
Care pathway extract
variance register

Lincolnshire Healthcare NHS

NHS Trust

INTEGRATED CARE
PATHWAY FOR EARLY
INTERVENTION IN
PSYCHOSIS

Variance Record Sheet from: *Derby Rd Clinic*

Date	Activity Code	Variance Code	Action to be Taken (If you need to repeat an intervention then fill in the blank rows in the appropriate time frame)	Sign
2.3.03	*1.1*	*2.3*	*John's referral has been placed on the waiting list and the assessment will be offered in 2-3 weeks*	*J Smith*

VARIANCE SOURCE CODES

User/carer codes	System codes	Other agencies
1.1 User unavailable 1.2 Carer unavailable 1.3 User refused 1.4 Carer refused 1.5 Intervention inappropriate 1.6 Deterioration of mental state: intervention inappropriate 1.7 Improvement of mental state: intervention inappropriate 1.8 User refused due to poor motivation 1.9 Intervention repeated due to lack of understanding or skills 1.10 Other (please state)	2.1 Date and time of intervention changed 2.2 Awaiting consultation from others 2.3 Staff/Service unavailable 2.4 Lack of time 2.5 Intervention postponed/ cancelled 2.6 Information results not available 2.7 Dept closed/room not available 2.8 Appointment not available /delayed 2.9 Other (please state)	3.1 Accommodation not available 3.2 Community support not available 3.3 Day services not available 3.4 Funding/benefits not available 3.5 Transport not available 3.6 Other (please state)

The list of variance codes is not exhaustive and the term 'other' is used to capture more infrequent causes of variation. The variance code is selected by the professional recording the variance. Added to this information is any action plan in relation to the variance. The process of using the pathway for managing care suggests the importance of the action plan. It is not sufficient to identify a variance. The need to take possible action in relation to a variance may be crucial. Professionals use this register to inform them of variances and activities yet to be offered. This register stays with the pathway as part of the clinical record and is available as verification of variances from the pathway and what action has been taken. The process of variance recording lends itself to a number of alternative formats; electronically, this may be facilitated by dropdown menus and programmatic reporting formats. An example of an electronic format is shown in Figure 2.3.

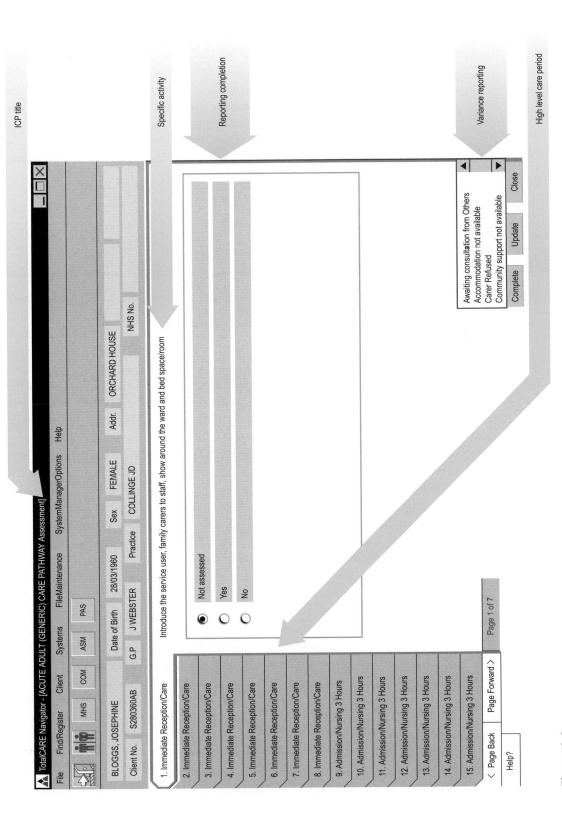

Figure 2.3

Example screen shot.

This figure is reproduced with the permission of McKesson Information Solutions UK, European Headquarters, Warwick Technology Park, Warwick CV34 6NZ, England. The data shown on the screenshot are fictitious.

Most care pathways involve recording the variances at intervals during the care pathway and often on a central register. However, the issue of who records a variance is not always straightforward. Ideally, the person to record the variance would be the person responsible for the activity. Under most circumstances this is appropriate. However, there are instances where an activity is not provided because the staff or service is not available; therefore the variance could not be recorded by the person responsible. Consequently, although it is often assumed that the person responsible for managing care during that time will record the variance, in reality this will most likely be the care coordinator, the named nurse or their deputy.

USING VARIANCE REPORTING

Variance reporting has two main purposes. The first is the day-to-day management of the service user journey. Wood et al (1992) argue that clinicians are at the core of managing care and therefore are accountable for service users' outcomes. The clinician thus uses the care pathway and the daily variance analysis to manage each stage of the service user's contact episode. This involves ongoing comparison between planned care and the reality of what actually happens. The outcome of the comparison is to enable early identification of problems and to take appropriate action. This specific information is used to facilitate decision-making and shape individual interventions.

Failure to meet outcomes can also be identified from the expected interventions and the causes of variation. In case management this information is used to discuss with the service user what possible actions should be taken. Some variations may be avoidable and action is needed to find the steps required to resolve variation or prevent the situation from recurring. During day-to-day care, identifying variances thus helps to evaluate what is effective and what needs to change. This helps to provide individualised care and is useful within supervision processes. Pathway content therefore provides the structure to review practice and care outcomes for particular cases.

Pathways reflect the norm of a care process and as people are unique there is and should always be variation. Using variances is a dynamic process, highlighting the need for alternative action. Information about interventions or activities which have not occurred is valuable information based on day-to-day practice. Inherent in this process is a built-in system for audit. The other main use of variance information is for the collective review of care outcomes and the exploration of avenues for improving quality. This involves identification of patterns and trends in variances across care settings and different service user journeys. This information can be used in longer-term planning to improve services.

VARIANCE ANALYSIS

Kitchener (1997, p 26) describes the purpose of variance analysis as to:

1. determine the goals, and variations from the goals of treatment
2. determine the cause of variation
3. find solutions to avoidable delays
4. investigate and analyse specific problems identified
5. redefine the pathway in light of the most recent experience.

Indeed, identifying patterns and trends from the information from variance registers offers significant opportunities for audit activity. The analysis of variances begins by examining the volume of variances for specific activities in the pathway. An example of this is shown graphically in Figure 2.4 for an acute adult inpatient care pathway, where activities and variances are represented in terms of volume by their activity codes along the horizontal axis.

It can be determined from the graph in Figure 2.4 that activities 5.1 and 5.2 occur as variances on more occasions than the other activities. Activity 5.1 is 'the service user knows who their care coordinator is and has their contact details (prior to discharge from acute inservice user care)'. Activity 5.2 is 'the service user has an appointment for 7 day follow-up and a copy of their care plan (prior to discharge from acute inservice user care)'.

Considering further activities 5.1 and 5.2, the shading patterns in the columns represent the different variance codes, i.e. the cause of the variance. These are explained in the key to the figure, and the codes relate back to Figure 2.2. For example, the dominant variance code in the column for activity 5.2 is 2.3. Looking back to Figure 2.2 it is seen that a variance code of 2.3 suggests that the staff/service

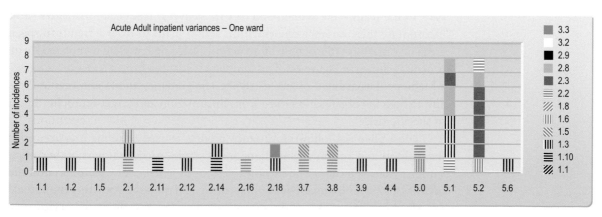

Figure 2.4
Graphical portrayal of patterns and trends in variances

were not available. Thus it can be determined that on eight occasions in this period service users were discharged from acute inservice user care without an appointment for 7 day follow-up and a copy of their care plan (activity 5.2). On five of these occasions, this occurred as there were no staff/service available to offer this activity. This information would form the basis of the variance report for that particular team.

CONTINUOUS IMPROVEMENT

Reports like this can be offered to teams on a regular basis. This identifies significant problems in pre-discharge processes and working relationships between wards and community mental health services. The benefit of this information is that it is contextual and meaningful to those with responsibility for managing the service user journey. Consequently, this information provides a basis from which to scrutinise working processes, and in this case issues related to use of the care programme approach.

Systematically collecting variance data is a credible and reliable method for developing changes in practice which are clinically led (Kitchener & Wilson 1995). It enables organisations to identify interventions which are ineffective, or which have not been delivered, and the reasons why. The information is analysed to determine how omissions and errors can be minimised. In the example of discharge planning and aftercare, it was possible to see how corrective action should be planned. Such omissions could have had significant consequences for vulnerable service users following their discharge from hospital care. Indeed, this is the basis for the current performance targets related to the provision of 7 day follow-up after discharge and reducing re-admission rates, and illustrates the close relationship between care pathways and performance.

To ensure improvement however, it is essential that variance information is fed back to the team – the actual point of care delivery. Teams and managers should incorporate their variance report within action plans to reverse trends in specific areas of variation. An example of an action planning template completed for this process is shown in Figure 2.5. This template is adapted from An Organisation with a Memory (Department of Health 2000). The guidance and the process used here aim to help the organisation learn from information and target action in response to specific risks.

Action planning following variance reports is used to refine practice, update the pathway and inform organisations about service needs. It is possible to compare variances across locations and teams to establish whether any patterns and trends occur across organisations. For example, one could determine whether the variances described in Figure 2.4 are common problems regarding discharge planning and aftercare which occur in several inpatient areas. This information can be used in the review of pathway content. The supporting evidence base and current processes should be re-considered to inform practice improvement and training

Figure 2.5

Learning the lessons template

Adapted from Department of Health (2000)

AUDIT ACTION PLAN

| Audit Title: |
| Return to Audit Dept By: |
| Date of Variance Report: |
| Lead Person: |

Audit Findings	Recommendations	Action Taken

needs. It is easy to identify common patterns in variances in different teams who are using the same care pathway. Sometimes there are isolated issues although common trends can be identified. As the structures and strategies to increase corporate accountability rapidly grow, this information is a highly suitable vehicle for making known quality problems and refining clinical governance mechanisms. This variance analysis process enables the collective review of care outcomes and the exploration of avenues for improving quality. Evaluative action leads to:

- continual re-monitoring of care provision
- a focus upon quality improvement
- changes in the pathway
- problem solving
- improved risk management
- individualised care provision.

The whole process of using variance information for quality improvement is shown in Figure 2.6.

LESSONS LEARNED FROM IMPLEMENTATION

Recording and examining variances can be stressful and frustrating for individuals (Hall 2001). Professionals are not accustomed to making known what they are

Figure 2.6
The quality improvement
cycle using variance
information

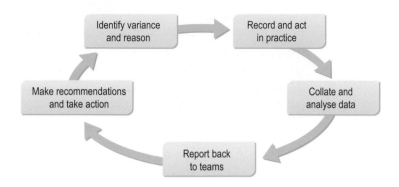

unable to deliver or identifying the interventions that they cannot facilitate due to lack of time or skills, and organisations need to be supportive towards this. Often there are recruitment, training and resource implications associated with significant variance trends. Variance data have an objectivity which is difficult to dispute and are credible evidence for teams to cite in support of claims for increased resources or new ways of working. Thus, if variance information is going to be integrated into an organisation's governance and performance processes, it is essential that care pathways are supported at all levels and in all areas (Wakefield & Peet 2003). It is crucial that care pathway development and variance information are tabled regularly at forums and that the links are drawn between governance, performance and modernisation. In particular, there is the need for high-profile supporters as this greatly influences how variance information is viewed and used. The support of clinicians in the development of care pathways and securing any variance information is also vital for success. A useful approach to secure this is to identify two champions for each team and enable those individuals to promote and support colleagues in using the pathway.

In turn, there must also be readily available training and guidance on how to use the pathway (and record variances). To support this, the front page of many pathway documents contains instructions on recording and this can be supplemented by a printed guide available in the practice setting or base. Securing a commitment to variance reporting is important to viable reporting. A level of understanding is essential otherwise the quality of variance information gained is poor. Experience has shown that the amount and quality of reporting increase over time. This is enhanced by confidence in using the pathway, training and assurance that the information is being used. The role of the care pathway facilitator is essential to this process, visiting and supporting staff through implementation as much as is feasible.

Although professionals are concerned about variance reporting, organisations who do not use variance information carry greater risks than individuals. Practitioners have information provided in the pathway which has usually been validated by the organisation. The pathway is required to be of sufficient quality and up to date. The professional knows that the service user journey has been pre-considered (which is often helpful in terms of standards, consensus and communication). Pathways though are no substitute for clinical judgment and are often accompanied with a disclaimer to that effect. Organisations should be aware of resource implications which can affect the implementation of care pathways. Where activities are not completed due to resources or systems these circumstances should be reviewed. Organisations who do not respond to variance information increase their culpability. To reduce risks to the organisation it is vital to consider how variance information should be used, and who should be responsible for the action planning as in Figure 2.5. Implementation has shown that responsibility for the causes of variance falls across different levels of hierarchy or responsibility. Effective action planning to improve care processes spans a range of positions in organisations. Some aspects of care are easily influenced at a ward or team level. However, variances which may have a financial or system origin may require action at different levels within an organisation. This is where the use of existing performance frameworks is needed to assure that the information is correctly used. Failure to use the information is largely related to an inability to achieve improvement in practice, or failure to reassess the effects of action taken. Persistence, high-level organisational support and recurrent measurement are obvious keys to success. Unfortunately the historically poor use of audit information by organisations is still applicable to variance information. The benefits and limitations of the described approach to variance reporting are summarised in Table 2.1.

SUMMARY

The successful development of care pathways in mental health care using variance information provides a fresh set of challenges. Zander (2002) describes variance as the most misunderstood mechanism of care pathways. The work of the Centre for Case Management indicates that variances should be documented and addressed as they arise; although retrospective use of the information warrants careful consideration. The use of a small number of critical indicators for retrospective analysis is felt to improve the quality of data. The use of variance information differentiates a care pathway from a care plan. This quality of information has been elusive in mental health audit. Assurance regarding the implementation of emerging guidance is valuable to all stakeholders. It is essential that the information is fed back to the team and through management and governance structures.

Nevertheless, applying the information to make meaningful improvements in care requires an organisational desire to improve quality at all levels. There are huge benefits to be realised in terms of outcomes and the effective utilisation of resources. A number of mental health trusts are moving towards making this idealistic state an actual prospect. Analysis of variance provides information which is high-quality, contextual, relevant and prospective. The manual and electronic

Table 2.1
Summary of the benefits
and limitations of
variance information

Benefits	Limitations
Information for day-to-day management of care	The quality of variance information can vary
Identification of risk and unmet needs or outcomes	The amount of variance reporting can be variable
Triggers clinical decision-making and action planning	Variance reporting takes time to develop
Contextual audit information	Training and support can be time consuming
Increased professional ownership of the care process	The process competes with many competing priorities
Enables individualisation of care	Professionals have concerns about how the information will be used
Information for identification of patterns and trends within care processes	The information may not be used, or used incorrectly
Information for benchmarking and monitoring performance	The information is used in isolation from other sources i.e. that from risk registers or other forms of audit
Less duplication of activities and reduced errors	Systems can be time consuming to develop and clinicians require support
Evidence of implementation of clinical guidelines	
Improved access to clinical information	
Process which contributes to organisational learning and continuous quality improvement	
An improved experience of receiving care as improvements are incorporated into routine practice and then re-evaluated	

systems to secure the gathering of this information are becoming increasingly common. The mechanics differ slightly between organisations but the philosophy of the process is the same. Many stakeholders are increasingly interested in this information. Service users and carers anecdotally confirm its validity and it is highly meaningful to professionals also. The remaining challenge is for organisations to realise the potential of this information and to invest in systems to support its delivery and then performance manage its use.

REFERENCES

Bridge GE, Norris AC, Melhuish PJ 2002 Care pathways in the quality management of UK healthcare. http://www.sis.port.ac.uk/~norrist/hic97gb.html accessed 24/09/02

Department of Health 2000 An organisation with a memory. HMSO, London

Edwards JNT 1998 Clinical care pathways: a model for the effective delivery of health care? Journal of Integrated Care 2:59-62

Hall J 2001 A qualitative survey of staff responses to an integrated care pathway pilot study in a mental healthcare setting. Nursing Times Research 6 (3):696-705

Johnson S 1994 Service user focused care without the upheaval. Nursing Standard 8:20-23

Kitchener D 1997 Analysis of variation from the pathway. In: Johnson S, Pathways of care, ch 3. Blackwell Science, London

Kitchener D, Wilson J 1995 Multidisciplinary pathways of care series – analysis of variance in service users. Healthcare Risk Report September pp16-17

Wakefield S, Peet M 2003 Developing integrated care pathways in mental health: the critical success factors. Journal of Integrated Care Pathways 4:47-49

Wilson S 1995 Multidisciplinary pathways of care – a tool for minimising risk. British Journal of Health Care Management 14:720-722

Wood RG, Bailey NO, Tilkemeier D 1992 Managed care: the missing link to quality improvement. Journal of Nursing Care Quarterly 6(4):55-65

Zander K 2002 Integrated care pathways: eleven international trends. Journal of Integrated Care Pathways 6:101-107

CHAPTER
3

Integrated care pathways and the mental health modernisation agenda

David Howard

THE STRUCTURE AND FUNDING OF SERVICES	**SAFETY**
QUALITY	**THE SHIPMAN INQUIRY**
CHANGES IN WORK PRACTICES	**CONCLUSION**
ACCOUNTABILITY	**REFERENCES**

This chapter identifies the policy context within which integrated care pathways are located in contemporary mental health services. The major policy developments leading to the current operational structure of mental health services in the United Kingdom are outlined. The move from institutional-centred care to community-based care, together with the shift in financial power, is considered, and the position of integrated care pathways in clarifying these processes is introduced. The chapter goes on to discuss how, within this environment, quality is addressed and the contribution of integrated care pathways to set and monitor quality standards as an integral component of governance.

With changes in the structure of contemporary mental health services have come radical new ways of working, incorporating redefined roles and extending the skills of differing grades of staff. The implications of these are considered in the next section of this chapter where the difficulties in maintaining adequate numbers in the mental health services workforce are examined. It is shown how integrated care pathways can assist in workforce planning by providing data to identify the numbers of staff that are required to operate a service, the skill mix requirement and, consequently, areas of staff development.

Finally, within the context of *Building a safer NHS for patients* (Department of Health 2001), and the implications arising from the Shipman Inquiry (Smith 2004), the chapter considers how integrated care pathways can be used to monitor the standards of care that are delivered within a mental health service, and how they can help to identify adverse events occurring within a service, or within an individual's caseload.

THE STRUCTURE AND FUNDING OF SERVICES

Historical context

From the late 19th century until the latter part of the 20th century, mental health care in the United Kingdom (UK) was developed around an institutional, medically dominated model. This was a convenient system for providers of care as the centralisation of madness permitted a powerful, effective control over its management. However, from the service users' perspectives the system was not particularly enabling, and the combination of the damaging effects of their illnesses with that of institutionalisation led to a poor prognosis and a consequent improbability of discharge back into society. In turn, the asylum system became 'silted' with those suffering from long-term mental illnesses.

The advent of the phenothiazine group of drugs during the 1950s gave hope to this dire outlook. This was the first group of drugs to offer relief from many of the severe distressing symptoms of major psychoses – the group of disorders that was so prevalent in those suffering from long-term mental illnesses. Consequently, by using this group of drugs, it became possible to think of treating people who suffered from these conditions outside hospital. Even if they required admission, phenothiazines would reduce their length of stay dramatically, ameliorating the effects of institutionalisation. This colossal pharmacological development was soon reflected in policy with the introduction of the Mental Health Act 1959. Most notably, this Act facilitated the community-based care ideal by simplifying the process of admission and discharge to hospital for short periods of treatment under Section 4 (informal admission). To complement this, the Act required community resources to be developed. The intent of these initiatives was to provide an infrastructure to enable individuals who would benefit from the new phenothiazines to return to, or remain within, their local community for as long as possible. Local authorities and health authorities were encouraged to plan facilities jointly, with the local authorities employing specialist social workers and providing resources such as sheltered accommodation and day centres. Further support for this strategy was seen in the 1962 Hospital Plan (Department of Health and Social Security 1962) which set a target to almost halve the number of mental illness hospital bed provision to 1.8 per thousand population by 1975.

The tradition of the 19th century, upon which the UK mental health system was developed, had been to build county asylums. However, because of the lower ratio of mentally ill per head population compared with those who would require hospitalisation for a physical illness, and because of a reluctance to invest in mental health services, whole counties would only have one or two asylums. This policy made it very difficult for individuals living on the boundaries of a county to access services. For those requiring hospitalisation for a physical illness however, within a county there would probably be general hospitals in several major towns, making them much more accessible for their local population. The 1962 Hospital Plan promoted the development of these provincial hospitals into district general hospitals. Because it was now possible to treat individuals suffering from mental illnesses within the local community though, district general hospitals were to develop their range of services to deliver acute psychiatric inpatient units supplemented by outpatient day-care facilities.

The embryonic move to community-based care thus began, although nationally the growth of services was variable. A major barrier to progress, and joint working between health and social services, was funding. Local authorities argued that they had not received a corresponding increase in their central support grant to develop services. The Joint Finance Scheme, introduced in 1976 (Department of Health and Social Security 1976), attempted to address this by paying an allowance from the health authority to the corresponding local authority for every long-stay patient that was discharged from hospital. In this scheme though, the grant payable was finite, reducing by a fifth annually after 5 years and expiring fully after 10.

Joint finance was reviewed by the House of Commons Committee of Public Accounts (1981) which recommended expansion of the scheme, but to provide the finance, hospital land and buildings should be sold. Thus, following the election of the Conservative government in 1979, a very rapid closure of inpatient facilities occurred and increasing reliance was placed upon community-based services. Additionally, the underpinning motive of the scheme was now to develop a service which used taxpayers' money more efficiently, rather than one that prioritised patients' and carers' needs. It followed the then popular 'return to family values' philosophy, making the family rather than society responsible for caring for their sick. Indeed, in the report *Growing older* (Department of Health and Social Security 1981) community care was redefined:

> *Care in the community must increasingly mean care by the community*
> (Department of Health and Social Security 1981, para.1.9)

The policy of inpatient closures thus accelerated. However, major concerns were being raised about the provision of adequate services. In particular, the media focus was on dangerousness and (lack of) supervision. This was illustrated in 1984 with the murder of social worker Isabel Schwarz by a former inpatient Sharon Campbell. Initially, the government introduced the Care Programme Approach (Department of Health 1990) which formalised aftercare provision from Section 117 of the Mental Health Act 1983. However, the tragedies continued, particularly with the case of Ben Silcock who was mauled badly after he climbed into a lion's cage in London Zoo, and in the case of Jonathon Zito who was murdered by recently discharged Christopher Clunis. The government's response was the Mental Health (Patients in the Community) Act 1995, which amended the 1983 Mental Health Act by introducing a new status of 'supervised discharge' under Section 25, and placed more emphasis on statutory services to ensure the public's safety.

The Thatcher years thus saw significant changes in the provision and delivery of mental health services; however, this was located within an environment that was moving the managerial planning and provision of health care away from hospitals and health authorities and towards a market-led service which co-ordinated and bought in services from various health and social care providers.

This strategy followed the Griffiths review into community care (Griffiths 1988). In it, the report argued for more care to be delivered in the community; however, instead of the traditional centrally controlled health and social care services providing this, more use was to be made of alternative providers of care such as voluntary (including informal carers), not-for-profit and commercial sectors. To enable this, local authority social service departments would contract and purchase health, domiciliary and social care services rather than providing any themselves, and this included taking over funding for nursing home and residential care from the Department of Social Security.

The Griffiths report into community care (Griffiths 1988) in turn became the foundation upon which the NHS and Community Care Act 1990, which infamously introduced the free market economy into the National Health Service (NHS), was built. The service was divided into those who provided services (NHS trusts, private and voluntary contractors) and those who purchased services on behalf of their local population (health authorities, GP fundholding practices and social services). Full implementation occurred on 1 April 1993 when the controversial funding for commissioning and contracting domiciliary, residential home and nursing home care fell to local authorities.

This system was reviewed by New Labour on their election to office in 1997. Their response was the White Paper *The new NHS* (Department of Health 1997) and was followed by the Health Act 1999. This continued with the purchaser/provider model, although to reduce the amount of paperwork involved with contracting, GP fundholders were amalgamated into fewer but larger primary care trusts. Their role was to negotiate with local authorities and user groups to produce health action plans aimed at meeting the health needs of their local population. In respect of funding however, this continued with the underlying framework of the radical changes introduced 9 years previously, whereby control of the health budget and commissioning of services had been relocated from centralised control into primary care. Indeed, by 2004 primary care trusts controlled 80% of the health service budget (Department of Health 2004a).

So, the contemporary context for mental health trusts is primarily that of provider, contracting with primary care trusts to provide a range of services to meet the needs of the local population, and it is here that integrated care pathways provide an invaluable management tool. The major cost within most contracts in health and social care is that of the workforce. Many contracts are based upon workforce projections from existing sources, many of which derive from data collected over a period of years. However, the change in nature of service users, and in the form of services' engagement deriving from recent changes in policy (Department of Health 1998) such as early intervention, assertive outreach and crisis intervention, and associated staff skill-mix reviews can reduce these data to little more than an educated guess. In chapter 1, the provenance of integrated care pathways was traced back to the insurance-based systems in the United States of America. In this instance, they were used to provide a contracted cost for a patient episode. Conversely, in the UK, the use of integrated care pathways in mental health has been as a tool to improve the quality of care by basing the pathways on contemporary theory. However, as pathways develop and variances are analysed, data will be generated from patient episodes that can be used to clarify how many staff are required, their grades, roles, expected frequency of, and duration of, contact time. In turn this will generate data that can be used to develop accurate contracting costs.

QUALITY

The delivery of mental health services locally

Traditionally, within the NHS, assurance of quality relied heavily on the professions and their associated regulatory bodies. It was assumed that altruistic professionals would always act in the best interests of their clients and so ensure quality of service. Unfortunately, this system was open to abuse and the professions often acted in their own interests and against those who questioned the quality of practice (Kennedy et al 2001, Redfern et al 2001, Smith 2004).

It was not until the introduction of general management following the Griffiths (1983) reorganisation of the health service that this situation was challenged. Following its implementation, the previously autonomous professionals became accountable to general managers who in turn were required to ensure high-quality, effective and efficient services that would compete within a health marketplace. Various Total Quality Management (TQM) initiatives were introduced, culminating in the BS 5050/ ISO 9000 systems. Their success was limited, though, because of their limited ability to engage the whole workforce. Integrated Care Pathways, however, afford an opportunity to develop the quality of services. Developing pathways locally should involve contributions from all stakeholders (Department of Health 1998). Thus, instead of the top-down approach set by TQM systems, individuals have ownership of the pathways they create. Furthermore, the clarity of the terms of engagement afforded by integrated care pathway documentation permits appropriate targeted interventions to be made, resulting in an improved quality of care (Burnett et al 2002, Jackson et al 2003, Nott 2002, Tarling et al 2002).

The delivery of mental health services nationally

Whereas the TQM initiatives focused on service delivery, little progress had been made in monitoring the effect of the services on the health of the population. One of the conditions of being a member of the European Union is that the country subscribes to the Treaty of the European Union 1992 (the Maastricht Treaty), within which article 129 sets targets for public health (this subsequently became article 152 in the Treaty of Amsterdam 1999). UK health policy initially reflected these within the document *Health of the nation* (Department of Health 1992), which, following the election of the New Labour government in 1997, re-emerged within the White Paper *Saving lives: our healthier nation* (Department of Health,

1999a). Of particular interest for mental health services was chapter 8 which addressed suicide, mental health promotion, early and effective intervention. In turn, these areas became the major focus of modernising mental health services (Department of Health 1998) and the National Service Framework for mental health (Department of Health 1999b) which subsequently set the targets for all mental health services to achieve.

The National Service Framework set national service delivery targets. However, within local budgetary management in the health service there was a long history of inequitable distribution of resources, with more popular areas, such as acute medicine and surgery, receiving very generous funding at the expense of less popular areas such as mental health and the elderly (Department of Health 1998). Furthermore, inconsistent service delivery was compounded by the difficulty in ensuring that clinicians updated their practice to incorporate the latest research-based evidence. The combination of these issues had led to a 'postcode lottery' where, depending on an individual's address, services were likely to be better, or worse, than adjacent areas.

To address this, the New Labour government's pursuit of standardising quality throughout the UK was strengthened by the Health Act 1999, which set up the National Institute for Clinical Excellence (NICE). The role of NICE was to advise on the latest good practice and produce standard clinical and practice guidelines. This was supplemented in 2002 by the National Institute for Mental Health in England whose role was to assist trusts to develop and implement good practice and policy. Furthermore, to ensure the national guidelines were enacted, they were incorporated within the clinical governance auditing process. This is monitored independently by the Commission for Health Improvement, which was also created by the Health Act 1999 as an independent inspector of governance arrangements within trusts. [Following the Health and Social Care (Community Health and Standards) Act 2003, the Commission for Health Improvement was amalgamated into the Healthcare Commission.]

Within this context, integrated care pathways afford a particularly responsive and proactive method of incorporating both policy and clinical guidelines into practice, particularly in their electronic formats, which can be amended rapidly. This is complemented by the detailed workforce analysis they afford which can be used to calculate the size and skill-mix of the workforce that are required to meet governance targets. Thus, by monitoring variance analysis integrated care pathways can be fine-tuned to reflect local conditions and, in turn, demonstrate the local attainment of quality standards (Bryan et al 2002).

CHANGES IN WORK PRACTICES

Fundamental to contemporary policy in mental health has been the concept of integrated working between a variety of stakeholders, but primarily between health and social care (Department of Health 1998). Although this ideal has been promoted since the Mental Health Act of 1959, a combination of differing priorities, conflicting professional interests, inconsistent accountabilities and independent budgets has invariably led to unsuccessful outcomes. This was set to change with the introduction of the NHS Plan (Department of Health 2000a) which created and promoted the development of care trusts. These were formed by the amalgamation of local authority social services and health service trusts, and were formalised under Section 45 of the Health and Social Care Act 2001. In addition to pooling management and budgets, what was particularly challenging within these new trusts was the appraisal of traditional job roles and boundaries, an issue that was to occur subsequently throughout health care in general.

It is the Wanless report (Wanless 2002) that drew attention to the impending crisis in the health service workforce. The population of the UK is ageing and the proportion of elderly, the largest users of health and social care services, is set to increase significantly. Additionally, recruitment into the health service reduced during the 1980s and 1990s, a situation compounded by a high number of staff who are projected to end their health service careers by the year 2012. Wanless was briefed to determine the requirements of the health service in 2022. In addition to improvements in ICT (information and communication technology) and hotel services, he projected an increase in the size of the NHS workforce that will entail recruiting a further 300,000 staff and this will include:

- 62,000 doctors
- 108,000 nurses
- 45,000 therapists and scientists
- 74,000 health care assistants.

The cost of recruiting such a large number of staff was minimised by examining traditional roles and boundaries. It was argued that less expensive staff could take on roles that were traditionally performed by more expensive staff by taking a radical review of skill mix. Suggested figures were:

- 20% of the work of GPs/junior doctors to be undertaken by nurse practitioners
- 12.5% of the nursing workload to be undertaken by health care assistants.

Agenda for Change, and the Knowledge and Skills Framework (Department of Health 2004b), was the first major step in reviewing traditional job boundaries and, for example, in nursing, advanced practitioner roles such as nurse consultants were created to undertake a range of skills that would traditionally have been carried out by medical staff. By defining clearly the responsibilities of all involved in care delivery, integrated care pathways provide a vehicle for this process, mapping the precise terms of engagement and, in turn, the skills that are required of all stakeholders involved in care. Thus, when identifying and developing roles for multi-professional staff, and reviewing existing role developments, integrated care pathways provide a tool that can be used to identify workforce requirements for planning and recruiting, and when identifying the educational/professional development needs of existing staff. It should be cautioned however, that should staff be unprepared, or unwilling to engage with this process, less successful outcomes will occur (Gibbon et al 2002, Rees et al 2004).

Inter-professional rivalry can be particularly problematic in multi-professional working (Gibbon et al 2002, Rees et al 2004). Often, however, it is the attitudes of staff, rather than the integrated care pathways, that are problematic, a situation that is compounded if there is a top-down approach to implementation. By way of contrast, Logan (2003) and Hall (2001) found that integrated care pathways enhanced multi-professional working. The significant difference though was ownership. In particular, Logan (2003) documented how all stakeholders were involved in developing the service, an issue that is emphasised in chapter 4 of this book where Simon Wood and Barrie Green report on their experiences of culturing a milieu of ownership within a multi-professional work environment. Furthermore, there is scope to involve both users and carers in this process, broadening ownership of the resulting pathway to all stakeholders in the healthcare community.

ACCOUNTABILITY

In an environment where there are changes in the roles of professional staff, and increasing demands are being placed upon informal carers, the quality of service that is provided to the individual is open to extreme scrutiny. Earlier in this chapter, the role of the media in sensationalising homicides committed by individuals who had suffered from mental illness was discussed and the policy that followed was seen to place an increased responsibility on local service providers. The principles from the cases of Bolam and Bolitho, as discussed in chapter 5 of this book, demonstrate that a minimum standard of care is expected from the responsible trust and that Courts will find them negligent should such care be unforthcoming. Consequently, it may be argued that placing responsibility on informal carers, or substituting the care usually offered by one grade of staff with that from another (perhaps less qualified) member of staff, amounts to a negligent act. Evidence is therefore required to demonstrate that such changes do not dilute the standard of services offered, and this is where the use of integrated care pathways assists by documenting who will do what with whom, when and to what standard. This then demonstrates the quality of services that are delivered, both to an individual and by the mental health services in general.

It is the clear concise documentation afforded by integrated care pathways that forms a key component of effective multi-professional working (Burnett et al 2002). They clearly identify individuals' roles and functions and, through the process of variance analysis, identify whether or not pathway objectives were achieved and to what extent. In turn, this provides the evidence to demonstrate the quality of service delivery.

SAFETY

As integrated care pathways specify the roles of all stakeholders involved, they also enable the contribution of each team member to be examined, enabling analysis of the effectiveness of their involvement. Inevitably, it is this aspect that creates suspicion amongst practitioners; however, this needs to be balanced by their ability to show good practice, identify areas for professional development, and highlight areas of excessive workload.

The report into patient safety *An organisation with a memory* by the Expert Group on Learning from Adverse Events in the NHS (Department of Health 2000b) came about in the wake of several major scandals in the NHS which had resulted in patients being put at risk, or not informed of issues. Two major incidents were also under investigation at this time:

- The Report of the Inquiry into the Royal Children's Hospital, Liverpool (Redfern et al 2001), otherwise known as the Alder Hey Inquiry, where body parts from deceased children had been retained without the parents' consent, and
- The Report of the Public Inquiry into children's heart surgery at the Bristol Royal Infirmary 1984-1995 (Kennedy et al 2001) where at least 29 babies had died following heart surgery at the Royal Infirmary.

Each reported on a culture of intimidation within the health service, from coercion within the employing organisations, and from fear of litigation, both of which had led to adverse events going unreported. Included within the recommendations were the following:

- a national system of incident reporting and a clear emphasis on the role of all staff within this area
- an open 'no-blame' culture to encourage the reporting of, and subsequent learning from, adverse incidents.

To enable this to occur, suitable reporting systems were developed which in turn supported the open organisational culture and attempted to ensure that the lessons learned reached practice. These were implemented more fully following *Building a safer NHS for patients* (Department of Health 2001) which stated that all organisations within the NHS must develop:

- agreed definitions of adverse events and near misses for the purposes of logging and reporting
- a minimum data set for adverse events and near misses, and
- a standard adverse event report format.

It also established the National Patient Safety Agency to coordinate, collect and analyse information on adverse events from all NHS organisations, NHS staff, patients and carers, and to disseminate the findings back to clinical practice.

The introduction of integrated care pathways affords several opportunities to incorporate error tracking. By monitoring the variance analysis of individual patients, those that deviate from the norm will automatically trigger further investigation and, in turn, this may uncover an event that ordinarily might proceed unnoticed for a longer period of time, or develop into one with more serious outcomes. In addition, several patients failing to respond to a pathway as expected may not simply indicate a problem with a pathway, but detailed analysis may identify failure of a system within it. Of course, with adverse event reporting integrated within clinical governance, there is a danger that a more sensitive diagnostic system, as is afforded by variance analysis, may initially reveal higher numbers of incidents occurring. In turn, this may show adversely within a trust's governance assessment and it is therefore essential that, should this occur, this is recognised by trust managers and Healthcare Commission inspectors.

More proactively, the speed by which integrated care pathways can be updated and, particularly in the case of electronic integrated care pathways, disseminated to clinicians, enables changes to be made to reflect both local and national findings. Indeed, with electronic care pathways, the speed of variance tracking is such that it is possible to flag and update errors simultaneously. In turn, care pathways thus become an extremely efficient vehicle with which to disseminate the contemporary findings of adverse incidents and amend practice accordingly. This integrates into the objectives of *Building a safer NHS for patients* (Department of Health 2001) and, as the use of integrated care pathways develops, it is expected that their use in this way will become more extensive.

THE SHIPMAN INQUIRY

Following the harrowing inquiry into the conduct of Harold Shipman (Smith 2004), many criticisms were levelled at the medical profession, and the closed, introspective conduct of the General Medical Council (GMC). The inquiry found that far from protecting the public, the GMC was reactive to adverse events and primarily acted in the interests of doctors. It also found that the GMC failed to monitor doctors' competence adequately, supporting what had been reported in the Bristol Inquiry 4 years previously. Arguments were made for the publication and comparison of individual doctors' mortality rates. However, the use of statistical analysis alone is an extremely crude method of identifying at-risk doctors. With some justification, doctors have argued against monitoring competence based on patient outcomes as the more expert doctors are often referred more severely ill patients who, in turn, have a poorer life expectancy. Indeed, as Mohammed et al (2004) show, when monitoring general practitioners statistical aberrations can be generated simply by the inclusion of a high number of nursing homes within a practice's catchment area. Consequently, they argue that more detailed analysis is required.

It is precisely this level of detail that analysis of the variance from integrated care pathways provides. In addition, it flags potential difficulties early, hopefully before a patient dies. As a part of medical audit therefore, this goes some way to addressing the monitoring requirement resulting from the Shipman Inquiry. Integrated care pathways are multi-professional tools; therefore, they could well be adapted for use within institutional audit procedures to assure the safe practice of all staff involved with patients' care.

CONCLUSION

The original intention for using integrated care pathways within the UK was to assist the implementation of the latest research and policy developments within contemporary practice and in both general medical services and mental health services; they generally have received positive evaluation. Within the context of contemporary mental health service delivery, they offer much more than this though. Their power lies in the evidence they generate during their operation and they provide a means of transformation and modernisation of mental health services. Consequently, in addition to their primary purpose of enabling practitioners to deliver optimal care, integrated care pathways can be used to assist in costing, to provide evidence of defensible practice and become an integral component of quality assurance. The move from institutional-run to primary care commissioned services is unlikely to change in the foreseeable future, bringing with it a new approach to care delivery that embraces many modernisation and policy themes such as choice, payment by results, integrated working and governance. Contracting will therefore continue between purchasers and provider trusts to deliver mental health services within agreed budgets and at a quality that will meet governance targets. Furthermore, in a political climate where equity of service provision, accountability in the form of evidence that quality and health targets are met, and efficiency in the use of resources remain high on the health and social care agenda, integrated care pathways provide continuous contextual information for performance monitoring. Consequently, it is expected that they will continue to develop, particularly in their electronic forms, as a fundamental component of contemporary mental health service delivery.

REFERENCES

Bryan S, Holmes S, Postlethwaite D et al 2002 The role of integrated care pathways in improving the patient experience. The first in a series of two articles. Professional Nurse 18(2):77-79
Burnett VW, Cavanagh S, Shearer J 2002 Multidisciplinary documentation in care of the elderly. British Journal of Therapy and Rehabilitation 9(10):382-385

Department of Health 1990 The care programme approach for people with a mental illness referred to the specialist psychiatric services (90)23/Lassl(90)11. HMSO, London

Department of Health 1992 The health of the nation. A strategy for health in England Cm 1986. Stationery Office, London

Department of Health 1997 The new NHS: modern, dependable. Stationery Office, London

Department of Health 1998 Modernising mental health services: safe, sound, and supportive. Stationery Office, London

Department of Health 1999a Saving lives: our healthier nation Cmd 4386. Stationery Office, London

Department of Health 1999b National service framework for mental health: modern standards and service models. Stationery Office, London

Department of Health 2000a The NHS Plan: a plan for investment, a plan for reform Cmd 4818-I. Stationery Office, London

Department of Health 2000b An organisation with a memory. Report of an expert group on learning from adverse events in the NHS, chaired by the Chief Medical Officer. Stationery Office, London

Department of Health 2001 Building a safer NHS for patients: implementing 'An organisation with a memory'. Stationery Office, London

Department of Health 2004a NHS improvement plan 2004: Putting people at the heart of public services. Stationery Office, London

Department of Health 2004b Agenda for Change final agreement (December 2004). Stationery Office, London

Department of Health and Social Security 1962 Hospital plan for England and Wales Cmnd 1064. HMSO, London

Department of Health and Social Security 1976 Priorities for health and personal social services. HMSO, London

Department of Health and Social Security 1981 Growing older Cmnd 8173. HMSO, London.

Gibbon B, Watkins C, Barer D et al 2002 Can staff attitudes in team working in stroke care be improved? Journal of Advanced Nursing 40(1):105-111.

Griffiths R 1983 NHS management inquiry. Report to the Secretary of State for Social Services. HMSO, London

Griffiths R 1988 Community care: agenda for action. HMSO, London

Hall J 2001 A qualitative survey of staff responses to a pilot study in a mental healthcare setting. Nursing Times Research 6(3):696-706

House of Commons Committee of Public Accounts 1981 Joint financing of care by the National Health Service and local government; disposal of surplus NHS land and buildings. HMSO, London

Jackson D, Turner-Stokes L, Williams H et al 2003 Use of integrated care pathway: a third round audit of the management of shoulder pain in neurological conditions. Journal of Rehabilitation Medicine 35(3):265-270

Kennedy I, Jarman B, Howard R et al 2001 The report of the Public Inquiry into children's heart surgery at the Bristol Royal Infirmary 1984-1995: Learning from Bristol. Stationery Office, London

Logan K 2003 Indwelling catheters: developing an integrated care pathway package. Nursing Times 99(44):49-51

Mohammed AM, Rathbone A, Myers P et al 2004 An investigation into general practitioners associated with high patient mortality flagged up through the Shipman Inquiry: retrospective analysis of routine data. British Medical Journal 328:1474-1477

Nott A 2002 Introducing an integrated care pathway on an acute mental health in-patient trust. Mental Health Practice 5(6):12-15

Redfern M, Keeling J, Powell E 2001 Report of the Inquiry into the Royal Children's Hospital, Liverpool. Stationery Office, London

Rees G, Huby G, McDade L et al 2004 Joint working in community mental health teams: implementation of an integrated care pathway. Health and Social Care in the Community 12(6):527-536

Smith, J 2004 The Shipman Inquiry fifth report – safeguarding patients: lessons from the past – proposals for the future, command paper Cm 6394. Stationery Office, London

Tarling M, Aitken E, Lahoti O et al 2002 Closing the audit loop: the role of a pilot in the development of a fractured neck of femur integrated care pathway. Journal of Orthopaedic Nursing 6(3):130-134

Wanless D 2002 Securing our future health: taking a long-term view. Stationery Office, London

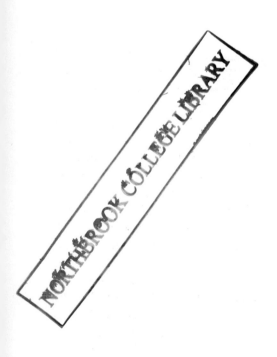

Integrated care pathways and integrated working

Simon Wood and Barrie Green

Modern transport systems and clinical practice have a lot in common. They have a number of component parts, many of which are very different in appearance and function, but they also have many similarities. In the process of getting from one place to another, a bus is different from a train, which in turn is different from a plane. One travels by road, one by rail, and another in the air. However, they are generally long multi-seated tubes (or boxes), designed to move groups of people. If you are travelling to Ibiza you cannot use one single vehicle; you need to integrate two or more. The end result is anticipated to be the same – a pleasant holiday destination, but getting there can be a very complicated process.

Clinical practice is not dissimilar. To a service user, doctors, nurses, occupational therapists and psychologists tend to look alike – human beings with similar physical features – but their modes of action or intervention have a diverse physical, social and biological basis. To the service user or carer they may all be one and the same, a healthcare professional, designed to cure, but in clinical practice they all contribute only part of the journey. What is vital is that the sum of the total parts equates to the same destination; it is pointless for one to head for Ibiza if another is aiming for Iceland. Clearly, they are both interesting places to be, but if you had anticipated speaking Spanish and had packed a bag full of beachwear then the latter is not really the expected outcome. Perhaps the analogy is a little crude, but the message for integrated working within integrated care pathways is the same. The destination should be agreed, the anticipated type of vehicle identified in advance, the route planned, and the resources (fuel, spending money and food) prepared. When we finally arrive, we should review which were the better parts of the journey, and make plans for both the return home and any future trips to the same place.

THE ORIGINS AND PURPOSES OF INTEGRATED CARE PATHWAYS

Integrated clinical (care) pathways (ICPs) have a basis within the 'managed care' environment of the United States of America (USA) (Jones et al 1999, 2000). This approach evolved by virtue of the insurance-based funding of the American healthcare system. As is the case with motor insurance in the United Kingdom (UK), the companies funding the bill need to be sure that they are getting what they pay for and are neither being overcharged nor being the victim of shoddy workmanship (hence, in the motor trade, approved repairers are often the path down which the damaged car is directed).

Consequently, in the USA, the funders required greater precision than had previously been the case in respect of diagnosis, evidence-based treatments for that diagnosis, expected duration of hospitalisation, and other related factors. An expected pathway could therefore be devised which was procedure based, whether for removal of an appendix or for implantation of an artificial hip joint. Until relatively recently, however, it had not been thought possible to adopt this approach in the field of mental health care. In contrast to physical health conditions and treatments, there are limits to diagnostic precision, and some overlap of treatments from one condition to another. It was therefore perceived that the innate variability within each person would colour his or her response to treatment to such an extent that no adequate average plan could be devised.

As contemporary clinical practice evolved though, there have been a number of attempts towards applying the principles of condition-specific integrated clinical pathways to the field of mental health care (Aitken 2000, Brett & Schofield 2002, Jones 2001, Nott 2002, Smith et al 2000). The authors' approach to this (Green et al 2001, Jones & Coyne 2001) has been to avoid developing a condition-specific pathway, but rather one which has pathways dependent upon a service user's legal status. This is because our work in a regional medium secure unit entails differing approaches for those subject to differing legal constraints, timescales and demands. Within this context however, coordination of a range of internal clinical disciplines and additional external agencies is essential.

MULTI-PROFESSIONAL WORKING

To return to the motoring analogy, the multi-professional team and the processes which drive it are akin to a gearbox. An efficient gearbox is designed with differing cogs which intermesh and relate to each other freely but within constraints. The cogs must transmit one to the other without undue impediment, and process force and motion from input to output. Similarly, in clinical practice, an integrated care pathway describes just these issues. It defines what is done, by whom, to whom, why, when and how. Middleton et al (1998) elaborate this by defining an integrated care pathway as:

> *A set of expected interventions placed in an appropriate timeframe written and agreed by a multi-professional team to help a service user with a specific condition or diagnosis move progressively through a clinical experience to positive outcomes.*

Multi-professional teams are not purely a healthcare phenomenon. The approach is also used in another high-cost, high-risk and low-volume world, that of oil exploration. Here, as in mental health, the benefits of integrated team, and agency, working are seen as a vital component of the organisational agenda. It is beneficial and superior to uni-professional strategies (Sneider 1999) because:

> *... individuals commonly have a limited view of overall objectives and goals, and communication among disciplines is generally only fair. In contrast, multi-professional organisations usually have shared objectives and goals, better communication among disciplines, and good integration of technical skills and knowledge.*

This form of team functioning is thus an acknowledged solution to complex organisational dilemmas. It develops the synergy associated with the skills of a range of individuals towards the overall goal. However, relationships within such a team are notoriously difficult to gauge, and unfortunately there are no reliable measures of the 'health' of the multi-professional team. A multi-professional team commonly comprises individual professionals from several different disciplines, working together yet towards discipline-related goals (Webster 2002). In poorly developed teams though, they can be ploughing individual parallel furrows. Within such teams, members are less likely to be inter-reliable or to gel well, since divided duties lead to divided loyalties and almost inevitably to reduced effectiveness. The authors have found that in their practice arena, forensic mental health, inappropriate referrals to an unnecessarily higher level of security stem largely from teams dominated by uni-professional or bi-professional approaches, indicating a narrowness of clinical repertoire that works against service users' needs.

In addition, there have recently been several significant changes to the roles of clinicians working within mental health. Professions allied to medicine are now taking on roles formerly seen as the exclusive province of the medical doctor, much of which has resulted from the increasing realisation that the demands for services are rising, and the availability of medical staff is finite. Tasks have therefore been redistributed, under the guise of enhancing practitioners' roles, while in truth the driver has been to make the system work. For some practitioners, and indeed services, a focus on justifying why and how they examine their skills, in the interests of effective care delivery, is a wake-up call. It is the authors' contention however, that integrated working is far removed from redistribution of workload, and is in fact a re-engineering of clinical roles and responsibilities.

MULTI-AGENCY WORKING

Multi-agency working is widely advocated as the nirvana to which modern clinical and organisational structures should aspire. However, the approach has a number of problems, particularly between formal agencies (Wood 1996). Often there is conflict between different bureaucratic structures, concerns over confidentiality, competition for funds between agencies, lack of clarity regarding roles and expertise, inadequate communication, conflicting expectations, scepticism, mistrust and rivalry. Frequently, structural re-organisation within individual, or groups of, organisations tends to create further confusion and reduces the potential for coordinated working. This creates an environment which is littered with the fragmented carcasses of well intentioned uni-agency strategies.

The absence of a common unifying thread is often the catalyst for failure though. A solution to this is the development of integrated inter-agency care (and management) pathways. If we return to the transport strategy outlined in the introduction to this chapter, one can envisage the 'joining up' of a series of short hops by a single ticket which incorporates all aspects into one long journey. Each agency can develop its own journey, or care pathway, but the critical success criterion is the use of the same map and planning from timetables which use the same clock and same days of the week.

In addition to 'the coordinated timetable' is the delivery of a sequence of routes which are planned to meet the needs of the passenger, or service user and carers. It is pointless defining the most integrated travel structures, combining the various components of road, rail and air, if the buses, trains and planes have insufficient capacity or do not stop at places that passengers either want to go to, can access easily or at times of day that are inconvenient. Therefore, user consultation, feedback and partnership are essential to the development of successful multi-agency strategies, strategies which are tailored to meeting their needs and not primarily those of the providers.

In the authors' field, there is recognition that service users and carers not only have a view, but a valid and useful view. In effect, one may see them as another discipline whose ' take' on a set of circumstances will be from a different angle and therefore potentially enriching to the overall consideration. In the National Institute for Clinical Excellence *Guidelines for schizophrenia* (National Institute for Clinical Excellence 2002) there is an explicit role for users and carers which extends into arenas previously thought the exclusive province of the expert professional. The concept of the 'expert patient' has arisen and user groups have produced research material which influences drug treatments (National Schizophrenia Fellowship 2001). This concept was incorporated within the development of ICPs within the authors' own service; user views were sought and the ideas generated were incorporated into revisions to the process map.

INTEGRATED WORKING

A number of centrally generated frameworks have been developed for mental health (Jones et al 2000). These include the Care Programme Approach (Department of Health 1990), supervision registers, supervised discharge (Department of Health 1996), and more recently proposals for changes to mental health legislation (Department of Health 2004). Over the past two decades, legislation for mental health has moved from an institutional model towards community care, and from uni-professional to multi-professional recognition. Elements of government thinking have thus contained frameworks similar to some elements of an integrated care pathway (Aitken 2000, Jones et al 2000, Smith et al 2000). However, integrated working has been aimed towards, and perhaps described, but not necessarily achieved. More recently, emerging legislative change (Department of Health 2004) has recognised that some labels on former roles may be unhelpful and even an impediment: for example, the replacement of the term RMO (responsible medical officer) with a more realistic/plural descriptor – that of clinical supervisor. This reflects a more inter-professional/inter-agency scenario whereby multi-agency working is both the norm and essential, particularly as the clinical load is able to be formally shared more widely. There is evidence from the user perspective that indicates increased satisfaction with the development of more specialist roles for nurses and other disciplines. For example, user satisfaction with nurse prescribing demonstrates the desire for more extended roles with respect to prescribing and medication management (Latter & Courtney 2003).

The Care Programme Approach (Department of Health 1990) is recognised as being an effective mechanism for integrating health and social service aspects of a care package in specialised mental health care (NHS Health Advisory Service 1996). In effect, the Care Programme Approach was a government-driven structure aimed at improving information sharing, recording and tracking. While falling short of being an actual pathway, it may perhaps be seen as prescribing elements of an integrated care pathway. It is disappointing though that it took a government to impose this and that the professions did not themselves combine to agree a common framework approach to describe what should already have been good practice. It remains the case, however, that the professions were handicapped by their separation. The integrated care pathway is thus a means of bridging this separation by converting the hierarchical content-driven approaches into a flatter process framework which not only binds professionals together but has some useful outcomes for the individuals using it.

INTEGRATED CARE PATHWAYS, MULTI-PROFESSIONAL TEAMWORKING AND RISK MANAGEMENT

Recently, there has been an increased drive towards caution and accountability within the area of risk management. A number of high-profile mental health inquiries into community care highlighted a need for increased communication and collaboration between professionals and agencies to reduce 'risk'(Zito Trust 1996). This placed unrealistic expectations upon the shoulders of statutory agencies, each having to justify the intricate minutiae of each decision in anticipation of failure. In turn, this redefined risk from a concept that contained both positive and negative potential, to the anticipation and elimination of danger.

It is no longer realistic for individuals to shoulder solo burdens of risk or care. It can however be difficult for some, especially those in numerically small number or in roles traditionally seen as powerful, to legitimately acknowledge the need for others, that they lack the complete view within themselves, or even that they might be mistaken. A positive example of risk-taking from a team perspective is a lottery syndicate. One person can buy a lottery ticket and expose themselves to the risk of winning the jackpot; however, if they work together with others and spread the range and combinations of numbers, the 'risk' of winning is increased. Conversely, the same principles apply to the management of negative risks (danger). The more widely teams share information and skill, the more likely is the potential for successful management of the risk.

Post-incident investigators always have the advantage of hindsight and will examine critically what a practitioner has done, and whether their actions were reasonable (Carson 1996). However, there is a powerful advantage for practice to be derived from integrated working. This is protective of staff, demonstrating that ideas were canvassed from a range of clinical and managerial viewpoints, and that the decision in contention is one to which all were signed up. This provides insulation, which is comforting in a litigious world, always of course providing that the process can be demonstrated to have taken place. So what is it that provides this evidence? It is the documentation of the integrated care pathway.

IMPLEMENTATION

Mental health practitioners are supposed to have expertise in human nature and behaviour. What we know of this in relation to working lives is that however dedicated and committed an individual may be, there will be an element of 'what's in it for me?' present somewhere in their psyche. The protective role of an integrated care pathway is not obvious at first glance; however, those who have come into the process from a different professional model usually develop a realisation of this. The authors suggest that bringing this to the attention of staff should be via subtle means since to do otherwise suggests, wrongly, that the prime purpose of the approach is defensive. Properly conducted, however, integrated care pathway based delivery of care does offer a measure of defence for its participants. This arises from being able to show a process, due consideration, and a description of why a decision took the direction it did. It offers a route to demonstrate that the care decision was reasonable and one which a responsible body of professionals would have taken. The legal case that underpins the notion of what is reasonable is Bolam (Bolam v Friern Hospital Management Committee [1957] 1 WLR 582) (described in chapter 5 of this book). Although the boundaries of this have been pushed and tested over the years (Young 2003), it remains the principal guiding case and one to which many individuals and professional bodies return. At its heart is the concept of comparison of the decision in question against what a responsible body would have done in the circumstances. The integrated care pathway provides this.

The authors' experience is that not only do practitioners, unsurprisingly, not move overnight from uni-professional to plural practice, but also this transition is not a continuous process as might be assumed. It takes place on a stepped basis as the individual moves from appreciating theoretical constructs to practical integration. The steps and their sequence will vary between individuals but generally include:

1. 'Realising safety in numbers' – professional isolation need not be countered by joining a cohort of same-type professionals.
2. Understanding the language, values and constructs of another profession – perhaps only one other as a starting position.
3. Appreciating the benefits to risk management of a shared approach.

The authors have successfully used this approach in multi-disciplinary training and development programmes to enhance the common understanding of relevant concepts and frameworks across agencies (Green & Wood 2002). Staff who do not grasp these key progression points are unlikely to work easily in an integrated setting or to comfortably and effectively handle clinical risk.

DEVELOPING A PLURAL LANGUAGE

The language of clinical activity is an essential part of the work of a team. Equally essential however, is that it is understood by all members of the team. We need not all be completely fluent, but it is vital to have a working knowledge sufficient to be able to understand the daily business.

The traditional stereotype of the English abroad is that they expect others to understand English, and in case of difficulty they shout slowly and loudly, in the belief that this helps communication. In health care, there are professions that traditionally have taken this approach in their communication with others. In addition though, when this is enacted within the clinical environment involving multiple disciplines, each profession needed to be seen to be valuable. Thus they promoted this by using their professional vocabulary to argue that they were best placed to decide upon and provide the care for the service user. Each profession then vies to be seen to have the best 'take' in a game of professional one-upmanship. Often, in such circumstances, the service user becomes secondary to the relational games, and their needs distorted or compromised. Therefore, it is essential that such opportunities are reduced, and an effective way of doing so would be to ensure full and active participation of the service user in the decision-making processes.

The integrated care pathway addresses this by producing content which must be understandable by all stakeholders. The culture of working within a pathway fosters readiness to question, which itself pre-empts others to give their input in an understandable manner. The practitioner who can avoid complex terminology and present a complex construct in an understandable way is likely to be best understood by all. Indeed, feedback from service users and carers completes the loop on practice reflection and monitoring, which is an integral part of the expectations within the pathway. It provides a check on understanding and is a further aid to flattening the hierarchy so that there is true plurality of work.

TRANSLATING MULTI-PROFESSIONAL PATHWAYS ACROSS AGENCIES

The difficulties and obstacles experienced by some individuals working multi-professionally extends into inter-agency working (Wood 1996). However, the development and introduction of integrated care pathways within and across agencies provide opportunities for enhanced cooperation and coordination of, and with, different teams and organisations. An example can be seen within forensic mental health and learning disability services. As a distinct specialty, it is forced to confront the wide spectrum of challenges posed by the various stakeholders that operate within Mentally Disordered Offender (MDO) agencies. The primary, and perhaps most obvious, examples are secure hospitals and prisons, although there are a number of other very closely involved agencies, e.g. court liaison and diversion teams, social and probation services, primary care participants (trusts and professionals), the police and legal representatives, and the generic community and hospital-based mental health and learning disability services (Birmingham 2001, Riordan & Wix 1999). Other involved groups may include the voluntary sector, support groups (carer and service user), academic institutions, the media, politicians and the general public. Each brings its own perspective into the clinical and organisational arena and each perspective has an influence upon clinical interventions and management strategies which must operate along an already complicated criminological and healthcare continuum. This continuum has a number of basic inherent tensions and competing priorities. For example, a fundamental care versus custody dilemma results in enough complications for clinical planning alone without the added dimensions of a number of other stakeholder perspectives added to the mix.

How does one integrate these dimensions? Are integrated care pathways a solution? As described earlier, there are a number of existing statutory frameworks which replicate a number of dimensions of integrated care pathways (Department of Health 1990, Jones et al 2000). Although these do not receive equal priority within each agency, they impose certain parameters upon inter-agency functioning. In addition, there are a number of natural inter-agency benchmarks at the point where the service user is handed from one to another.

Traditionally, when a service user leaves one part of the system they tend to 'belong' to someone else. The challenges include different philosophical service designs, finite resources, agency or professional conflict/competition, and an inherent cross-dimensional inertia caused by lack of shared ownership of the service user or their problems (Wood 1996). For example, the forensic service user's journey from offence to hospitalisation often involves a number of stopping-off points (arrest, police station, court, prison and/or hospital), and a number of professional contacts (police officers, lawyers, custody diversion teams, court officials, private prisoner transport officers, prison officers and/or nursing and medical staff). Each of these points, and contacts with professionals, involves a number of micro-journeys (hops) within the overall process. For example, placement within a medium secure unit (MSU) can involve all of these micro-journeys as well as liaison and integration with community mental health teams, acute hospitals, prison health care and prison in-reach teams. Their individual part of the process needs to be coordinated to reach a satisfactory outcome.

DEVELOPING HIGH-LEVEL PROCESS MAPS AND VARIANCES

Two of the major components of any integrated care pathway, high-level process mapping and variance tracking, are vital to producing satisfactory outcomes. The former is a means of bringing the various stakeholders together whereas the latter, more threatening, component is a means of exploring the potential structural weaknesses.

High-level process maps

The high-level process map is a strategy that brings together a range of professionals from each agency involved in the service user's journey to agree common objective(s), and the shared benchmarks within and between each stakeholder (Jones et al 1999). The map itself begins as a flow chart with boxes diagrammatically describing the key stages in the clinical journey for the service user and care providers. Decision trees can be incorporated to identify the points at which the progress will take one of several different routes dependent upon test results, treatment response, and so forth. If there are pieces of care provided as an identifiable sub-package with the main process, perhaps by means of an intervention principally from one staff group or discipline, or within one establish-ment, then those identifiable pieces would themselves be formed into smaller pathways. Each has a starting point at some place along the main pathway and a point of re-connection to it. Thus is born the branch pathway (Figure 4.1).

From the high level map one can begin to incorporate timescales and to describe expectations of what should occur within each box in the diagram in order to progress to the next. The components which form each box, who delivers them, and the success/failure or entry/exit criteria can be delineated. This is a straightforward process which can provide an opportunity for the range of stakeholders to 'join up' their thinking towards plurality; the leap into developing

Figure 4.1
Humber Centre clinical pathway, high-level process map (referral) (Jones et al 1999)

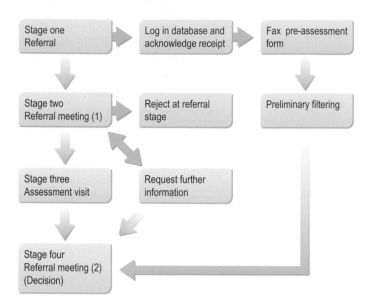

a fully fledged integrated care pathway is inappropriate, but such integration of the various stages of the service user's journey can be used as a means of developing protocols and processes for linking services. As success tends to breed success, the next step, that of developing truly integrated inter-agency care pathways, is not such a huge and complicated task. Should the leap into an integrated care pathway be too great a move for an agency or service to make at the outset, a similar approach can be used to develop protocols for linkage between the agencies. This offers less of a perceived threat to the internal working of each organisation involved, as in the first instance it will be largely unchanged. What will alter, however, is the processes by which the organisation engages with and relates to other organisations with which it has dealings. Changes in process at the margins do not radically alter the core at the outset, but they do act as a Trojan horse to inject concepts of pathways and processes into the organisation, and can thereby demonstrate that the threat is limited and the benefit high. Once pathways are demonstrated to be appropriate and relevant, the height of the hurdle to an integrated care pathway will have been reduced considerably.

Variance

The concept of variance can cause anxiety among staff if they perceive it is to monitor shortcomings in their performance. The health and social care arena is however now more familiar with audit, appraisal, and other performance management measures, and variance can be set within a context of being another aspect of these same, familiar, processes.

A much more tangible benefit to staff can be emphasised, which offers the potential to draw in members of the wider team and act as a tool for resource planning and delivery. This is the use of variance coding to identify episodes where the planned care or intervention took place in a manner different from that envisaged, or not at all, by reason of an individual or discipline being overloaded or in short supply. Consequently, variance helps in workforce planning, and in making a case for more or better use of members of staff.

Alternatively, variance coding can identify specific areas of unmet need, or needs that would benefit from specialist input. If an overview is taken of such needs within a service, it can inform managers and supervisors of the areas which require developing and how, offering a facility to deploy and encourage the skills of individuals within the service who have an interest in specialist areas of practice. Similarly, if an individual within the service is known to have particular skills, the integrated care pathway allows ready identification of areas of clinical activity which would most benefit from that professional's input. A scenario is therefore created which allows practitioners to select particular niches of skills or interests, and allows the service to select from the portfolio of specialist interests offered by its practitioners.

Now the tricky part – introducing variances across agencies. Dictionary definitions and general perceptions tend to emphasise the disintegrative nature of the term 'variance'. Therefore, the use of such terminology between professions and agencies can be threatening, invoking images of disagreement. Even sharing of the main functions of variance recording, an audit cycle which acknowledges system, professional or service user centred alterations to a planned clinical journey, can suggest that 'big brother' is checking on individuals or teams. Poor outcomes can be perceived as resulting in loss of organisational face. It is therefore important to emphasise the benefits of variance tracking/recording as a means of accurately identifying structural weaknesses across inter-agency structures, not as a means of apportioning 'blame', but as an opportunity for identifying resource and service opportunities. If variance tracking repeatedly shows instances where therapy x has not been delivered, this may not be due to personal failing or laziness of a therapist. Rather, it may be that there is a mismatch between the times when they are available and the times when they are needed, or alternatively because the demand for that therapy is higher than the staffing resource can support. In these instances, therefore, variance data from an ICP can be used to support a business case for more staff or changes to improve patient care. These are poles apart from the personal threat which practitioners may feel as their first response to variance coding.

Another less obvious benefit of variance recording is the ability to accurately reflect changes to risk management strategies. As discussed earlier, in the event of an adverse incident, variance tracking can provide an audit trail that demonstrates subtle or dynamic changes to treatment and management plans which are not always obvious from traditional clinical or other agency-based records. The comprehensive and evidence-based nature of integrated care pathways not only demonstrates the actual outcome for any one service user, but in such an incident, also the intent behind the plans. It allows the service and those within it to show that they had thought prospectively about various possible options, and actively chose one rather than allowing passive drift.

DEVELOPMENT OF PATHWAYS

The essence of developing multi-agency integrated care pathways is to organise a number of stakeholder events, which encourage active participation of multi-professional, inter-agency teams, their managers and service users/representatives. The primary aim of these events should be to produce solution-focused developments that bring benefits towards integrated care, rather than as a managerial imperative. In other words, service user focus is the driver of managerial initiatives to facilitate empowerment and a reduction in individual or team resistance. In the current climate of partnership, the statutory agencies and the service user groups are becoming more conversant in the social 'norms' of such active collaboration. However, partnership must be facilitated in a way that balances the sometimes controversial relationship between participants and can acknowledge the limitations that exist in certain legal, clinical or organisational situations. Clarity of purpose, openness and honesty is undoubtedly the best approach.

Within each integrated care pathway, high-level process maps of each micro-system (hospital, prison, court) should be developed, each identifying potential cross-over points, benchmarks or points of concordance. These 'micro-maps' can be brought together subsequently into a coordinated 'visual' representation of the whole system. This can be compared with an expected or ideal service user journey (Jones et al 2000), any deficits identified by the multi-agency group can eventually form the basis of variance codification, and are then followed by solution strategies.

The process described above could also be approached by using a meta analysis of the whole system. Potentially, this could create momentum towards strategic service redesign. However, a risk associated with this approach is that smaller stakeholders may be overlooked, or feel undervalued and disempowered, resulting in subsequent lack of ownership and/or disengagement. Another risk is that without a starting point which is seen by all as legitimate, the development of strategic thinking towards pathways is likely to be fractured, inefficient, and slow. Both of these approaches can result in integrated care pathway development, but in the structured approach where pathways are designed with a more local focus, attention to detail and individualised (hence more valuable) variances, there is greater scope for joint ownership and subsequent success.

CONCLUSION

As with any journey's end, those who have experienced the trip often express their thanks to the driver of the vehicle. For an integrated care pathway a driver is required in the form of product champions. These individuals have an understanding of the benefits of integrated care pathways and integrated working, and can express these in a non-threatening way to an audience which will initially contain both supporters and wreckers. Champions must have credibility as practitioners in a field seen by most as having relevance to the core business of the team or organisation.

Be in no doubt though that there will be attempts at wrecking, whether by active opposition or passive inertia. The integrated care pathway development process is one which can form a momentum however, which can take the majority with it and even early successes can be contagious. The product champion should therefore be alert to the possibility of making the journey towards the integrated care pathway in one of several different ways. The opposition will either be left behind as the transport departs, or voluntarily leave the tour. Rather than restricting organisations, integrated care pathways can energise towards enhanced and coordinated clinical inter-professional and inter-agency practice. The opportunities at journey's end are considerable and offer benefits to the participants and organisations both in their own professional health and that of the system in which they practise. As with many journeys, the travel may prove scary but interesting at the first pass. As one grows familiar with the route and the fellow passengers, subsequent trips provide the opportunity to enjoy more of the scenery whilst learning more about the surroundings and the other travellers.

REFERENCES

Aitken P 2000 An integrated care pathway for severe mental illness in primary care. Public Health Medicine 2(4):140-145

Birmingham L 2001 Diversion from custody. Advances in Psychiatric Treatment 7:198-207

Bolam v Friern Hospital Management Committee [1957] 1 WLR 582

Brett W, Schofield J 2002 Integrated care pathways for patients with complex needs. Nursing Standard 16(46):36-40

Carson D 1996 Risking legal repercussions. In: Kemshall H & Pritchard J (eds) Good practice in risk assessment and risk management. Jessica Kingsley, London, pp 3-12

Department of Health 1990 The care programme approach for people with a mental illness referred to the specialist psychiatric services (90)23/Lassl(90)11. HMSO, London

Department of Health 1996 Guidance on supervised discharge (after-care under supervision) and related provisions HSG(96)11/LAC(96)8. Stationery Office, London

Department of Health 2004 Draft Mental Health Bill Cm6305. Stationery Office, London

Green B, Green C, Wood SM 2001 The implementation of an integrated clinical pathway into a medium secure forensic psychiatric unit. In: Landsberg G & Smiley A (eds) Forensic mental health: working with offenders with mental illness. Civic Research Institute, Kingston New Jersey, USA

Green B, Wood SM 2002 Training for plurality. Conference paper, 5th Forensic Mental Health Symposium, Aberdeen Conference Centre, October 2002. Royal Cornhill Hospitals

Jones A 2001 Hospital care pathways for patients with schizophrenia. Journal of Clinical Nursing 10:58-69

Jones T, Coyne H 2001 Modernisation and care pathways. ICP symposium, Association of Chartered Certified Accountants, London

Jones T, de Luc K, Coyne H 1999 Managing care pathways: the quality and resources of hospital care. Association of Chartered Certified Accountants, London

Jones T, Hardwick A, Carruthers I 2000 New commissioning: applying integrated care pathways. Association of Chartered Certified Accountants, London

Latter S, Courtney M 2003 Effectiveness of nurse prescribing: a review of the literature. Journal of Clinical Nursing 13:26-32

Middleton S, Roberts A 1998 Clinical pathways workbook. Kings Fund, London

National Institute for Clinical Excellence 2002 Clinical guideline 1: schizophrenia. Stationery Office, London

National Schizophrenia Fellowship, Manic Depression Fellowship, MIND 2001 That's just typical. NSF, London

NHS Health Advisory Service 1996 Mental Health Services Heading For Better Care. London. HMSO

Nott A 2002 Introducing an integrated care pathway in an acute mental health inpatient unit. Mental Health Practice 5(6):12-15

Riordan S, Wix S 1999 Diversion of mentally disordered offenders – to what and when? British Journal of Forensic Practice 1(3):23-26

Smith C, Embling S, Lyons C 2000 Integrated care pathways in acute psychiatry at the Gatehouse Assessment Centre. Mental Health Practice 3(9):20-21

Sneider R M 1999 Challenging to build, easy to use: geo-teams prove their E&P value. AAPG Explorer 11/99. Online. Available: http://www.aapg.org/explorer/1999/11nov/multi-teamexpl/html

Webster J 2002 Teamwork: understanding multi-professional working. Nursing Older People 14(3):14-19

Wood H 1996 Inter-agency working in developing local services. The CMHT Manager 4:1-2

Young A 2003 When things go wrong. Mental Health Practice 6(8):22-26

Zito Trust 1996 Learning the lesons (2nd ed). Zito Trust, London

Legal aspects of integrated care pathways

Ashley Irons

INTRODUCTION	**NEGLIGENT PATHWAYS**
PROFESSIONAL AND OTHER GUIDELINES	**CONCLUSION**
THE STATUS OF CARE PATHWAYS	**LIST OF CASES**
DEPARTURE FROM CARE PATHWAYS	**REFERENCES**
SWORD OR SHIELD?	

INTRODUCTION

The intention of this chapter is to look at how courts interpret legal duties and whether they have been breached or not when something goes wrong. It seeks to extract from legal cases the way in which courts determine whether there has been any fault at all – and if so, whether this may create legal liabilities on authors of care pathways, or service providers adopting them. In other words, what both should have in mind before putting a care pathway into practice.

Duty of care and negligence

If 'something goes wrong', any claim that follows will always include an allegation that there has been a breach of duty of care and/or negligence (without which there would have been no incident). What follows is a summary of principles relevant to this book.

> *Once a patient has been received into hospital, a duty of care arises – a duty to provide and go on providing treatment.*
>
> (R v GMC & Others ex p Burke [2004]
> Lloyd's Medical Law Reports 476)

A patient is entitled to expect a 'reasonable' standard of care (quite apart from being within Bolam/Bolitho principles that are discussed under the next heading below). If there is a breach of this duty, it may become the subject of a court challenge, either by way of a compensation claim or judicial review. Perhaps one of the clearest expressions of what amounts to 'reasonable' skill and care, is from a former Australian Chief Justice who said:

> *It is easy to overlook the all important emphasis placed on the word 'reasonable' in the statement of the duty. Perfection, or the use of increased knowledge or experience embraced with hindsight, after the event, should form no part of the components of what is 'reasonable' in all the circumstances.*
>
> (Barwick CJ & Maloney v Commissioner for Railways NSW [1978] 52ALJR292)

A duty of care can be regarded as a contract under which the service provider undertakes to provide certain services for the patient. This duty is illustrated by *Kent v Griffith* [1996] Lloyd's Medical Law Reports 424, where an asthma sufferer (K) required admission to hospital. The delay meant that K suffered respiratory arrest and, in consequence, suffered brain damage. Proceedings were brought against London Ambulance Service and it was accepted that the Ambulance Service owed a duty of care. It was held that once it had taken the details of an emergency, an ambulance must be provided within reasonable time (having regard to traffic conditions and other unavoidable factors). If it had arrived at K's home within a reasonable time, brain damage would have been avoided. Therefore, judgment in favour of the claimant was given. In other words, the moment a duty of care arises, there can be a claim where the provider has fallen short.

Negligence may arise out of fault, regardless of the existence or otherwise of a 'contract'. This is why negligence and duties of care go hand in hand and commonly appear in a claim together. There is no such thing as 'strict liability' in the UK. In other words, if a patient has a relapse whilst in hospital, it does not follow automatically that anyone, or any process, is to blame or that compensation is payable. An adverse outcome to surgery would be a most unfortunate outcome, but it does not mean that the surgeon was negligent. The same applies in mental health. The key principle of negligence is whether the treatment given (or not given) falls sufficiently short of an acceptable standard, so as to render the service provider liable to the patient for the consequences of that negligence. Mishaps, therefore, do not always mean negligence, as judgments in the leading cases of Bolam and Bolitho demonstrate.

Bolam and Bolitho

In *Bolam v Friern Hospital Management Committee* [1957] 1 WLR 582 it was held that the proper test was whether the standard of care given was that of the ordinary skilled man or woman, exercising and professing to have that special skill. A doctor is not negligent if he or she acted in accordance with a practice accepted as proper by a responsible body of medical opinion. As the judge in this case said:

> *I myself would prefer to put it this way, that he is not guilty of negligence if he has acted in accordance with the practice accepted as proper by a responsible body of medical men skilled in that particular art... Putting it the other way round, a man is not negligent, if he is acting in accordance with such a practice, merely because there is a body of opinion that would take a contrary view.*

This is important because in psychiatry contrary views are not difficult to find. That is to say, there can be perfectly respectable opinions that are complete opposites. One cannot look at the outcome of a clinical decision and claim it is negligent simply because it went wrong. Courts recognise that 'being wise after the event' is an unfair way of looking at matters. This means that if there is a negligence claim where there has been breach of a care pathway, the court might decide that there were perfectly proper reasons for departure – if it is persuaded that a minority, but 'responsible', opinion would have acted in the same way.

The test was tightened in *Bolitho v City & Hackney HA House of Lords* [1997] 3 WLR 1151 where it was held that in applying the above test, experts must direct their attention to the question of comparative risks and benefits to reach a defensible conclusion. If professional opinion was incapable of withstanding logical analysis, a judge was entitled to decide that a doctor's conduct fell below the benchmark.

> *The use of these adjectives, responsible, reasonable and respectable, all show that the court has to be satisfied that the components of the body of opinion relied upon, can demonstrate that such opinion has a logical basis. In particular in cases involving, as they so often do, the weighing of risks against benefits, the judge, before accepting the body of opinion as being responsible, reasonable, or respectable, will need to be satisfied that, in forming their views, the experts have directed their minds to the question of comparative risks and benefits and have reached a defensible conclusion on the matter.*

Consequently, judges may decide whether there has been any wrongdoing after listening to expert evidence tested by oral evidence in court, rather than simply relying upon their written reports. This is relevant to care pathways where, for example, there is a dispute as to whether it was a sensible approach in a particular case. This is illustrated by the Court of Appeal in a case where procedures were followed, but nevertheless the Court of Appeal ordered that the medical evidence should be tested by cross-examination to decide whether the hospital doctor's approach was appropriate. In *R v Broadmoor Hospital ex p Wilkinson* [2002] 1 WLR 419 a patient complained that he was being medicated compulsorily on the basis that his disorder did not warrant it. Although the hospital followed the Section 58 procedure in obtaining a second opinion (confirming that it was appropriate in this case), the court nevertheless was entitled to examine whether this was a proper approach for this patient. They ordered that doctors should attend court so that the conflict of opinion between the hospital and an independent doctor, instructed on behalf of the patient, could have its evidence tested. In other words, following a care pathway gives no guarantee of immunity from judicial scrutiny in any particular case.

A claimant must establish five things when alleging clinical negligence:

1. that there has been fault
2. that fault reached the threshold of negligence or failure of duty of care
3. that Bolam/Bolitho tests are not met
4. that damage/injury had been suffered

5. causation – that the injury was directly due to the above negligence or failure of care (and not due to anything that was not negligence).

Thus, even though there may be an unfortunate outcome, negligence claims do not succeed where a service provider can show that it took into account the risks and benefits and made a properly reasoned decision about a course of treatment. The golden rule is to consider, and above all to record, factors justifying a decision at the time. No record of such invites claims and makes them difficult to defend (especially where there is departure from a care pathway).

Causation

Causation is extremely important in claims. If there is negligence, a service provider will be liable to compensate for the consequences of that negligence, but not for any other consequences that might be due to anything not negligent. For example, if a patient is given inappropriate medication for depression to the extent that it was negligent, the service provider will be liable for that consequence. However, if part of the relapse that follows is due to another cause (e.g. death of a close relative), the service provider will only be liable for that part of the consequence that is due to its negligence, as distinct from any consequence arising from how the patient responds to the death of a near relative. Causation is thus the link between the harm complained of and the negligent act or omission.

Many claims fail because causation cannot be established (the test is upon the 'balance of probabilities').

PROFESSIONAL AND OTHER GUIDELINES

Professional organisations are increasingly providing guidance and, as set out elsewhere in this chapter, they carry considerable weight. Similarly, the Department of Health issues guidelines for good practice, for example via the National Institute for Clinical Excellence (NICE). These may be written into integrated care pathways to ensure local and national guidelines are incorporated within everyday practice, to assist in the management of clinical risk and to meet the requirements of clinical governance.

One view of these guidelines, however, is that they constrain individual clinical assessment of what is best for a patient. Even so, compliance with them may occur as a result of a fear of potential liability if something goes wrong when a guideline is not followed.

Thomson v James & Others [1996] 31BMLL reinforces this view. Here a claimant claimed compensation for brain damage induced by measles where the general practitioner (GP) had advised the child's parents, for various reasons, not to have a vaccination. As the GP failed to follow the Department of Health guidance that children who had suffered fits should be inoculated against measles at 2 years of age, it was held that the GP was negligent. He had not fulfilled a duty of care. The significance of this case for care pathways is that the judge was prepared to find the defendant negligent, even though there was a respectable body of opinion that would have done the same as the GP. But the court said that it would be wrong if 'the decision of negligence or no negligence is left in the hands of doctors, whereas the question must at the end of the day, be one for the courts'. The judge said that the GP 'owed a duty to explain that DHSS guidelines advised that special precautions could be taken, so a child (with a history of convulsions) could be vaccinated against measles'. That is, for the parents to make an informed choice as to the course of treatment, they should have been told about this advice. This assertion of authority of the courts over the medical profession in determining negligence is significant. It moved away from Bolam, in favour of an approach that permitted consideration of professional guidelines as indicative of the standard of care expected.

Similarly, the case of *R v London LB Sutton ex p Tucker* [1998] 40 BMLR 162 concerned a patient fit for discharge from hospital and who was awaiting community care, the provision of which according to Department of Health guidelines (Department of Health 1989) was the responsibility of the Borough. Unfortunately, the Borough did nothing and in consequence the patient remained confined in hospital. Thus, the court held that the Borough had acted unlawfully as they had 'departed, without good reason, from the policy guidance issued by the Secretary of State' (which guidance was held to be binding on local authorities).

That guidance is available does not mean that following it guarantees immunity though. Occasionally, the professional guidance itself may be criticised by the court. This was the case for the General Medical Council's (GMC) guidance *Withholding and withdrawing life-prolonging treatments: good practice in decision making* (General Medical Council 2002). In *R v GMC & Others ex p Burke* [2004] Lloyd's Rep Med 451 the claimant complained that his life could be brought to an end as a result of this guidance. The High Court agreed with the claimant that the guidelines were inappropriate and in part unlawful and should not be followed. However, after a much publicised appeal, the Court of Appeal reversed the decision, stating that the GMC guidance did not put the patient at risk as had been claimed, and that the guidance had been misinterpreted by the High Court Judge. The Court of Appeal gave the GMC guidance very considerable weight and indeed the litigation assumed that doctors would certainly follow the guidance of their professional body. They did so without disagreeing with the High Court Judge, who said (p. 497) 'Guidance is not a legal text book or statement of legal principle. It consists primarily of professional and ethical guidance for doctors, provided for them by the professional body which is responsible for such matters'.

Nevertheless, as much earlier noted by another author, 'there is certainly evidence that the courts are prepared to accept guidelines produced by the medical profession and to elevate them almost to the status of rules of law' (Harpwood 1994).

The absence of a protocol, or pathway, was criticised in *Temple v South Manchester Health Authority* [LTL 21/10/2002]. A 10-year-old claimant was diagnosed as suffering from diabetic ketoacidosis (DKA) by a paediatric registrar. The claimant lapsed into unconsciousness and suffered a cerebral oedema, causing him severe and permanent brain damage. It was alleged that the paediatric registrar failed to consult the consultant shortly after the claimant's admission, to monitor the condition properly, and failed to make appropriate adjustments to the claimant's management during the night.

The court said it was negligent not to have involved the consultant earlier, as the claimant's condition was critical with real risks of fatal or other devastating consequences. Secondly, the court criticised the absence of a clear protocol in the hospital for DKA (later noting that the registrar's management did not reflect appropriate clinical practice). Despite such criticism, however, the claim failed because of a dispute between experts as to whether the cerebral oedema was actually the direct consequence of the faults identified (causation).

As can be seen from the above, where something goes wrong, there has to be justification for the course adopted by clinicians in line with the Bolam/Bolitho principles. This will relate both to the care itself and also to any guidance that exists. The rest of this chapter examines the status of care pathways and their impact, one way or the other, when a claim is made.

THE STATUS OF CARE PATHWAYS

Care pathways are assumed to set out benchmarks for best practice incorporating the latest research and guidelines. If a pathway sets itself out as a process that should be followed, however, then the court will usually make this interpretation, regardless of whether it is called a guideline or a procedure or anything else. This is especially so if falling short of the pathway leads to harm, that would otherwise have been avoided. Therefore, variance from pathways needs to be justified by entries in the notes that set out the reasons for departure with clarity.

But are pathways mandatory? As noted elsewhere in this chapter, there are examples of varying degrees of expectation as to compliance. As noted below, for example, the NICE guidance is prescriptive on electroconvulsive therapy (ECT) (National Institute for Clinical Excellence 2003) whereas, generally, clinicians are not constrained to that extent. For example, in relation to communication detoxification pathways 'This guide offers an outline pathway, providing information to inform consistent evidence-based practice in the planning and delivery of community based detoxification…' (Effective Interventions Unit 2005). The offender mental healthcare pathway expresses a similar view 'This care pathway document lays down valuable best practice templates…to guide the practice of people who directly deliver services, and support decision-making for those who commission them' (National Institute for Mental Health in England 2005).

However, courts will make their own decision as to whether guidance is mandatory or otherwise. This is illustrated by *R v Mersey Care NHS Trust ex p Munjaz* (2005) UK HK 58. The issue at stake was the status that should be given to the Code of Practice whose introduction stated that it was intended as 'guidance'. The case concerned a reduction in the number of doctors' reviews for patients secluded over 7 days, as a result of a new hospital policy. Reversing the Court of Appeal decision in 2003, the Court noted that the Code was a broad church applying to all patients admitted to all mental hospitals within England and Wales. Consequently, there could be departure from the Code as a matter of policy, but per Lord Hope at paragraph 74 '[t]he reasons for any departure from the Code which puts the patient's Convention rights at risk must be subjected to particularly careful and intense scrutiny'. In the leading Judgment, Lord Bingham at para 21 stated that the Code was 'not instruction, but it is much more than mere advice which an addressee is free to follow or not as it chooses. It is guidance which any hospital should consider with great care, from which it should depart only if it has cogent reasons for doing so.'

It was held that the policy justified the reasons for departure and provided ample safeguards for patients. This is in contrast to the Court of Appeal, which said that any departure could never be justified as a matter of policy, but only by individual consideration of each patient's situation.

Whilst the case concerned a seclusion policy departing from the Code, the Judgment can be applied to a wide variety of other guidance and the basis upon which there can be any departure. Those writing procedures that depart from authoritative guidance must take great care to ensure that a patient's domestic and Convention rights are protected, quite apart from justifying the reasons for departure.

It can be seen then, that guidance, whether from professional organisations, the Department of Health or from other government bodies, is taken seriously by the courts. Whilst not mandatory, falling short of a care pathway without good reason may render a service provider liable for an adverse outcome. This chapter now looks at the implications of departures.

DEPARTURE FROM CARE PATHWAYS

The experience elsewhere

Care pathways are, in reality, standard-setting processes for delivering high (or higher) standards of care. However, as has been shown, a clinical guideline does not change the legal responsibilities and duties of care owed to patients. The mere existence of a guideline '...does not itself establish that compliance with it is reasonable, or that non-compliance is negligent' (Hurwitz 1999). Nevertheless, there is not the slightest doubt that compliance with a guideline discourages negligence claims. Equally, non-compliance gives encouragement. Consequently, departure from guidelines could be seen as prima facie evidence of 'a case to answer' (Harpwood 1994).

There is a real problem with a plethora of procedures though, because the more policies a service provider has, the more likely it is that some will be overlooked (as has been noted by more than one public inquiry), whether excusable or not. Not being aware of a policy or protocol, and therefore not taking it into account when making a clinical decision, is a sure way to encourage a finding of fault.

In France, in view of escalating expense and demand for health care, the French medical profession and health insurance organisations produced regulations, the product of some 50 working groups involving 670 experts. The guidelines produced are considered to have improved clinical practice. What is interesting about them is that they do not set out what clinicians should do in particular situations, but what they should not do. These guidelines usually begin with the words 'It is inappropriate to...'. Whilst these are virtually mandatory, the regulations accept that there are uncertainties such as to diagnosis, and then there can be departure (Maisonneuve et al 1997).

An Australian research paper considered the evidence upon which clinical practice guidelines were based and noted that:

> they pertain to the 'usual' case, as they are based primarily on evidence from randomised trials which, because of inclusion and exclusion criteria and controlled clinical environments, produce an average result for the condition studied. However, there may be many reasons for a clinician to provide care to an individual that departs from guidelines' recommendations. The clinician may be aware of evidence other than that included in the guidelines, appraise the evidence differently to the guideline developers, managing a person whose situation is different from that within the guidelines, or be treating a person who selects management outside of the guidelines.
>
> (Pelly et al 1998)

The Australian National Health and Medical Research Council regards 'clinical practice guidelines' as one component of good medical decision-making (National Health and Medical Research Council 1999, p 10). In other words:

> Guidelines assist clinical decision-making. They do not replace it. Guidelines are not prescriptive and do not cover all of the myriad variations in a clinical situation.
>
> (Coates 1998)

Nevertheless, per the above case of *Munjaz*, the clinician departing from guidance must identify persuasive reasons to justify a different course of treatment.

Generally, courts condemn departure from guidance when it cannot be justified. For example, in *Sookia v Lambeth, Southwark and Lewisham Health Authority* [LTL 19.11.01] a 12-year-old girl received damages for bilateral hearing loss, sustained following her premature birth in 1989. She was born with rhesus haemolytic disease. Her condition was satisfactory at birth and she was treated appropriately with phototherapy in an exchange transfusion. However, 4 days later, the claimant's bilirubin levels rose to a concentration that was above the Health Authority's criterion for triggering further exchange transfusion. Action was delayed for 32 hours and as a result injury was caused. One of the allegations of negligence was that the hospital failed to adhere to its own guidelines or protocol, as to the bilirubin levels at which exchange transfusion became mandatory, or make any reasoned decision for departing from them. The Health Authority agreed and admitted liability.

It is the author's view that if care pathways are stated to be not mandatory, it must follow that individual departures by clinicians are anticipated. If so, there should be no initial presumption of fault when that departure takes place, especially so when the reasons for departure are clearly set out in the clinical records. However, experience of litigation in the USA, where the concept of care pathways originated, is that 35-40% of malpractice claims in the USA cannot be defended due to documentation problems. It is therefore essential that for a record of departure to be defensible, it must be legible, accurate, timely and comprehensive.

Departures from guidelines that lead to suicide/ self-harm

Cases in a Coroner's Court illustrate the attention that courts do give to procedures that exist, particularly where the consequence of not following them has caused or contributed to a fatality. For example, in the case of *R v HM Coroner for Inner West London Ex p Scott* [2001] 61 BMLR 222, a prisoner who suffered from schizophrenia was recognised to be a suicide risk, but was allowed to retain his shoelaces. In addition, he received no special observations, neither was he given medication. This was in breach of internal procedures, which, had they been followed, might have prevented his death, as he subsequently used the shoelaces to hang himself. The High Court ordered a fresh inquest because a jury should have been allowed to consider a neglect verdict, given that there was evidence of a failure to provide medical attention, and there was a direct connection between the absence of this and death.

More recently, the House of Lords changed the Coroner's Court process substantially as a result of two cases in March 2004. In one case, the equivalent of a care pathway was not followed. In this instance, a single mother of two children, who was also a drug addict, had been placed on a detoxification programme. She presented as extremely depressed, stating that she had 'nothing to live for'. The Magistrates' Court Custody Officer had assessed her as a suicide risk and as a result the At Risk procedure was commenced. Unfortunately though, the document and the information contained in it did not travel to the prison; contrary to procedure. As a result, the prison was unaware and conducted no particular risk assessment. Furthermore, she was seen by at least one clinician, who was unfamiliar with the risk assessment procedures. The woman subsequently killed herself in her cell.

The following words of the House of Lords underline the scrutiny that established procedures will have in the future at Coroners' Courts:

The purpose of the investigation is to open up the circumstances of the deaths for public scrutiny. This ensures that those who are at fault will be made accountable for their actions. It also has a part to play in the correction of mistakes and search for improvement. There must be a rigorous examination in public of the operation at every level, of the systems and procedures which are designed to prevent self-harm and to save lives.

(R v HM Coroner for West Yorkshire ex p Sacker [2004] 2 All ER 495)

Whilst referring to prison procedures, these words will also apply to deaths in hospitals. Hence, managers responsible for systems and operations may find themselves called to give evidence to explain the existing procedures, whether they were followed, and if not, why not.

Furthermore, for the first time jurors may 'by one means or another…be permitted to express their conclusion on the central facts explored before them' (*R v West Somerset Coroner ex p Middleton* [2004] 2 All ER 484). What will happen now is that the general circumstances of someone's death will be considered much more carefully, and the scope for critical verdicts greatly increased. Departures from established procedure/care pathways will receive critical comment in a much more public form than has ever been the case before (unless good reasons were established for departure).

The implications for service providers are that they must not create for themselves care pathways unless they are robust, practical and realistic. Otherwise, managers in the witness box will have a very uncomfortable time explaining why they adopted a process that was not achievable. It will be assumed that if there is a process, it is because it was thought necessary and, therefore, there will be scant sympathy from any court if it is breached. Coroners' Courts may well examine why a hospital thought it necessary to have a procedure and may call those responsible to give evidence for operations and procedures. Risk managers and directors of operations are obvious candidates. It is the author's experience that sometimes those writing policies are not responsible for the operation of them, and often draft policies on the basis of their view of undefined 'best practice', rather than that which is realistically achievable. Policies and procedures should underpin improvements in clinical practice and should not be written in the hope that setting a higher standard will encourage and improve practice, in the knowledge that adherence will be patchy.

Departures from guidelines on prescribing

Guidelines do not displace proper consideration of an individual patient. Medication is an area where psychiatrists may arrive at a number of different treatment options in any particular case. What matters is that decisions can be justified on Bolam/Bolitho principles and that evidence of appropriate consideration is recorded at the time.

Or as the National Health Service (NHS) Executive put it 'The critical point is whether the clinical care choices made were reasonable, having regard to all the circumstances of a particular case' (National Health Service Executive 1996 p 10).

An Australian GP was accused of misconduct having prescribed injectible diazepam to heroin users, contrary to the Australian National Methadone Guidelines. He was initially found guilty by his professional body of 'infamous and improper conduct'. However, when the Supreme Court of Western Australia heard of a responsible minority medical opinion supporting such treatment of addicts within a harm reduction framework that was followed by Dr Cranley, his appeal succeeded (*Cranley v Medical Board of Western Australia* SUP Ct WA [1992] 3MLR94-113).

In *Vernon v Bloomsbury Health Authority* [1995] 6 Med LR 297 the claimant was given a course of gentamicin therapy as treatment for an infection of the heart valve. The claimant brought a claim for negligence. It was held that whilst the dosage exceeded the manufacturer's guidelines, 'the dosage was a proper one'. The guidelines 'erred on the side of caution' – the use of a high dosage on a patient with a long history of culture negative endocarditis, whose condition was deteriorating, was appropriate.

Cases like these will assist when, for example, British National Formulary (BNF) guidelines are exceeded by a doctor recording his or her reasons to justify this.

In mental health, the BNF guidance is sometimes departed from, but the clinician is unlikely to be found negligent if it can be proven that the risks and benefits were considered adequately at the time. The author has had cases where, at an inquest, questions were asked of the doctor as to why BNF guidance was exceeded and its potential impact upon the cause of death. Invariably, BNF levels are quoted as the benchmark, often with the implication that exceeding such is indicative of fault. In no case attended by the author did the doctor have much difficulty in justifying the reason for higher-dose medication, for example in the treatment of resistant schizophrenia.

Departing from NICE guidelines

A good example of the issues and controversy that can arise from guidance can be seen from the application of guidance upon electroconvulsive therapy (ECT) (National Institute for Clinical Excellence 2003). This provides an analogy for potential care pathway issues in quite different areas of care.

The NICE guidance (paragraph 1.1/2) states that:

It is recommended that ECT is used only for rapid and short-term improvement of severe symptoms after an adequate trial of other treatment options has proved ineffective and/or when the condition is considered to be potentially life threatening in individuals with:

- Severe depressive illness
- Catatonia
- Prolonged or severe manic episode.

The decision as to whether ECT is clinically indicated should be based on a documented assessment of the risks and potential benefits.

As it is a 'recommendation', it must follow that it is not mandatory and yet it continues (at paragraph 7.1) – 'NHS trusts should ensure that ECT is carried out in accordance with the recommendations… Local guidelines or care pathways involving ECT should incorporate the guidance'. In other words, it is intended to be prescriptive. This is reinforced by the next paragraph in contrast to that above, 'ECT is used only for an individual with...' (paragraph 7.4) the three illnesses referred to in paragraph 1.

The Australian Royal College of Psychiatrists (National Health and Medical Research Council 1999, paragraph 7.4) said on continuation (maintenance) ECT:

> *We feel there is sufficient evidence from clinical experience and case studies to support the view that a small proportion of patients can only stay well, when continuation ECT is used, and that although it is possible to gain a short-term improvement with ECT, this cannot be sustained by other available treatment such as lithium, anti-depressants, or psychotherapy, and that only continuation ECT allows such patients to stay well (National Health and Medical Research Council 1999).*

The Royal College of Psychiatrists also disagree with some other NICE guidance: 'One of the grounds on which the committee did not agree with NICE, was that ECT should only be reserved for the treatment of severe depression' (Psychminded News 2003a).

Similarly, Dr Donny Lyons, consultant in ECT at Leverndale Hospital in Glasgow, has warned that he will ignore the new guidance:

> *If I have a choice between following these guidelines and doing what I think is best for my patients, then I will do the latter. I am not going to tell my patients that they cannot have this treatment because NICE advises against it. My duty to patients will take precedence. I have no difficulty deciding not to follow the guidelines because I do not think they are correct. I would be very unhappy if my ability to help people is impeded by guidelines that do not make any sense' (Psychminded News 2003b).*

Support for this view has been expressed by others (Cole & Tobiansky 2003):

> *Our clinical experience is that many patients who may benefit from ECT will be denied it under these guidelines. Apparently the NICE appraisal panel did not include a single psychiatrist, which may partly explain why clinical experience of the potential benefits of maintenance ECT seems to have been discounted.*

They go on to point out that in severely depressed patients, ECT might be considered 'a first line treatment' (Cole & Tobiansky 2003).

Reflecting on these observations, the author had the experience of asking psychiatrists at an ECT conference which of them had ever prescribed maintenance (or continuing) ECT for a patient. The answer was every single one! The NICE guidance on ECT is thus especially contentious. As yet though, there has been no legal case where a decision not to follow this guidance has been before the courts or the General Medical Council. It therefore seems clear that there is a responsible body of opinion who would take a quite contrary view to NICE on ECT and consequently it would not be taken as negligent to adopt such a course (provided the explanation is recorded adequately). In considering whether a minority opinion is that of a 'responsible' minority, courts will look at not simply the research justification for the protocol, but the research justification/clinical experience that supports departure. As with all guidance, the freedom of a clinician to act according to his or her best judgement is not prevented – it is simply that the quality of that judgment will be examined and the first paperwork a judge will look at is the evidence of that assessment in contemporaneous notes.

SWORD OR SHIELD?

Whether in respect of itself or professional bodies, the NHS has stated that:

> *Clinical guidelines can still only assist the practitioner; they cannot be used to mandate, authorise or outlaw treatment options regardless of the strength of evidence. It will remain the responsibility of the practising clinicians to interpret their application, taking account of local circumstances and the needs and wishes of individual patients… It would be wholly inappropriate for clinical guidelines to be used as a means of coercion of the individual clinician by managers and senior professionals.*
>
> (National Health Service Executive 1996 p10).

Despite its assumption that clinical judgment trumps any guidance, it is easier to sail with the wind than against it. Hence, clinicians are likely to feel more assured when following professional guidance than in departure. In the event of a dispute, it will boil down to the courts' view of expert evidence as to whether a clinical judgment was justified as it was, for example in *McFarlane v Secretary of State for Scotland* [1998] SCLR 623.

Courts usually find guidelines influential, but not determinative. But, protocols will always be quoted in support of one case or the other. It is for this reason that any departure needs to be considered carefully and recorded clearly. Courts are sympathetic to the dilemmas facing clinicians, but this sympathy evaporates in the absence of any evidence of appropriate consideration (at the time the decision was taken).

In the USA, a study found that guidelines played 'a relevant role in the proof of negligence' in less than 7% of malpractice actions (Hyams 1995). It is likely that the position has now moved on. However, Pennachio (2004) stated that:

> *Although clinical practice guidelines can be used by both plaintiffs and de-fendants, one notable study, published in the mid 1990s, shows that guidelines are more commonly used by claimants. Of the 37 cases studied, plaintiffs used guidelines to back-up their charges in 29 cases, and were successful in 22 of them. Similarly, doctors defended themselves successfully in six cases out of just eight using guidelines in the defence.*

As to why doctor defendants use clinical guidelines so infrequently, the article quotes a New York plaintiff's attorney – 'This is because guidelines are rarely specific enough to provide a good shield'. Pennachio comments – 'You are more likely to be sued for not following guidelines than for following them. But you can never count on what a jury will do'. She goes on to make a comment that applies in the UK every bit as much as in the USA – 'If you follow appropriate guidelines and prove it, that might not only help you in court, but it could ward off a malpractice suit in the first place. Claimants' attorneys often hesitate to file suit when a physician clearly followed clinical practice guidelines. For sure, if you choose not to follow a particular guideline, make sure you can demonstrate that you were aware of the guideline and had good reason for not using it' (Pennachio 2004).

Jhawar (2004) arrived at a similar conclusion, stating that 'Integrated care pathways can be invaluable in minimising clinical risk, and thereby litigation, since they incorporate complete documentation. As this is done against the current best practice norms, and 'accounted for' variations, the hospital and its staff base are well protected'. The paper acknowledged that 'ICPs act as the template of care to be provided and are not intended to compromise clinical judgment. The clinical team can deviate from the pathway if there is a valid reason for doing so'.

Pelly et al (1998) note that the legal status of protocols has been unclear and that 'in particular, there is confusion about whether doctors will be more, or less, vulnerable to a successful lawsuit if they follow guidelines or depart from guidelines for clinical reasons'. On surveying 150 surgeons concerned with the early management of breast cancer, it was found that 37% felt the guidelines increased their exposure to medico-legal problems, whilst 41% felt that they would protect clinicians from legal problems. The same survey notes that such a long time passes before malpractice claims come to court, that 'there is virtually no judicial comment on their legal status' (Pelly et al 1998).

Another Australian study concluded that 'It is likely that departure from the practice advised in a guideline would be subject to the same tests as any other departure from a generally accepted standard of care. Departure from practices recommended in guidelines, because of ignorance of the guidelines, would seem more likely to expose a doctor to risk of litigation, if a patient is damaged by breach of the guidelines. Conscious departure from guidelines because of specific circumstances in a particular patient, may be much easier to defend as consistent with appropriate standard of care'. In other words, any practice outside guidelines must ensure that the reasons are well documented (Tito & Newby 1998).

An Australian barrister's view is that 'In an appropriate case, a medical witness called to give expert opinion evidence on behalf of a plaintiff might refer to clinical practice guidelines, offering the opinion that the defendant doctor wrongly departed from the guidelines and the treatment of the patient. It would be open to a defendant doctor to counter this with evidence that the guidelines were not available at the time, or were not updated or relevantly endorsed, or that clinical practice justified departure from the guidelines and the exercise of professional judgment, or that the treatment given did in fact comply with the guidelines. Ultimately, care may well come to be regarded as less than reasonable should clinical practice guidelines be available but not followed, unless this can be justified on appropriate clinical grounds' (Dwyer 1998).

In the UK, however, it is unlikely that claims against a service provider will get off the ground, if appropriate guidance was competently followed on the face of the clinical notes. These are the first papers that a potential litigant/expert will examine. This is because the majority of funding for litigation is invariably either through Legal Aid, or Conditional Fee Agreements underpinned by an insurance policy. Neither will fund a claim in these circumstances. But any evidence of fault can only be reinforced if, on the face of the documents, a care pathway was not followed.

NEGLIGENT PATHWAYS

The above has considered the impact of the existence of a care pathway where a clinician is facing a claim. It has already been noted that pathways themselves can be challenged as being inappropriate, but what if the guidance itself is at fault?

Is the pathway negligent?

Unless a medical procedure adopted by service providers is patently unsafe, or against acceptable practice, the courts should not find its adoption was negligent. It therefore provides protection as it will have been subject to assessment beforehand.

Where there is an allegation that the pathway is at fault, the courts will expect to hear from either the author or, more likely, the service provider adopting it. The research and evidence underpinning the pathway will be examined to assess their appropriateness or otherwise – the court will decide on the basis of Bolitho described earlier in the chapter. However, the main focus of court attention is whether the actions of clinicians are appropriate. An existing care pathway will be considered as part of the process of reaching a decision to that central question.

Where a pathway is followed, a claimant may allege that the pathway itself is at fault. For example, in *Early v Newham HA* (1994) 5MEDLR the claimant (P) woke up in the middle of an operation. The anaesthetist followed the procedure laid down by the Health Authority and did not attempt re-intubation, but allowed P to wake up. P claimed that the failure to re-intubate was negligent. The claim was dismissed, as the court accepted that the risk of waking up was less than the greater harm that could occur if re-intubation had taken place. In other words, the procedure was a sensible one.

Who is liable?

Where a claim includes an allegation that a pathway was negligently created, who will have to defend such a charge?

Liability of the author to service provider/clinician

The service provider would have to demonstrate that they were misled as to the appropriateness of its use, or that the pathway was prepared in such a way that was plainly negligent, in circumstances where the author of the pathway knew that it would be relied upon and that, in so doing, harm might result. That is a very high threshold.

It is doubtful whether there can be any legally enforceable duty of care between the author of a pathway and the multitude of those who may adopt it. It would be unlikely in the extreme that an author would be liable when he or she has no control over the circumstances of the use of the protocol. A protocol is, after all, 'guidance' and does not absolve clinicians of their duties of care. No court would excuse a service provider/clinician blindly following a pathway without checking its appropriateness in any particular case.

Authors will usually be employed by a service provider and therefore, if there was any neglect, the employer would be held responsible. If the author is an independent consultant who wrote a pathway specifically for the provider, there could in theory be a claim against the author by the service provider, but for the reasons discussed below, it would be hard to establish.

Authors/defences to claims

The author will have to show that the care pathway was developed taking into account numerous different considerations. Ultimately, the author will need to demonstrate that the pathway was a sensible response to them (or even to conflicting opinions). Also that it was intended as general guidance, and was the type of guidance that would be accepted under Bolam/Bolitho principles.

It is essential that authors keep evidence of their research consideration and discussions leading to the preparation of the pathway. This is to demonstrate that there is a reasonable and up-to-date information base upon which to draft the guidance (with the date clearly stated). Contemporaneous documents carry a great deal of weight with courts.

A further defence for the author is to show that the pathway was not followed in circumstances for which it was intended, or it was otherwise changed or applied inappropriately. The bottom line, however, is that the author of a pathway should not put it forward unless it is supported by other practitioners or relevant opinions that stand up to logical analysis (applying the Bolitho test), including a risk benefit analysis. There is nothing wrong in writing a care pathway that carries risks provided these are openly acknowledged and clearly set out. After all, a pathway may be created to give the best route for clinicians to take when there are risks in whatever route is taken. It is wise to acknowledge contrary opinions to the pathway recommended.

Authors are also advised to include a disclaimer. Although these do not grant immunity, they will assist if properly written. Also there should be a clear statement that every treatment decision is for the practitioner to make upon the circumstances applying to each individual patient. Consequently, advice is not mandatory.

Or, as stated by an Australian publication, 'guidelines should not be unduly prescriptive and must allow for cases that call for management that differs from what is recommended' (National Health and Medical Research Council 1999, para 6.3).

Liability of author to service user

In theory, the author of a negligent pathway may be liable to the service user if it can be shown that he or she knew service users would rely on the pathway. It is most unlikely, however, that the author would be liable to service users directly. A claimant will sue the service provider concerned and not the author.

The Australian NHMRC *Guidelines for the development, implementation and evaluation of clinical practice* state 'Normally a general publication, even when negligently collated, does not give rise to liability because the author does not owe a duty of care to the general public at large'. The same publication notes that 'guideline developers need to be able to demonstrate that the information in the guidelines has been properly developed and ratified' (National Health and Medical Research Council 1999, para 6.2).

It has been reported by the Scottish Intercollegiate Guidelines Network (www.sign.ac.uk/guidelines/50) (SIGN) that a successful claim against an author of a guideline 'is very unlikely, because developers of clinical guidelines in general do not owe a duty of care to patients. It is also recommended that any significant departure from the guidelines and the reasons for these should be fully documented in the patient's case notes at the time the relevant decision is taken'. Similarly, the NHS Executive has said 'While an action can be taken against a clinician for not keeping up to date, one against a college is probably not actionable, as it would be difficult to show it owes a duty or obligation directly to the patient' (National Health Service Executive 1996 p 10). In other words, an author or college proposing a pathway is unlikely to be liable to a patient.

In *Caparo Industries Plc v Digman & Others* [1990] 1 All ER 568 the House of Lords examined the liability of the maker of a statement to 'strangers' in a purely commercial context. They held that there was no relationship, 'proximity', between the maker of the statement and the person reading it; that is, unless it was shown that the maker knew that the statement was very likely to be relied upon for the purposes of deciding whether to enter into a particular transaction. This case offers some comfort to authors of care pathways.

The above Australian view echoes the 'proximity' point. A professional organisation, for example, issuing guidance:

> *Could be held liable, if a relevant close relationship can be established between them and the person who suffers a loss. If guidelines purport to be a definitive statement of the correct or appropriate procedure, there would be a greater risk of liability, than where the guidelines are expressly stated to be provided as a general guide, subject to the medical practitioner's expert judgment in each case'* (National Health and Medical Research Council 1999).

Liability of the practitioner/ employers

The service provider/trust or practitioner will usually be liable if they follow a procedure or pathway in a way that departs from good practice and cannot be justified for an individual patient. If so, the courts are likely to find the practitioner (or rather the employer) liable, regardless of any fault on the part of the author. Under the principle of vicarious liability, an employer is usually legally responsible for the actions of its staff and will indemnify its staff if there are proceedings against them.

Where clinicians do not agree with a particular care pathway applying, they should check to see whether it is up to date, as it may not be. Secondly, if they do not agree with it, there should be evidence of adequate consideration of its merits or otherwise. This might, for example, include getting the opinion of another doctor within the trust or beyond. What courts expect to see, as a minimum, is consideration of the pathway and the greater arguments for departure as recorded in contemporaneous notes; in other words, justifying the different approach. It is quite possible for a service provider to be deemed negligent when following a care pathway that is inappropriate to a particular case.

Where a care pathway was appropriate for a patient's care, but not followed, the service provider/practitioner will be liable for any harm resulting. The Australian NHMRC acknowledges that guidelines could be produced as evidence of what constitutes reasonable conduct by a medical practitioner, for the purposes of assessing whether the practitioner's duty of care has been breached in a medical negligence action. However, as noted earlier in this chapter under the heading *Sword or shield*, it is the case that 'the existence of clinical practice guidelines will provide a measure of protection for practitioners who use the guidelines' (National Health and Medical Research Council 1999, para 6.1).

Standard setting and writing care pathways

It will be apparent that if standards are set, there will be criticism and sometimes liability in failing to meet them. If a service provider decides that a standard is appropriate, it must follow that, in failing to reach that standard, the conduct may be blameworthy. Sometimes those who write policies do not have sufficient regard to the real world, with the result that a pathway can be a triumph of hope over reality. 'Doctors and managers who draft guidelines of any kind should be aware that these might be used in litigation' (Harpwood 1994). The problem arises when the author has no experience of the inevitability of things going wrong, or being cross-examined upon the reason for a standard, and why it was not met. Where there is a requirement for standards to be raised, the author suggests that, from a legal perspective, the proper vehicle for this is through other measures such as training and audit. A pathway setting a standard that will not be attained is an open invitation to litigation and liability.

In other words, a care pathway should underpin raised standards and not set unachievable targets.

The author once questioned a pathway developer:

Q: The purpose of a procedure is to avoid avoidable errors?
A: Yes.
Q: If you write a policy, it is intended that staff will follow it?
A: Yes.
Q: As it is necessary for safe practice?
A: Yes.
Q: If it is not followed, errors are more likely?
A: Possibly.
Q: Has the pathway been followed here?

Setting a standard amounts to an assumption that (at its most modest) falling short of it is undesirable. This will undoubtedly be argued as being the same thing as being negligent, or failing in the duty of care that is properly owed by a service provider to its patients.

So what should authors have in mind?

Make clear that there could be departure from the pathway; i.e. that it is not mandatory, but indicative of generally accepted good practice for most patients, most of the time. In other words, the author should not be over-prescriptive, to the extent that there could be no considered departure in individual cases.

Additionally, a care pathway should acknowledge that, in some individual cases, departure would be the only sensible path to take.

Referring to developing clinical guidelines, the Department of Health states that 'the objectives of the guidance must be clearly stated, as should its intended use and applicability; they should make clear for whom they are intended and should be constructed in such a way that allows deviation' (National Health Service Executive 1996 p 10).

Consequently, care pathways need to emphasise the importance of individual consideration being properly documented. Clinicians should always be aware that a wider audience may read their notes in the future – whether as the basis of a negligence claim, a judicial review challenge, a complaint or an inquiry.

As to the influence of litigation on the writing of procedures, one American view is that claimant lawyers are complaining that, for example, the American College of Obstetricians and Gynecologists' guidance appears designed to shield doctors from liability, rather than to improve care. An example is given whereby that College discourages caesareans even when labour has gone on too long. Arnold Rosoff, Professor of Legal Studies at Pennsylvania University, states 'A professional society should have a duty to improve the quality of care. Instead, each time a claimant's attorney wins a case by proving that a doctor did not follow one of their guidelines, they may simply weaken the guideline'. Whereas in previous years a guideline might have said 'in this situation, the doctor should do the following…' now they are written more defensively, carefully avoiding prescriptive language, to become 'in this situation, a doctor might consider doing the following…' (Pennachio 2004).

A contrary view referred to in the same article states 'Yes, we leave leeway for styles and settings of practice, but that is not to shield members from liability – it is because there is no right way to practice'. The article refers to the AMA (American Medical Association) House of Delegates saying that all medical societies should include disclaimers on their guidelines, reaffirming that they are not a substitute for the experience and judgment of a physician, and are developed to enhance a physician's ability to practise evidence-based medicine. The Association states that guidelines 'shall acknowledge the ability of physicians to depart from the recommendations…when appropriate in the care of individual patients' (Pennachio 2004).

An Australian paper came to a similar conclusion in referring to the NHMRC early breast cancer guidelines: 'Following them to the letter would not be possible or desirable; as such, words like 'must' or 'should' are not appropriate, and are not used in these guidelines' (Pelly et al 1998). In other words, they provide leeway for clinical judgment taking into account the circumstances and preferences of the patient and a range of other factors.

When setting standards and writing care pathways, authors (and providers adopting them) will need to have these points in mind when balancing the desire to raise standards with the desire not to encourage litigation.

CONCLUSION

In conclusion, it can be seen that policies and procedures of all sorts can help to avoid litigation by being a feature of improving clinical practice; in other words, to reduce the number of errors. The other side of this coin is that determination of whether or not there has been fault may adopt as a benchmark the standards set out in a procedure. For this reason, it is essential that day-to-day practice is not remote from standards that a provider seeks to achieve. The introduction of any pathway needs to be preceded by training to reduce the potential for non-compliance and for this to be maintained by ongoing audit and further training.

Where a care pathway relates to the exercising of clinical judgment, training must make clear to doctors and other clinicians that an adequate record of the reasons for departure must be kept. These reasons must demonstrate that the pathway has been properly considered.

It would be wise to assume that it is easier to defend a process or decision that follows a pathway than one that does not – even with a pathway acknowledging that there can be individual departure where justified. Where a mishap has occurred that might have been prevented by following a pathway, claimants will be confident of establishing liability.

LIST OF CASES

Barwick CJ & Maloney v Commissioner for Railways NSW [1978] 52ALJR292
Bolam v Friern Hospital Management Committee [1957] 1 WLR 582
Bolitho v City & Hackney HA House of Lords [1997] 3 WLR 1151
Caparo Industries Plc v Digman & Others [1990] 1 All ER 568
Cranley v Medical Board of Western Australia SUP Ct WA [1992] 3MLR94-113
Early v Newham HA (1994) 5MEDLR
Kent v Griffith [1996] Lloyd's Medical Law Reports 424
McFarlane v Secretary of State for Scotland [1998] SCLR 623
R v Broadmoor Hospital ex p Wilkinson [2002] 1 WLR 419
R v GMC & Others ex p Burke [2004] Lloyd's Medical Law Reports 476
R v GMC & Others ex p Burke [2004] Lloyd's Medical Law Reports 451
R v GMC & Others ex p Burke [2005] EWCA CIV 1003
R v HM Coroner for Inner West London Ex p Scott [2001] 61 BMLR 222

R v HM Coroner for West Yorkshire ex p Sacker [2004] 2 All ER 495
R v London LB Sutton ex p Tucker [1998] 40 BMLR 162
R v Mersey Care NHS Trust ex p Munjaz [2003] Lloyd's Medical Law Reports 549
R v West Somerset Coroner ex p Middleton [2004] 2 All ER 484
Sookia v Lambeth, Southwark and Lewisham Health Authority [LTL 19.11.01]
Temple v South Manchester Health Authority [LTL 21/10/2002]
Thomson v James & Others [1996] 31BMLL
Vernon v Bloomsbury Health Authority [1995] 6 Med LR 297

REFERENCES

Coates A 1998 Evidence-based health advice workshop, Australian Cancer Society, Menzies Foundation, November 1998

Cole C & Tobiansky R 2003 Electroconvulsive therapy: NICE guidance may deny many patients treatment that they might benefit from. British Medical Journal 327(7415):621

Department of Health 1989 Policy guidance. Community care in the next decade and beyond

Dwyer P 1998 Legal implications of clinical practice guidelines. Medical Journal of Australia 169:292-293

Effective Interventions Unit 2005 Integrated care pathways guide 5: community detoxification pathways. Scottish Executive 2 February

General Medical Council 2002 Withholding and withdrawing life-prolonging treatments: good practice in decision making

Harpwood V 1994 NHS reform, audit, protocols and standards of care. Medical Law International 1:241-259

Hurwitz B 1999 Legal and political considerations of clinical guidelines. British Medical Journal 318:661-664

Hyams AL, Brandenburg JA, Lipsitz SR et al 1995 Practice guidelines and malpractice litigation: a two-way street. Annals of Internal Medicine 122(6):450-455

Jhawar S 2004 Outlining integrated care pathways. Express Healthcare Management 16 June

Maisonneuve H, Codier H, Durocher A et al. 1997 The French clinical guidelines and medical references programme: development of 48 guidelines for private practice over a period of 18 months. Journal of the Evaluation of Clinical Practice 3:3-13

National Health and Medical Research Council 1999 Guidelines for development, implementation and evaluation of clinical practice guidelines. NHMRC, Canberra

National Health Service Executive 1996 Clinical guidelines. NHSE, Leeds

National Institute for Clinical Excellence 2003 Guidance on the use of electroconvulsive therapy. NICE, London

National Institute for Mental Health in England 2005 Offender mental health care pathway. January

Pelly JE, Newby L, Tito F et al 1998 Clinical practice guidelines before the law: sword or shield? Medical Journal of Australia 169 (6):330-333

Pennachio DL 2002 Abortion. A right or an outrage? Medical Economics 79(19):77-78, 81, 85

Pennachio DL 2004 Malpractice: clinical guidelines – sword or shield?. Medical Economics 81(12):22-24

Psychminded News 2003a http://www.psychminded.co.uk/news/news2003/may03/RCP%20launches%20new%20accreditation%20service%20to%20raise%20standards%20for%20ECT%20.htm 3 May 2003

Psychminded News 2003b http://www.psychminded.co.uk/news/news2003/may03/I%27ll%20defy%20NICE%27s%20ECT%20guidelines,%20vows%20Glasgow%20psychiatrist.htm 17 May 2003

Tito F, Newby L 1998 Medico legal implications of clinical practice guidelines. NHMRC – National Breast Cancer Centre, Sydney

Integrating care pathways into the Care Programme Approach

Ruth Page and Rafael Sorribas

INTRODUCTION

How do we know that the care provided to a user of specialist mental health services is applicable to their needs, does not vary from practitioner to practitioner or from provider to provider? How do we know that the management of care on the frontline, in people's homes, in the community in general and in hospitals is of good quality? Is the collection of items of mandatory information, and ordering them in a particular way, a good indicator of effective practice? Do we know why the plans we make with our users do not always work? Could we do things differently?

These questions, and I am sure you can think of many more, are increasingly more difficult to answer in today's specialist mental health services. The area and practice of specialist mental health care is an interpersonal information-rich environment, which in an information age should flourish and grow ever more effective through the use of technology, and the opportunities it presents. This chapter applies the principles of care pathways to the Care Programme Approach, highlighting that the same high standards and best practice which are evident in clinical care (treatments, procedures and processes) can be applied to the information-processing requirements of managing care.

THE CARE PROGRAMME APPROACH

The requirement of a framework through which care could be coordinated began after the move from the centralised hospital model of care, to a community-based model of care. For patients of adult working age, the Care Programme Approach (CPA) (Department of Health 1990) is the de facto framework which is used to manage, document and communicate the care provided by specialist mental health services for an individual patient.

The principles of the CPA began life in a health circular (Department of Health 1990) which came into effect on 1 April 1991. This required the then district health authorities to implement the CPA for people who were suffering with a mental illness, the nature of which led them to be accepted for treatment by specialist mental health services. It also required the local authority Social Services departments to collaborate with their respective health authorities to expand social care services to support CPA patients being treated within the community. The success of the CPA consequently relies on joint working and training between social services and health to achieve integration of care.

The inquiry into the care and management of Christopher Clunis after the stabbing and subsequent death of Jonathan Zito (Ritchie et al 1994) highlighted the importance of formalising a duty of care, and ensuring adequate communication and cooperation exist between health and social care organisations. In the subsequent report *Building bridges* (Department of Health 1995) the principles of the CPA were upheld; however, the importance of risk assessment prior to discharge was emphasised. Attention was also drawn to patients to whom Section 117 of the Mental Health Act 1983 applied and the need in their case to implement the CPA fully in order to carry out aftercare duties effectively.

Most recently, *Effective care coordination in mental health services: modernising the Care Programme Approach* (Department of Health 1999) brought about procedures for the integration of CPA and care management, known as the Integrated Care Programme Approach (ICPA).

Currently, there are four components to the CPA:

1. A systematic assessment of health and social care needs, including a detailed risk assessment, for everyone accepted into specialist mental health services.
2. A care plan which identifies the care required to meet each individual's needs. This must contain details of who will be involved in providing the care and include risk management, crisis intervention and contingency plans.
3. A nominated care coordinator who will be available to the patient and who will monitor and evaluate the care provided.
4. Regular reviews of care with changes to the care plans as appropriate.

Furthermore, depending on the complexity of an individual's needs, the Care Programme Approach may be delivered in standard (low level of help) or enhanced (high level of help with multi-agency involvement) format (Department of Health 1990).

The CPA thus promotes consultation with patients and their carers during planning and evaluation of care. Therefore, using the CPA to formalise the management of care enables patients to negotiate and take control of their care package. It also decreases the variability of care that is delivered and provides a defensible record, via detailed documentation of the care, that it will be provided, when it will be provided, and by whom.

Arguably, in light of the original premise of the CPA to record and communicate information across organisational boundaries, it is good practice to collect, record and process this information for all individuals who have been accepted for specialist mental health services. In so doing, the need for a care pathway directed towards the information-processing requirements for delivering multi-disciplinary, multi-agency care is explicit.

Across the country there are huge differences in how the CPA is implemented though, from organisations using almost totally paper-based processes (although an electronic CPA register is mandatory), to complex electronic solutions that can interface with local social services' information systems. Furthermore, the local 'choice' of how to implement the CPA has led to differing prioritisation of the information that is recorded. For example, instead of adopting a comprehensive multi-professional approach, some systems emphasise the contribution and ownership of one profession (e.g. systems that focus on care plans are often seen as the domain of nurses and therefore not truly multi-disciplinary). In other systems, the major focus is not on a particular profession, and they are prioritised simply on what is required for reporting purposes. Indeed, clinical governance driven audits of CPA information are concerned more with the presence or absence of a document/data item rather than the quality and completeness of the information. Through this disparity then, a process emerges that does not truly live up to the expectations of national policy or stakeholder requirements.

A GENERIC SERVICE MODEL OF THE CPA

A generic service model is a high-level representation of a service and its actions. It is concerned with organisational processes rather than the care activities; but does allow processes to be mapped out beyond the constraints of the CPA. It is this understanding of how the CPA fits with existing processes, and activities that are not directly governed by the CPA, which provides the linkage to other activities, as a whole systems approach rather than a framework to be used in isolation (Figure 6.1).

THE CARE PROGRAMME APPROACH AS A CARE PATHWAY

There is much to be gained by moving from traditional CPA methods towards the functionality of care pathways. Care pathways are usually health and/or social

Figure 6.1

A generic service model detailing stages that can be used to determine linkages to other pathways

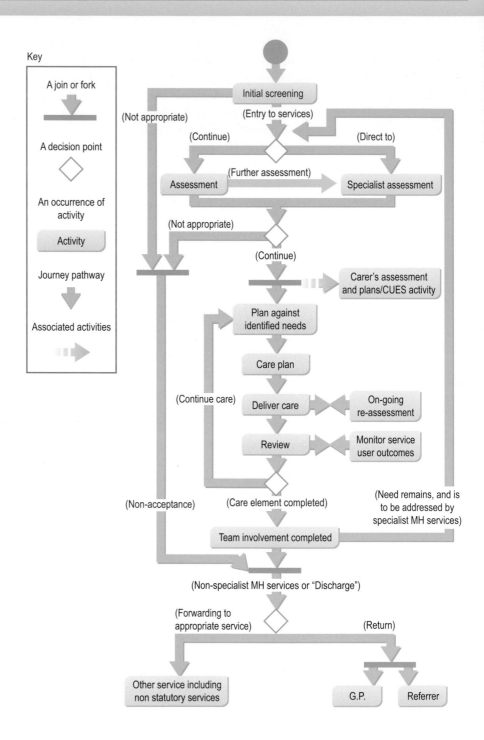

need driven (it is this that defines the care activity) and they are underpinned by standardised frameworks of best and agreed practice. In turn, a care pathway that is developed and owned by an organisation both removes the feeling of personal risk from an individual and ameliorates the risk to the organisation.

Figure 6.2
The central nature of a CPA or information-oriented care pathway

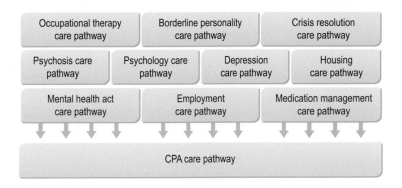

Furthermore, by shifting the administrative burden from a system laden with extensive documentation, to one which records basic core information, a great deal of clinical time can be recovered for other care activities.

A patient is likely to have more than one issue that requires addressing, however, each requiring its own set of activities and interventions. These can be incorporated within a CPA care pathway as detailed in Figure 6.2 which, in turn, supports a person-centred approach to care: eclipsing the somewhat rigid methods that are associated with the traditional implementation of the CPA.

In order to incorporate the activities of single-issue care pathways into a CPA care pathway, and to do so in a uniform way, there needs to be a standard way of defining and agreeing what these activities are and what they do within the care process. By having just one way to define a care pathway and the constituent elements, it is possible to improve the understanding and application of care pathways in the care process and, in turn, the communication about the care that is delivered. The CPA helps to establish standards of care. Thus, logically, there is an expectation to have a standard way of incorporating the CPA within care pathways. But to do this, care pathways must also be based on a standard understanding of their composition and application.

STANDARDISATION AND THE NATIONAL PROGRAMME FOR INFORMATION TECHNOLOGY (NPFIT) IN THE NHS

To understand how care pathway related concepts associate and fit together, the Clinical Design Group, at a meeting in September 2004 (National Programme for Information Technology 2004), identified the need for clear unambiguous explanations of the terms used for electronic care pathways and related subjects, particularly the distinction between care pathways and care plans. In response, they produced a set of draft definitions to be used as a standard for NPfIT system developments (Page 2004).

The initial task of the Clinical Design Group was to clarify and agree on what exactly constitutes a care pathway, keeping in mind how care pathways are expected to work electronically, and what can become the standard reference for NPfIT and system development. The group agreed on the following draft definition:

> *A care pathway maps out a consistent set of decisions and activities relating to one or more issues or problems. The aim is to define a structured process of care in order to achieve specified goals. Care pathways comprise the current best practices that are supported by an evidence base. A care pathway enables the variance between proposed and actual care to be audited, and best practice to be refined accordingly.*

The Clinical Design Group agreed that there are differences between care pathways that are developed and authored by the team of clinicians responsible for delivering care which exists as a template ready to use, and care pathways that are applied to a patient modified in some way to meet a patient's individual needs. The following definitions were agreed by the group:

- *care pathway templates* have a tightly controlled authoring and versioning process
- *care pathway in-use* is a care pathway template applied to a patient, adjusted according to the requirements of the patient.

In respect of traditional care plans, although many of their components could be incorporated into a care pathway, the decision was made by the group to maintain care plans as a distinct entity from care pathways. This is because there are many instances when care planning is an established part of the care process. Consequently, the resulting care plan is an important component of the service provision.

The following definitions for care plan were thus agreed:

- Care plan template – the combination of a need, goal and a set of activities including decision-making; a (possibly) reusable chunk of a care pathway. Although it is often locally defined to agreed policy, it may be personally defined but reusable.
- When a care plan template is applied/personalised for a patient, it leads to a group of planned activities – a care plan, which becomes a subset of the care programme.
- A care plan may be designed from scratch with a patient for that patient only, or refined from an existing care plan template.

INCORPORATING THE CPA WITHIN A CARE PATHWAY

It is the cohesiveness of the care pathway procedure that is lacking in traditional clinical note recording. On its own, implementation of the CPA results in a set of activities that can be regarded independently from each other. Although assessments are initiated and completed, due to multi-professional involvement these often exist as separate documents. Consequently, the associated plans of care, records of the care delivered and ongoing monitoring also exist as separate documentation. Additionally, although each CPA review results in a new care plan, how the new plan is developed from the previous one is rarely explicit. As a result, these components of the care process are usually disjointed, particularly when they are documented within paper records.

The structure of care pathways demands the identification of activities and determining when they should happen, in what sequence, and who should perform them. Depending on the specific needs of the patient, the order and work flow of activities may be significant and it may be that certain activities should be completed within a certain time period, or stopped if a new one is introduced. As the evidence base for mental health practice develops, the demand for enacting and recording more specific care activity will also grow. When applied to the CPA, care pathways thus enable effective capturing of the cause and effect relationship between components of care.

Once activities are detailed and ordered, and relationships between them determined, the next step is to identify satisfactory parameters or tolerances for each activity. It may be that there is a period of time within which delivering an intervention is considered acceptable. Or, that it is acceptable to replace certain activities with others, to do them in a different order, or to have them performed by staff in different roles. When activity occurs outside of acceptable tolerances however, variance has occurred. Types of variance include variance between activities, the beginning and end of an activity or indeed the care pathway, between specified and actual roles of performers of activities, between patient objectives and outcomes, and between patient characteristics (symptoms, needs) as described in the model template and those with which the patient presents. By applying this level of detail to the CPA, and capturing variance in such a systematic way, extensive information about practice is obtained. In turn, this provides a means of auditing the care process.

Depending on the needs of the patient, the CPA may continue for a very long period of time. It can also be difficult to predict an individual patient's response to interventions. The CPA process therefore includes determining a date for the next review and it is these points of formal review that form natural endpoints for care pathways. The outcome of each review may result in new or repeated assessments, new information about a patient's needs, the ending or starting of interventions in the care plan, changes in the resource responsible for carrying out a particular intervention or changes in the patient's choice of care delivery. Consequently, the CPA care pathway consists of all of the planned activities and information gathered about the patient as the CPA process is enacted.

THE CARE PROGRAMME APPROACH AS THE HIGH-LEVEL CARE PATHWAY

Another way of aligning the principles of the CPA and care pathways is to think of the CPA as an umbrella of all care past and present. This idea of a generic care programme for all patients was introduced through the clinical design work of NPfIT (National Programme for Information Technology 2004). The care programme would be the very foundation of a patient's care record, and be the platform for creating various views of care pathways/plans/components that are being enacted for the patient. Furthermore, it would be possible to view any of these at any point in time. Figures 6.3 and 6.4 (created by Peter Borden from Sapient, a member of the NPfIT Clinical Design Group) help to explain this idea and can be found in the *Electronic care pathway definitions document* (Page 2004).

Care programme overview

Figure 6.3 shows how care plan and care pathway templates are applied to a patient. The guidelines, protocols and activities of the care pathway/plan direct the care process and state what needs to be done and by whom. Ongoing monitoring and evaluation follow, and a record of all of the care is documented in the patient's notes. The care programme is thus a record of all of this activity and includes the care pathways and plans chosen for the patient, the ongoing monitoring and evaluations.

The care programme is not limited to a single episode of care (whether it is hospital or community based, long-term or short). It has the potential of forming the structure in which all care plans/pathways/components that are applied to a patient are held. This is illustrated in Figure 6.4, the care programme overview,

Figure 6.3
The relationship of care plans and pathways contributing to a care programme

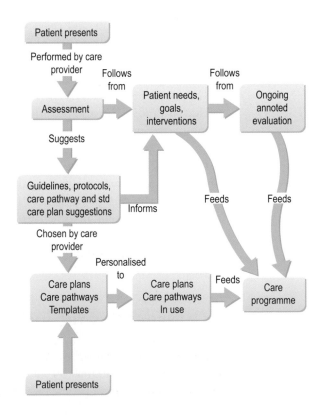

Figure 6.4

Relationship of the care programme within the care process. The dotted vertical line indicates the present point in time. The small arrows pointing down indicate that as care plans and pathways are applied to a patient, the resulting information is captured in the patient's care record. The boxes labelled *care plan a, b, c* and *d* represent care plans that have been chosen for a patient over time. The little tabs represent interventions or sets of tasks within the care plan. At the point of time indicated by the vertical line, care plans *a* and *b* no longer apply, care plan *c* is active and care plan *d* is scheduled to take place in the future

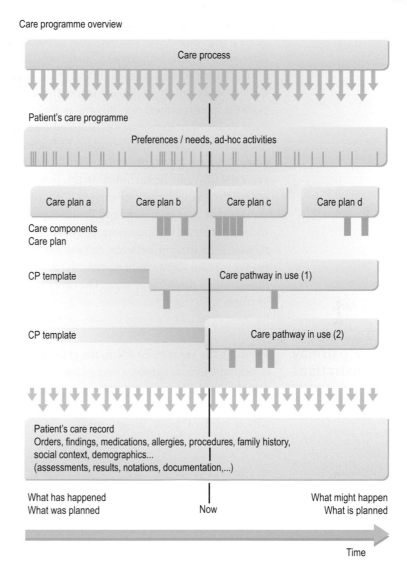

which shows that the information in a patient's care programme (regardless of whether it is an ad hoc activity, a care plan or a care pathway) is:

■ what was planned and has happened
■ the future; the care that is planned.

There are also two care pathways represented in Figure 6.4 that are currently active and in progress for the patient. To consider these within the context of a CPA care pathway, imagine that the care plans represent small packages of care such as anxiety management, assertiveness training, or some other psycho-social skills training that is of a short duration and set up as care plans. The patient might also be on a depression care pathway (e.g. pathway 1 in the diagram) and a medication management care pathway (e.g. pathway 2). The care programme thus provides a full picture of all activities taking place at the present point in time. However, the advantage of the CPA environment is that it provides the context for the planned interventions. So, looking at Figure 6.4, the record of active care at the 'now' point only shows care plan c, and care pathways in use (1 and 2) applied to the patient. In contrast, by using the full care programme model system, care plans a and b which have now finished and care plan d which is planned but has not yet started would be included. If the point 'now' represented a CPA review, this other information might be missed. Consequently, being able to have information on care that is past, present and future expands what is normally given in the CPA. Indeed, when this is incorporated within an electronic system, the user can easily request information between certain dates and the view of the care programme would contain all the information about the patient, both physical and mental for this specified duration of time. The care programme is thus essentially the patient's journey.

Care pathway illustrations

Planning the steps to be taken, the criteria to be applied and the resultant options is helpful when designing a care pathway which captures CPA-type data. Figure 6.5 attempts to demonstrate at a high level some of the elements which can be expected to be present within a care pathway for CPA and includes interventions, which type of team is responsible for those interventions, and the variance elements.

A CPA care plan, in its broadest sense, captures actions and interventions to address the issues, needs, or goals that are required to effect a transfer of care, or discharge from the specialist mental health service. While differing professions currently may plan care in a disjointed manner, the aim of the CPA is to draw these elements and activities together. Figure 6.6 represents the selection or addition of an anxiety management care pathway to a CPA care plan. (For clarity, in the following examples an electronic version is shown. However, the principles remain the same for traditional paper-based methods.)

Once selected, as shown in Figure 6.7, the person responsible for the care pathway is entered and this completes the high-level care plan. Naming the care plan as 'high level' indicates a lower level of detail that may include a great deal of information on how the issue is to be addressed, or on how the goal is reached.

Focusing onto the lower level of detail reveals the standardised activities (which could be added to or personalised) including variance recording (Figure 6.8). In turn, each of these may result in various additional actions, either linked to the high-level care plan or introducing other activities.

This approach both adds a richness of information to the ongoing assessment of an individual and provides opportunities for the quantification of the efficacy of the services offered.

Figure 6.5
High-level care pathway
plan

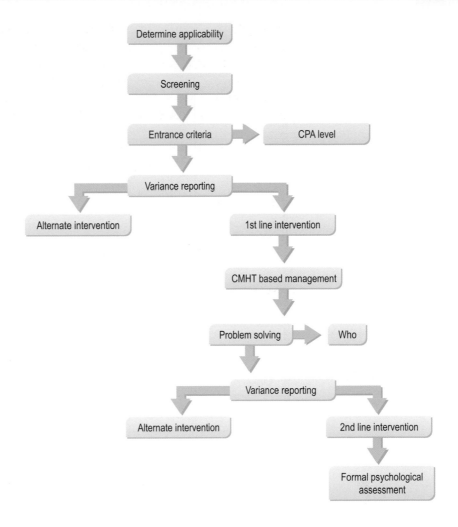

Figure 6.6
Selecting a care
pathway

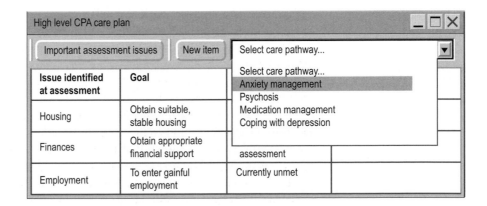

Figure 6.7
Care pathway merged
into care plan

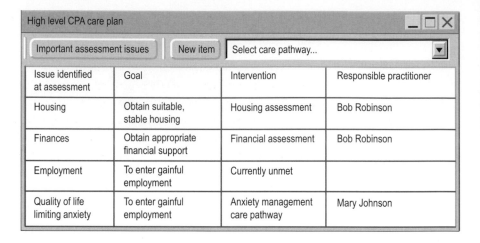

High level CPA care plan			_ □ X

Important assessment issues		New item	Select care pathway... ▼

Issue identified at assessment	Goal	Intervention	Responsible practitioner
Housing	Obtain suitable, stable housing	Housing assessment	Bob Robinson
Finances	Obtain appropriate financial support	Financial assessment	Bob Robinson
Employment	To enter gainful employment	Currently unmet	
Quality of life limiting anxiety	To enter gainful employment	Anxiety management care pathway	Mary Johnson

Figure 6.8
Lower-level care
pathway plan

Anxiety management care pathway				_ □ X
Intervention	**Frequency**	**Location**	**Responsible practitioner**	**Variance**
Problem free talk	Weekly	Sam's home	Mary Johnson	Select ... ▼
Exception finding	Weekly	Sam's home	Mary Johnson	Select ... ▼
Scaling	Weekly	Sam's home	Mary Johnson	Select ... / Achieved / In progress / Client unable to complete / Practitioner unable to complete / Other
Locating resources	Weekly	Sam's home	Mary Johnson	▼
Building strengths	Weekly	Sam's home	Mary Johnson	▼
Coping	Weekly	Sam's home	Mary Johnson	Select ... ▼
Stopping things getting worse	Weekly	Sam's home	Mary Johnson	Select ... ▼

SUMMARY

What we have shown in this chapter is a method of integrating care pathways into the Care Programme Approach. However, for effective implementation involving all stakeholders, it was shown that there must be a high level of standardisation. Much work has taken place across the United Kingdom to create standard templates for CPA assessment, care plans/pathways/components, monitoring and review. If it is possible to standardise these for large sections of the country, then it may be possible to agree on one standard for the whole country. In turn, this would improve cross-country communication and facilitate the sharing of records electronically. The real challenge is to determine the level of detail that can be standardised for all mental health specialist services and to retain clinical meaning and validity.

The trouble with developing a nationally agreed solution, however, is that geographic, cultural and demographic differences make it difficult to generalise content. A care pathway must therefore be constructed bearing in mind the most current thinking and guidance surrounding the subject, but within the context of the local care delivery environment and resources. The CPA has nationally defined guidance on the manner in which it should be applied to a person. It is, therefore, these principles which should be incorporated within care pathway development, but allowing sufficient interpretation to meet the needs of local implementation.

REFERENCES

Department of Health 1990 The care programme approach for people with a mental illness referred to the specialist psychiatric services. HC (90)23/LASSL(90)11. HMSO, London

Department of Health 1995 Building bridges: arrangement for inter-agency working for the care and protection of severely mentally ill people. HSG (95)56. HMSO, London

Department of Health 1999 Effective care coordination in mental health services: modernising the care programme approach – a policy booklet. 16736. The Stationary Office, London

National Programme for Information Technology Clinical Design Group 2004 Unpublished

Page R 2004 Electronic care pathway definitions V1. NPfIT, NPFIT-FNT-TO-DPM-0187.02.

Ritchie J, Dick D, Lingham R 1994 The report of the Christopher Clunis inquiry. North West Thames Regional Health Authority

Using integrated care pathways in forensic services

Karen J Jenkins

INTRODUCTION	**IMPLEMENTATION**
BACKGROUND	**OUTCOMES AND CONCLUSIONS**
PATHWAY DEVELOPMENT	**REFERENCES**

INTRODUCTION

The State Hospital is the main provider of forensic care in Scotland, with 255 of the total 520 forensic beds nationwide. Integrated care pathways (ICPs) have been under development at the Hospital since the late 1990s. At least two other hospitals with forensic beds have used the State Hospital admission ICP as a starting point for their ICPs. These include the Royal Cornhill Hospital in Aberdeen and the Murray Royal Hospital in Perth. Therefore, based on the number of beds, the majority of Scottish forensic care providers now use ICPs. Nationally, Scottish Executive Health Department (SEHD) policy has referred to the 'patient's pathway' in the *Services, care, support and accommodation for mentally disordered offenders in Scotland: care pathway document* (Scottish Executive Health Department 2001). Care pathway is a more general term than ICP, relating to the patient's journey of care. To support the development of ICPs for forensic mental health services the Managed Care Network was established in 2003. One of its aims is to develop protocols which will support the transfer of patients between the different levels of service. It is believed that the sharing of ICPs between services will help to achieve this.

Recently, the National Health Service (NHS) Quality Improvement Scotland (QIS) national report for schizophrenia standards recommended that NHS boards, in partnership with other agencies, should develop ICPs to implement the clinical standards for schizophrenia, effective interventions and good practice (National Health Service Quality Improvement Scotland 2004). In order to establish ICPs as an intrinsic element of forensic care at the State Hospital, they have been embedded in the hospital's policies, health improvement plans, clinical strategy, clinical governance success criteria and various action plans. The ICPs were designed to support existing processes in the State Hospital. For example, the NHS QIS schizophrenia standards require annual case reviews (Clinical Standards Board for Scotland 2001). The ICPs embedded in this service exceed this requirement and the presence of the ICP and variance reports provides evidence to NHS QIS that the case reviews and other standards are being adhered to.

BACKGROUND

The State Hospital provides treatment and care in conditions of special security for individuals with mental disorder who, because of their dangerous, violent or criminal propensities, cannot be cared for in any other setting. Patient referrals are received from three main sources: prisons, courts and other NHS hospitals. The organisation's purpose is to provide care and treatment of the highest standards in a safe and secure environment for patients from Scotland and Northern Ireland. The hospital aims to help patients recover from their illness, whilst managing the risks they may present, so that they can be transferred to services closer to their home and families. Located in rural Lanarkshire in central Scotland, the hospital can offer care for up to 255 patients, provided for by 550 staff. The campus consists of 11 wards covering admission, rehabilitation and continuing care. There are also dedicated services for females and those with learning disabilities. In terms of mental health problems, approximately 70% of patients suffer from schizophrenia, and 50% have multiple diagnoses. The average age of inpatients is 37, but the age ranges from 18 to 62. The average length of stay is around 6 years; however, the length of stay varies from 10 weeks to 36 years. Around 93% of patients are male and 7% are female.

ICPs have been in use at the State Hospital since 1998. They were initially developed on the male admission ward (McQueen & Milloy 2001) in response to the recognition that there was a lack of clarity about roles and responsibilities within the clinical team. Also there were varying views regarding interventions and the timescales within which they should be completed. After successful implementation, the development of ICPs spread to two further wards, which ultimately led to the commitment to implement ICPs hospital wide (Duncan & Moody 2003). In the initial stages, the clinical effectiveness department facilitated the development and implementation of ICPs in addition to other quality improvement activities. However, the hospital's commitment to ICPs manifested itself in the appointment of a dedicated ICP facilitator in 2000. One of the initial tasks of the postholder was to produce an ICP strategy that would establish the vision and means of using ICPs to improve the quality of patient care. This strategy provided the foundation for ICPs to be developed across the hospital. The successful roll-out of ICPs across the site means that every patient has had an ICP since 2002.

Traditionally, pathways had been used in general and acute hospital settings for procedures such as hip replacements where a patient's pathway to recovery may be relatively predictable with clearly definable milestones. However, in mental health, given the ranges of responses to treatment within even a single diagnosis, it can be more difficult to predict how and when a patient will recover. As a consequence of this, the ICPs developed at the State Hospital are based upon processes rather than outcomes. Process-based ICPs provide a description of interventions, when they should be completed and by which member of the clinical team. While these ICPs tend not to have delineated outcomes or milestones the interventions are evidence based where possible. ICPs have been developed around critical points in the patient's journey through the hospital:

- admission
- continuing care
- transfer between wards.

Indeed, the importance of these processes is recognised in the schizophrenia standards (Clinical Standards Board for Scotland 2001) with each having their own standard.

The admission assessment is a key juncture for all patients; once the assessment is completed, the decision is made whether the patient should remain in the hospital or leave. Development of an ICP around this process was a priority, ensuring the assessment is complete and the clinical team have all the information required to make the right decision with the patient. In continuing care wards, the case review process provides the focus of decision-making for planning care. The development of a treatment and rehabilitation ICP for use across the hospital was undertaken in response to a Mental Welfare Commission report (Mental Welfare Commission for Scotland 2000) into the care and treatment of a patient at the hospital. Transfer between wards is another key juncture in the patient's care. Any transfer between services has the potential for complications. Care should continue with the least disruption for the patient, with the new clinical team receiving all the information they need.

The admission assessment ICP

Admission to the State Hospital is often a result of other services being unable to cope; it provides the highest level of secure psychiatric services in Scotland. The assessment of new patients is key to deciding their future care at the State Hospital and beyond. Generally, clinical staff in 'admissions' determine whether the patient should stay or be treated elsewhere. In some cases, the clinician is required to determine whether the patient should return to prison or is fit to plead. The admission assessment process was translated into an ICP, with timescales and responsibilities clearly defined. With the ICP in place the Responsible Medical Officer (RMO) can be assured that the assessment has been completed ready for the case conference so that the most appropriate decision can be made to determine future care. This ICP is used for all admissions and can be found in Appendix 7.1.

The inter-ward transfer ICP

Patients in the hospital have complex needs, with care being delivered by a multidisciplinary team. To move a patient to another ward means that information about how to meet the needs of patients, risk areas, or effective treatment strategies needs to be passed seamlessly to the new clinical team. The process has to run smoothly for the patient, easing them through a difficult period as they have to settle into a new environment with new staff and patients. This ICP is used for all transfers between wards in the hospital. It covers preparation for the move, the first few weeks in the new ward and then links to the treatment and rehabilitation ICP.

The treatment and rehabilitation ICP

The patient's case review is the culmination of 4 months' work by ward staff and the clinical team. Here, a patient's progress is discussed. Treatment objectives are agreed and the need to stay in hospital is considered. The ICP plays an important role in organising the case review. It prompts: patient involvement in reports (by nursing and occupational therapy), carer/relative involvement (by invitation to case reviews), full and timely assessments (mental state reviews, Model of Human Occupation Screening Tool (Parkinson & Forsyth 2001)) and further reports (by various members of the clinical team). Once at the review, the ICP ensures key decisions are made, such as reviews of medication, planned activities, ground access, consent to treatment and the need for patient information. After the review, the ICP ensures the case review objectives and the plan are discussed with the patient. In short, this ICP ensures case reviews are well organised with appropriate decisions being made regarding future care. The good practice in this ICP is implemented across the hospital, helping to ensure consistent standards of care. The treatment and rehabilitation ICP is shown in Appendix 7.2.

At the State Hospital, ICPs do not replace case notes and treatment planning documentation, but they act in concert with existing paperwork. However, the care pathway development process does aim to reduce duplication where possible.

PATHWAY DEVELOPMENT

The ICPs at the State Hospital were initially developed within clinical teams, supported by clinical audit staff. When the ICP facilitator was appointed, the ICP strategy recommendations (see Box 7.1) provided the methodology for the roll-out of ICPs across the hospital. The strategy stated that ICPs should be used by clinical teams to monitor, coordinate and improve high standards of patient care. It was proposed that ICPs would improve patient care by:

- promoting the coordination of patient care
- improving multidisciplinary teamwork
- assisting in the process of evaluating patient care (through variance analysis)
- educating staff
- helping to ensure that patients receive up-to-date and appropriate care.

When the strategy was approved, the existing ICPs were developed so they could be used across the organisation. Three themes were embraced throughout

Box 7.1   RECOMMENDATIONS FROM THE STRATEGY

1. Continued commitment by directors and senior management
   - providing encouragement to staff to take ICPs forward
   - providing time and replacement costs for staff to take part in training and education
   - incorporation into department strategies or work plans
   - incorporation into job plans or personal development plans.

2. Pathways are owned and completed by clinical staff
   - ICP facilitator and the clinical team are jointly responsible for developing, implementing, completing and evaluating ICPs – for example, the clinical team is able to make changes to the ICP and decide on appropriate reports.

3. Pathways are based on available evidence and best practice
   - adherence to national standards.

4. Variations in practice are collated, analysed and fed back to clinical staff
   - reports will be collated for clinical teams
   - reports will also be available for the clinical governance committee as appropriate.

5. Programmes of training and education are provided as follows:
   - written information e.g. leaflets and articles
   - formal training sessions tailored to need, and
   - informal/unstructured training sessions.

6. ICP business to be discussed at every ward core group.
7. ICPs will be embedded within the structures and supports necessary for clinical governance.
8. An incremental approach will be taken for the implementation of ICPs. This will ensure issues are identified and addressed, lessons learned and applied.
9. A variety of approaches will be taken to identify and measure the impact of ICPs on practice.
10. Clear guidance will be provided on the priority areas for ICPs.
11. Additional support is provided for the ICP facilitator (it was suggested 0.75 post for an additional facilitator and an ICP assistant was required).

the development process: communication, consensus and consultation. This was demonstrated by staff being informed and involved, information materials being circulated at clinical team meetings and ICPs being raised as agenda items at department meetings. The final draft of the treatment and rehabilitation ICP was the result of gaining consensus across the hospital.

In retrospect, the starting point for ICP development was discussion about the scope of the pathway. Once this was agreed, discussions focused on how care was delivered, whether this was for the admission assessment, case reviews or ward transfers. Discussions were undertaken by an individual clinical team (for the admission assessment ICP) or by professional groups as a whole (for the treatment and rehabilitation ICP). The clinicians process mapped current care, noting when interventions were delivered and by whom. Once the care process was described, national standards and best practice guidelines were reviewed. These included the schizophrenia standards (Clinical Standards Board for Scotland 2001), generic clinical governance guidance and various relevant physical health standards. The smoking cessation standards (National Health Service Health Scotland 1998) and relevant Scottish Intercollegiate Guidelines Network (SIGN) resources were reviewed. The ICPs also provided the opportunity to include various tools such as ethnic screening, cultural screening, risk assessments, rating scales and blood risk screening. The inclusion of QIS standards into ICPs led to the State Hospital being commended in the national reports for schizophrenia and generic clinical governance.

Draft ICPs were prepared by combining current practice with the best practice from the standards. An iterative revision and review process was used to convert the draft into an effective ICP. This entails each intervention being assigned a due date (e.g. 3 days after admission) and a responsible discipline (e.g. nursing or occupational therapy). A space to record variances was also included. The ICPs were circulated to members of the clinical team, revised, re-circulated and revised until the team agreed that they were ready for pilot.

IMPLEMENTATION

In the State Hospital the pilot of ICPs is just one part of the implementation process. Preparation has been key to successful implementation. Training and education feature highly. Clinical teams and nursing staff are visited at ward meetings or during the handover period. An ICP link nurse is trained for each ward. Educational materials are also produced in the form of an information folder, ICP bulletin and emails. In the State Hospital all wards are locked and visits have to be arranged in advance, thus reducing the opportunity for informal discussion about ICPs. Financial constraints have also impacted on staff accessing training, so most training is conducted on the wards. Therefore, the ICP facilitator had to take a proactive approach to ensure staff were both involved with and informed about ICPs. By the implementation date, staff need to know what to do and when. When in use, the ICPs are stored in the ward office and staff record when they have completed an intervention (or a variance). The ICP is designed so it is possible to tell whether an intervention has been completed on time, late or not at all. For the latter cases, a variance code is written on the ICP. This enables

Table 7.1
Categories for variance codes

Variation category	Examples
Patient	Patient choice, illness and communication
Staff	Availability of staff, risk assessments
Relative/carer	Carer/relative choice, availability and contact
Hospital systems/information availability	Hospital systems and impact on the delivery of care
Care and treatment	Standard assessments are not appropriate for all patients

clinicians to determine whether an intervention has been completed and, if it has not, then the reason for this.

As described in Chapter 2, variances have been defined as 'the difference between how patient care and outcomes were defined on the critical pathway and what actually happened' (Dykes & Slye 1997 p 40). A variance record includes the reason why a clinician has been unable to deliver an intervention: for example, carer details are not available. Initially, variances were written as narratives on the ICP. However, when ICPs were rolled out to every ward, the process of analysing the many different variances became more problematic. In 2003, approximately 300 ICPs were examined and a pattern of variances emerged, which is described in Table 7.1. The table shows the variation categories developed and examples of variances common to each category. For example, in the patient variation category, interventions have not been completed due to patient choice, the health of the service user or for reasons of communication.

Within each category separate codes were defined, such as:

- patient declined
- patient communication problems
- staff – other commitments
- staff – risk assessment e.g. pregnancy.

The development of the codes was supported by a new intranet system, where minimal free text was permitted. This was easier for clinicians to use and helped to identify what prevents clinical staff from delivering care to the standard specified in the ICPs. This information is summarised in variance analysis reports.

For all the pathways in use, the variations are recorded, analysed and reported upon. Variance analysis is defined by Middleton & Roberts (2000 p 6) as 'Analysis of variations from the pathway through retrospective audit identifies trends in the delivery of care'. Pathways and the variance reports together provide the summary of care delivery for a set period, describing the interventions which have been completed and those that have not and the reasons why.

Variance analysis aims to:

- influence change
- improve patient care
- manage risk, and
- enable staff to reflect upon practice.

In order to collate ICP variance reports, the dates interventions were undertaken and the variances are manually entered onto an ICP intranet system by an ICP assistant. A computer reporting system compiles the data from each ward. The ICP facilitator then takes selected information from this and converts it into ward variance reports. These reports are based on the interventions relevant to the schizophrenia standards (Clinical Standards Board for Scotland 2001). Reports highlight areas where care is good and areas where there are still challenges. Contextual data are also provided. Variance analysis reports also contain an action plan, with clear responsibilities assigned for action that should occur after the report is considered by the teams. This is to ensure that the issues identified are followed up. Reports are circulated to wards and discussed with the clinical team and the ICP facilitator. This can be a difficult area as discussion on practice and evaluating how care has been delivered is not always welcome. The open discussion of clinical practice which is needed requires a 'blame-free' culture which is the goal of many hospitals, but present in few.

When the treatment and rehabilitation ICP was implemented, variance analysis reports highlighted inconsistencies in practice between wards, which the hospital had not been aware of. The hospital-wide summaries of profession-specific data were anonymised according to clinical audit good practice. The author believes that it is essential that this information is not used for performance monitoring but rather to provide a picture of care delivery across the hospital. After presenting this information, the ICP facilitator works with the clinical teams and professional groups to achieve greater clarity about the precise nature of key interventions, thus standardising practice across wards. An example of an action plan in response to differences in practice was an ICP protocol developed by the occupational therapy department. This provides explicit guidance on the specific interventions to be conducted, the timescales, and the circumstances under which it is permissible not to undertake an intervention. This has been implemented by the occupational therapy staff to reduce variation.

In addition to quality problems, these variance reports also highlight areas of good practice. For example, the treatment and rehabilitation ICP variance report revealed variations in key worker attendance at case review; this variance was further investigated. The ICP facilitator asked the ward managers of the wards where key worker attendance was good to outline the systems they had in place which developed such positive outcomes (and less variance). The good practice described by the ward managers was shared at directorate meetings, providing an opportunity to improve clinical practice across other settings. The provision of this contextual data generally reduces the potential for clinical teams to work in isolation from each other, helping to ensure improvements in care across the hospital.

Overall, ICPs and variance analysis have been found to promote clinical governance, in particular by:

- increasing the coordination of care
- improving multidisciplinary working
- assisting in evaluating care
- acting as an educational tool
- helping to ensure patients receive evidence-based care
- enabling audit to be integral to routine practice
- improving communication, and
- providing an opportunity to continually improve practice.

To secure implementation, the role of ICP link nurse was created to provide additional ICP support for ward-based staff. The ICP facilitator had traditionally attended clinical team meetings, but this only involved contact with one or two nurses. Information about ICPs was not always widely circulated and failed to reach the 20 or so nursing staff in each ward who use the ICPs. Networking with NHS colleagues suggested that ICP link nurses could provide additional support to ward staff who were implementing ICPs. They could help with day-to-day queries and would be available to give advice at the times when it is needed. Discussions with the senior nurses and ward managers helped to agree the detail of the role shown in Figure 7.1.

A nurse from each ward was selected to attend a half-day training session and take up the role. Nursing staff were also provided with an information pack. Back

Figure 7.1
The role of the ICP link person

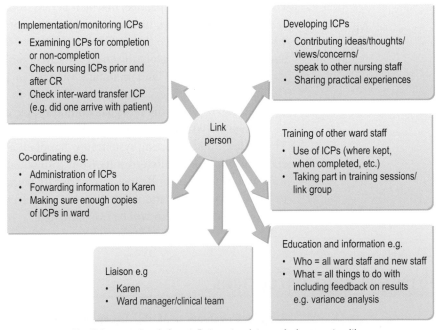

The link person's role is not: Data entry, data analysis, report writing

on the ward the amount of time the link nurse dedicated to ICPs was dependent on the individual and their ward manager, as there was no official dedicated time allocated. The ICP facilitator still provided support with regular visits to the ward. After some time, the role was reviewed from ICP link nurse to 'ICP link person' to provide additional support for other professional groups. In 2004 the first ICP link person forum was held. This aimed to get the link staff together as one group for discussions on various ICP matters. The meeting was well received and it was agreed that the link role required review. It was realised that initial expectations of the link person were too high and that not all aspirations had been achieved. For example, problems around completion of ICPs were still not regularly passed on to the ICP facilitator.

Implementation of the ICP was found to be relatively straightforward. Full integration into daily routines has been more challenging. The State Hospital ICPs have evolved and the hospital aims to continually improve practice using ICPs. At a basic level, this occurs by updating the interventions in the ICP. The admission ICP is updated many times each year and it is nursing staff who most frequently offer additional interventions to the ICP content. The treatment and rehabilitation ICP is reviewed annually. As standards of practice rise, some interventions are no longer required and new ones are added. Nearly every clinician in the hospital uses the treatment and rehabilitation ICP so changes have to be discussed and agreed within each professional group. The ICP facilitator ensures that ICPs are still in accordance with the hospital objectives.

Maintaining the enthusiasm of the lead facilitator and ICP link people is a challenge. One of the main focuses of the ICP facilitator's work is preparing and presenting variance analysis reports. Clinical teams do not always welcome these. From the author's perspective, maybe it is rare to have an organisation where staff readily discuss mistakes or practice which has not been ideal. ICPs and variance analysis is one initiative that is helping the State Hospital move towards this goal and become a learning organisation. In any organisation it takes time to change culture, to implement and maintain changes in practice. To this end the ICP facilitator is currently examining how ICPs can fit more closely with the agendas of clinical staff. Achieving this goal would provide a 'win win' for all involved.

In August 2003 the ICP intranet database was re-developed and implemented. The database and reporting system now handle ICP analysis for all wards. Reports are available which collate results from individual wards and patients, enabling variances to be tracked. Reports are currently being developed which enable data to be summarised for the whole hospital on selected ICP interventions. In 2005 a revised intranet system will be implemented.

OUTCOMES AND CONCLUSIONS

A formal evaluation of the treatment and rehabilitation ICP has been carried out. This aimed to review the implementation process and impact on patient care.

The evaluation was conducted by facilitated discussion using a question guide. Discussions took place at multidisciplinary business meetings or interviews with individual ICP link people. The findings showed benefits related to organisation and planning; and the ability of the ICP to highlight problems in care. It was also thought that the ICP improved communication between clinicians and acted as an educational tool for new staff. Staff noted that ICPs 'make sure things are done', 'provide evidence of care, the same standard of care for all patients', 'more equal spread of time with patients' and 'highlight areas where care is falling down'. The main problems identified with the ICP were related to the design and content. Staff pointed out that: 'it would be good to reduce the amount of boxes that need to be signed off'. Comments were made about the ICP content suggesting that it 'lacks qualitative aspects of care'. Some staff proposed that they 'still have problems with completion' of the ICP. The evaluation also identified a number of changes to practice that have occurred since using the ICP. For example, teams now use standard letters inviting relatives to case reviews and junior doctors now see patients prior to reviews. These were perceived as definite examples of improvements in practice.

Overall, conducting the evaluation was a very useful exercise and it was helpful to obtain views, either positive or negative ones. At the time of the evaluation (October 2002) the main challenges were to shift opinion and increase the number of ward teams to a 'pro ICP' way of thinking. It was suggested that this could be done by increasing the reporting of ICP results and ensuring appropriate feedback is given throughout the organisation. The majority of the recommendations of the evaluation report (see Box 7.2) were implemented; although further evaluation is still required.

Box 7.2 RECOMMENDATIONS FROM THE EVALUATION REPORT

1. Improve the link nurse system by providing training for new link nurses.
2. Improve the link nurse system by organising regular ICP link nurse meetings to facilitate the sharing of ideas in relation to ICPs.
3. Improve feedback loop and reports for clinical teams.
4. Report overall variance results to departmental meetings and the clinical forum.
5. Clinical teams should have regular core groups – to help with planning workload and visits to teams.
6. Explore alternative styles for the ICP.
7. The link between ICPs and treatment plans and nursing care plans should be explored and streamlined to avoid duplication.
8. Priorities should focus on improving current systems, before moving to new areas.
9. Patients to be given an information sheet about the continuing care ICP and given the opportunity to see their ICP (by their key worker).

Reflecting on 6 years of ICP development at the State Hospital, the recommendations from ICP strategy are still as relevant today as when they were written in 2001. To anyone considering developing ICPs, a strategy with recommendations provides a good starting point. The strategy has been reviewed on a regular basis, either in a specific annual report or as part of the clinical governance annual report. Within the strategy there is a section noting people, time and costs. Most of this has been discussed in this chapter with the exception of clinical champions. At the State Hospital clinical champions have been essential sources of support for ICPs as many clinicians are more likely to listen to influential colleagues regarding the benefits of ICPs, rather than a facilitator. The wards where ICPs have been most successful have a ward manager and/or a Responsible Medical Officer who are committed to ICPs. It has been very important to have key stakeholders who are supportive and can influence others. When this does not exist the ICP link person and ICP facilitator have to work much harder to gain commitment from staff. It is the author's view that it would still be possible to develop ICPs without an ICP facilitator. Networking with ICP enthusiasts will provide enough information to begin development. It is recommended that development begins with a small enthusiastic clinical team. If this is successful, the ICP sells itself and others will want to get involved.

Appendix 7.1
The State Hospital ICP
admission assessment,
Lomond version

THE STATE HOSPITAL
INTEGRATED CARE PATHWAY– ADMISSION ASSESSMENT
LOMOND VERSION

Patient details		Staff details	Print Name	Signature
Patient Name		RMO		
Hospital ID		SHO		
D.O.B.		Key Worker		
Admission Date:		Ward Manager		
Admission Time:		Psychologist:		
Date of Initial CTM		Social Worker		
Case Conference Date:		Security		
Disch/trans Date:		Pharmacist		
Disch/trans Loc:		PARS staff		
Patient Signature		Other		

Instructions for completion of ICP
If an intervention **is completed on time** – enter the date and sign in the box.
If an intervention is **late** (but is completed) – enter the date, sign and tick " **late**" box and write the reason why in the variance box.
If an intervention is **not done** – **DO NOT SIGN AND DATE** but tick box "**not done**" and write the reason why in the variance box.
If it takes several attempts to complete the intervention (e.g. taking bloods or contacting relatives/carers), enter the date when the intervention **was completed** tick "**late**" box and write the reason why in the variance box.
If the intervention is **not appropriate/not applicable** tick "**N/A**" box and write the reason why intervention is not appropriate/applicable in the variance box.

If you have any queries regarding the ICP please contact Karen Moody or Carole Campbell on extension 315
It remains each profession's responsibility to ensure that practice is safe

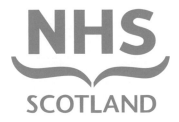

1

Patient Name...................................... Patient ID....................................... Admission date: ..../..../....
Admission ICP – Lomond Ward
July 04

VARIANCE CODES – NOT DONE		
Variance code to be entered on ICP	Meaning/Interpretation	EXAMPLES
Relative variances: *These relate to patient choice, illness, language etc.*		
P1	Patient declined	E.g. to invite relatives, to participate with a clinician, to having open door, to an outing etc.
P2	Carer/relative unable to attend	E.g. due to poor mental health, the patient doesn't engage well with staff.
P3	No carer/relative identified	E.g. patient at local hospital.
P4	Patient communication problems	E.g. patient doesn't speak English, interpreter required etc.
Carer / Relative variances: *These relate to carer/relative choice, availability, contact etc.*		
C1	Carer/relative declines	E.g. they don't want to attend meetings, case reviews or receive information regarding the patient.
C2	Carer/relative unable to attend	E.g. due to travelling time, on holiday. However they would've liked to attend.
C3	No carer/relative identified	E.g. no carer/relative identified by patient.
C4	Carer/relative not available	E.g. unable to get in contact with carer/relative.
C5	No regular contact with carer/relative	E.g. patient has no contact with relative/carer.
C6	Carer/relative – incomplete contact details	E.g. patient unsure of address/phone number.
Staff variances : *These variances relate to the availability of staff*		
S1	Staff not available	E.g. due to: Annual leave, sick leave, study/training leave, days off etc.
S2	Staff other commitments	E.g. at another meeting, workload, KW in numbers therefore, not able to attend, shift change etc.
S3	Staff – risk – assessment	E.g. the result of a risk assessment means that a staff member can't work with a patient e.g. if staff member is pregnant etc.
S4	Staff new to ward/induction period	E.g. new member of nursing staff or clinical team etc.
Care & treatment variances		
T1	Not clinically indicated at present	E.g. the patient might not be ready for the intervention, or a clinician could be waiting for a clinical team decision before working with the patient.
T2	No outstanding need	E.g. all relevant work has been done with the patient; there will be no more input with the patient at the moment.
Hospital systems / information availability		
R1	Information not available	E.g. treatment plan not on ward etc.
R2	Patient not available	E.g. patient gone to placement or appointment.
R3	Case review/conference date changed	E.g. staff unable to attend or do report because the date has been changed at short notice etc.
R4	Patient moved ward	E.g. interventions were not completed prior to patient moving to another ward.
R5 (Admission ICP)	External information not available	E.g. records from previous hospital/prison.
R6 (Admission ICP)	Emergency Admission/Court Referral	E.g. no pre-admission assessment/report.
VARIANCE CODES – LATE		
Patient Variances: *These relate to patient choice, illness, language etc.*		
LP1	Patient declines	E.g. patient declined at first but intervention was completed at a later date.
LP2	Patient unsettled presentation	E.g. had to wait until patient's mental state/health improved before intervention could be completed.
LP3	Patient physically unwell	E.g. patient at local hospital etc.
LP4	Patient communication problems	E.g. patient does not speak English, had to wait for an interpreter to complete intervention.
Carer / relative variances: *These relate to carer / relative choice, availability, contact etc*		
LC3	No carer/relative identified	E.g. on admission to hospital NOK is not always known etc.
LC4	Carer/relative not available	E.g. tried to contact but not available at first etc.
LC6	Carer/relative – incomplete contact details	E.g. patient unsure of address/phone number.
Staff variances: *These variance relate to availability of staff*		
LS1	Staff not available	E.g. due to: Annual leave, sick leave, study/training leave, and days off.
LS2	Staff – other commitments	E.g. another meeting, workload.
LS4	Staff new to ward/induction period	E.g. new member of nursing staff or clinical team etc
Hospital systems / information availability		
LR1	Information not available	E.g. treatment plan not available on ward etc.
LR2	Patient not available	E.g. gone to placement or appointment.
LR3	Case review/conference date changed	E.g. staff unable to attend or do report because the date has been changed at short notice etc.
LR5 (Admission ICP)	External information not available	E.g. Records from previous hospital/prison.

Other: If you feel that the variance doesn't fit into one of these categories, it can be written onto the ICP

2

Patient Name...   Patient ID...   Admission date: ..../......./.......
Admission ICP – Lomond Ward
July 04

Appendix 7.1   (*Continued*)

MEDICAL INTERVENTIONS – ADMISSION ICP

SAME DAY	Date and Sign	VARIANCE – Please tick box as appropriate, write reason for variance, action taken and final outcome
1. Admission mental state examination completed	../../..	☐ LATE ☐ NOT DONE
2. Ward copied with pre-admission report	../../..	☐ LATE ☐ NOT DONE
3. Physical examination (including neurological examination & general medical history completed)	../../..	☐ LATE ☐ NOT DONE
By DAY 7		
4.Folstein M.M.S.E. completed	../../..	☐ LATE ☐ NOT DONE ☐ N/A
5. Admission bloods (LFTs, U&E, FBC+ESR, glucose, syphilis serology, TFT) taken	../../..	☐ LATE ☐ NOT DONE
6. Preliminary assessment by allocated Consultant	../../..	☐ LATE ☐ NOT DONE
At CTM		
7. Initial strategic review completed	../../..	☐ LATE ☐ NOT DONE
8. CC scheduled for W8	../../..	☐ LATE ☐ NOT DONE
By Day 14		
9. Previous psychiatric admission/prison files requested	../../..	☐ LATE ☐ NOT DONE ☐ N/A
10. Request medication history from pharmacy (if indicated)	../../..	☐ LATE ☐ NOT DONE ☐ N/A
11. Referred for neurology opinion (if indicated)	../../..	☐ LATE ☐ NOT DONE ☐ N/A
By Day 49		
12. Admission history compiled and sent to ward	../../..	☐ LATE ☐ NOT DONE
At CC		
13. Patient referred to high dose antipsychotic patients to ECG clinic (if appropriate)	../../..	☐ LATE ☐ NOT DONE ☐ N/A
14. CC attended by Consultant	../../..	☐ LATE ☐ NOT DONE ☐ N/A
15. Carers attend CC	../../..	☐ LATE ☐ NOT DONE ☐ N/A
After CC		
16. Information about schizophrenia given to carer after CC (if appropriate)	../../..	☐ LATE ☐ NOT DONE ☐ N/A
17. Diagnosis discussed with patient	../../..	☐ LATE ☐ NOT DONE ☐ N/A

3

Patient Name.. Patient ID.. Admission date: ..../......./......

Admission ICP – Lomond Ward

July 04

Appendix 7.1 *(Continued)*

NURSING INTERVENTIONS

Prior to Admission	Date and Sign	VARIANCE – Please tick box as appropriate, write reason for variance, action taken and final outcome
18. Nursing pre-admission assessment completed	../../..	☐ NOT DONE ☐ N/A
PLEASE TICK IF THE PATIENT WAS AN EMERGENCY ADMISSION ☐		
On Admission		
19. Nursing pre-admission report available	../../..	☐ NOT DONE
20. External notes available at point of admission	../../..	☐ NOT DONE
SAME DAY		
21. Bloodborne virus risk assessment	../../..	☐ LATE ☐ NOT DONE
22. Pre-admission assessment report in MDT notes	../../..	☐ LATE ☐ NOT DONE ☐ N/A
23. Patient introduced to ward	../../..	☐ LATE ☐ NOT DONE
24. Patient assigned to keyworker	../../..	☐ LATE ☐ NOT DONE
25. Patient introduced to KW	../../..	☐ LATE ☐ NOT DONE
26. Admission profile completed	../../..	☐ LATE ☐ NOT DONE
27. At-risk register completed	../../..	☐ LATE ☐ NOT DONE
28. Care plan commenced	../../..	☐ LATE ☐ NOT DONE
29. NOK contacted successfully	../../..	☐ LATE ☐ NOT DONE
30. Patient with physical disability and minority grps. Referred to Clinical Nurse Spec. (if appropriate)	../../..	☐ LATE ☐ NOT DONE ☐ N/A
31. Risk assessment tool completed	../../..	☐ LATE ☐ NOT DONE
32. Cultural assessment tool completed as required	../../..	☐ LATE ☐ NOT DONE
By DAY 5		
33. Information booklets i.e.: Patient Info, Hospital Info, Section Info & MWC Info given to patient	../../..	☐ LATE ☐ NOT DONE
By DAY 7		
34. NOK letter with Clinical Team, visiting info. and info about CC sent	../../..	☐ LATE ☐ NOT DONE
35. Directory of procedures and services given to patient	../../..	☐ LATE ☐ NOT DONE
AT CTM		
36. Risk assessment discussed	../../..	☐ LATE ☐ NOT DONE

4

Patient Name... Patient ID... Admission date: ....../...../.....
Admission ICP – Lomond Ward
July 04

Appendix 7.1   *(Continued)*

NURSING INTERVENTIONS

By Day 14		
37. Complete LUNSER	../../..	☐ NOT DONE ☐ N/A
38. Referral to Occupational Therapy for assessment completed	../../..	☐ LATE ☐ NOT DONE
39. PECC assessment completed (includes EPSE assessment if appropriate)	../../..	☐ LATE ☐ NOT DONE

INTERVENTIONS PRIOR TO CASE CONFERENCE

By Day 42	Date and Sign	VARIANCE – Please tick box as appropriate, write reason for variance, action taken and final outcome
40. PECC assessment completed (includes EPSE assessment if appropriate)	../../..	☐ LATE ☐ NOT DONE
By Day 49		
41. Data entered on to computer (PECC)	../../..	☐ LATE ☐ NOT DONE
42. Substance use screening assessment & initial summary report completed	../../..	☐ LATE ☐ NOT DONE ☐ N/A
Prior to CC W8		
43. Substance abuse report sent to RMO	../../..	☐ LATE ☐ NOT DONE ☐ N/A
44. CC report prepared	../../..	☐ LATE ☐ NOT DONE
At CC		
45. Lorazepam reviewed at CC (if appropriate)	../../..	☐ LATE ☐ NOT DONE ☐ N/A
46. CC attended by KW	../../..	☐ LATE ☐ NOT DONE

5

Patient Name... Patient ID... Admission date: ....../....../......

Admission ICP – Lomond Ward

July 04

Appendix 7.1 *(Continued)*

PSYCHOLOGY INTERVENTIONS – ADMISSION ICP

BY DAY 7	Date and Sign	VARIANCE – Please tick box as appropriate, write reason for variance, action taken and final outcome
47. Initial patient interview conducted	../../..	☐ LATE ☐ NOT DONE
By DAY 14		
48. Compilation of background report commenced	../../..	☐ LATE ☐ NOT DONE
By DAY 28		
49. Formal psychology testing started	../../..	☐ LATE ☐ NOT DONE ☐ N/A
By DAY 42		
50. Formal psychological testing completed	../../..	☐ LATE ☐ NOT DONE ☐ N/A
51. Commence clinical interviews	../../..	☐ LATE ☐ NOT DONE ☐ N/A
By Day 49		
52. Psychological opinion formulated and report compiled	../../..	☐ LATE ☐ NOT DONE
At CC		
53. CC attended by Psychologist	../../..	☐ LATE ☐ NOT DONE

PARS INTERVENTIONS ADMISSION ICP

BY DAY 7	Date and Sign	VARIANCE – Please tick box as appropriate, write reason for variance, action taken and final outcome
54. Consent for FITECH from patient	../../..	☐ LATE ☐ NOT DONE
55. Patient seen by GP if indic.	../../..	☐ LATE ☐ NOT DONE ☐ N/A
56. FITECH completed	../../..	☐ LATE ☐ NOT DONE ☐ N/A

6

Patient Name.. Patient ID.. Admission date: ....../....../......
Admission ICP – Lomond Ward
July 04

Appendix 7.1   *(Continued)*

SOCIAL WORK INTERVENTIONS ADMISSION ICP

BY DAY 7	Date and Sign	VARIANCE- Please tick box as appropriate, write reason for variance, action taken and final outcome
57. Initial patient interview conducted	../../..	☐ LATE ☐ NOT DONE
BY DAY 14		
58. Letter of introduction to family	../../..	☐ LATE ☐ NOT DONE
Prior to CC W8		
59. Relative or carer contacted	../../..	☐ LATE ☐ NOT DONE
60. Carer's assessment arranged	../../..	☐ LATE ☐ NOT DONE
61. Liaison with hosp/comm/prison/SW	../../..	☐ LATE ☐ NOT DONE
62. Client seen re preparation of report	../../..	☐ LATE ☐ NOT DONE
63. SW report prepared	../../..	☐ LATE ☐ NOT DONE
CC		
64. Review child visit/child contact	../../..	☐ LATE ☐ NOT DONE
65. CC attended by Social Worker	../../..	☐ LATE ☐ NOT DONE
AFTER CC		
66. Client seen post CC	../../..	☐ LATE ☐ NOT DONE

PHARMACY INTERVENTIONS ADMISSION ICP

BY DAY 7	Date and Sign	VARIANCE – Please tick box as appropriate, write reason for variance, action taken and final outcome
67. Complete medication profile	../../..	☐ LATE ☐ NOT DONE
68. Register in Form 9/10 reminder system	../../..	☐ LATE ☐ NOT DONE
Prior to CC		
69. Complete pharmaceutical care plan report	../../..	☐ LATE ☐ NOT DONE ☐ N/A
70. Complete medication history review (if indicated)	../../..	☐ LATE ☐ NOT DONE ☐ N/A
AT CC		
71. Attend CC	../../..	☐ LATE ☐ NOT DONE

7

Patient Name... Patient ID.. Admission date: ...../...../.....
Admission ICP – Lomond Ward
July 04

Appendix 7.1   (*Continued*)

SECURITY INTERVENTIONS ADMISSION ICP		
WITHIN 24 HRS OF ADMISSION	**Date and Sign**	**VARIANCE – Please tick box as appropriate, write reason for variance, action taken and final outcome**
72. Take photograph of patient	../../..	☐ LATE ☐ NOT DONE
BY DAY 2	**Date and Sign**	**VARIANCE – Please tick box as appropriate, write reason for variance, action taken and final outcome**
73. Security Admission Assessment	../../..	☐ LATE ☐ NOT DONE
Prior to CC		
74. Provide updated Security Assessment	../../..	☐ LATE ☐ NOT DONE
AT CC		
75. Security Manager attends CC	../../..	☐ LATE ☐ NOT DONE

8

Patient Name.. Patient ID.. Admission date: ....../....../......

Admission ICP – Lomond Ward

July 04

Appendix 7.1   (*Continued*)

THE STATE HOSPITAL
TREATMENT AND REHABILITATION
ICP

Patient details		Staff details	Print Name	Signature
Patient Name		Key Worker	Name: Designation:	
Patient ID No:	/	Occupational Therapist		
DOB:	...../...../.....	PARS staff		
Patient Signature		Pharmacist		
		Psychologist		
		Psychology Associate		
		RMO		
Discharge/Transfer date: ...../...../.....		SHO		
		Security Manager		
Discharge/Transfer location		Social Worker		
		Ward Manager		

Treatment & Rehabilitation ICP Index	Page
Front Page	T&R ICP 1
Variance Codecs	T&R ICP 2
Nursing	T&R ICP 3
Medical	T&R ICP 4
Psychology Social Work	T&R ICP 5
Security/Pharmacy	T&R ICP 6
Occupational Therapy	T&R ICP 7
Table	T&R ICP 8&9

Abbreviations

ICP - Integrated Care Pathway

KW - Keyworker

CR - Case Review

MDT - Multi-disciplinary Team

PTS - Psychological Therapies Service

PARS - Patient Activity & Recreation Services.

INSTRUCTIONS FOR COMPLETION OF ICP

1. **SIGN AND DATE** - *if intervention has been completed on time*
2. **IF THE INTERVENTION HAS NOT BEEN DONE – DO NOT SIGN OR DATE** *Put a line through the intervention then tick* **"NOT DONE"** *and enter the variance code*
3. **IF THE INTERVENTION IS LATE –** *Date and sign only when it is completed. Tick the* **"LATE"** *box on the variance sheet and enter the variance code*
4. **IF THE INTERVENTION IS NOT APPROPRIATE/NOT APPLICABLE –** *Tick the* **"N/A"** *box*
5. **IF IT TAKES SEVERAL ATTEMPTS TO COMPLETE THE INTERVENTION**
   (*E.g. getting bloods or contacting carers*) – *Only date and sign when the intervention has been completed ;tick the late box and enter the variance code*

If you have any queries regarding the ICP please contact Karen Moody or Carole Campbell on extension 315
It remains each profession's responsibility to ensure that practice is safe

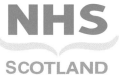

Appendix 7.2
The State Hospital treatment and rehabilitation ICP

VARIANCE CODES INDEX

VARIANCE CODES – NOT DONE		
Variance code to be entered on ICP	Meaning / Interpretation	EXAMPLES
Patient variances: *These relate to patient choice, illness, language etc.*		
P1	Patient declined	E.g. to invite relatives, to participate with a clinician, to having open door, to an outing etc.
P2	Patient unsettled presentation	E.g. due to poor mental health, the patient doesn't engage well with staff.
P3	Patient physically unwell	E.g. patient at local hospital.
P4	Patient communication problems	E.g. patient doesn't speak English, interpreter required etc.
Carer/Relative variances: *These relate to carer/relative choice, availability, contact etc*		
C1	Carer/relative declines involvement with patient	E.g. they don't want to receive information regarding the patient
C2	Carer relative unable to attend	E.g. due to travelling time, on holiday. However they would've liked to attend.
C3	No carer/relative identified	E.g. no carer/relative identified by patient
C4	Carer/relative not available	E.g. unable to get in contact with carer/relative.
C5	No regular contact with carer/relative	E.g. patient has no contact with relative/carer.
Staff variances : *These variances relate to the availability of staff*		
S1	Staff not available	E.g. due to: Annual leave, sick leave, study/training leave, days off etc.
S2	Staff other commitments	E.g. at another meeting, workload, KW in numbers therefore, not able to attend, shift change etc.
S3	Staff– risk– assessment	I.e. the result of a risk assessment means that a staff member can't work with a patient e.g. if staff member is pregnant etc.
Care & treatment variances		
T1	Not clinically indicated at present	E.g. the patient might not be ready for the intervention, or a clinician could be waiting for a clinical team decision before working with the patient.
T2	No outstanding need	E.g. all relevant work has been done with the patient; there will be no more input with the patient at the moment.
Hospital systems/information availability		
R1	Information not available	E.g. treatment plan not on ward etc.
R2	Patient not available	E.g. patient gone to placement or appointment.
R3	Case review/conference date changed	E.g. staff unable to attend or do report because the date has been changed at short notice etc.
R4	Patient moved ward	E.g. interventions were not completed prior to patient moving to another ward.
VARIANCE CODES – LATE		
Patient variances: *These relate to patient choice, illness, language etc.*		
LP1	Patient declines	E.g. patient declined at first but intervention was completed at a later date.
LP2	Patient unsettled presentation	E.g. had to wait until patient's mental state/health improved before intervention could be completed.
LP3	Patient physically unwell	E.g. patient at local hospital etc.
LP4	Patient communication problems	E.g. patient does not speak English, had to wait for an interpreter to complete intervention.
Carer/Relative variances: *These relate to carer / relative choice, availability, contact etc*		
LC1	No carer/relative identified	E.g. on admission to hospital NOK is not always known etc.
LC2	Carer/relative not available	E.g. tried to contact but not available at first etc.
Staff variances: *These variances relate to availability of staff*		
LS1	Staff not available	E.g. due to: Annual leave, sick leave, study/training leave, and days off.
LS2	Staff – other commitments	E.g. another meeting, workload.
Hospital systems/information availability		
LR1	Information not available	E.g. treatment plan not available on ward etc.
LR2	Patient not available	E.g. gone to placement or appointment.
LR3	Case review/conference date changed	E.g. staff unable to attend or do report because the date has been changed at short notice etc.

Other: If you feel that the variance doesn't fit into one of these categories, it can be written onto the ICP

T & R ICP JULY 03   Patient Name:...................................... Patient ID...

Appendix 7.2   (*Continued*)

NURSING				
INTERVENTIONS	**Case Review Date :-**			**INTERIM/ANNUAL REVIEW** (circle which review)
2 WEEKS PRIOR TO CASE REVIEW	**Date completed**	**Initials**	**Variance** (✔ box if appropriate)	**ENTER VARIANCE CODE – See Page 2** (if intervention is late or not done)
1. Request PARS report (if appropriate)	…./…./…		☐ NOT DONE ☐ N/A ☐ LATE	
2. KW liaise with ward staff re proposed recommendations for nursing report (interim & annual)	…./…./…		☐ NOT DONE ☐ N/A ☐ LATE	
3. Patient asked if they would like relative/carer invited to CR	…./…./…		☐ NOT DONE ☐ N/A ☐ LATE	
4. KW/Patient invite relative/carer to CR (if consent was given)	…./…./…		☐ NOT DONE ☐ N/A ☐ LATE	
5. Patient asked if they would like advocacy invited to CR	…./…./…		☐ NOT DONE ☐ N/A ☐ LATE	
PRIOR TO CASE REVIEW				
6. If CR date has changed and relatives/carers are attending – inform them of new date (if appropriate)	…./…./…		☐ NOT DONE ☐ N/A ☐ LATE	
7. Prepare Interim Case Review report (if appropriate)	…./…./…		☐ NOT DONE ☐ N/A ☐ LATE	
8. Prepare Annual Case Review report (if appropriate)	…./…./…		☐ NOT DONE ☐ N/A ☐ LATE	
9. KW/Associate worker discuss nursing report with patient	…./…./…		☐ NOT DONE ☐ N/A ☐ LATE	
10. Does patient smoke? (circle)	Yes / No			
11. Patient Prompted Re: giving up smoking (if appropriate)	…./…./…		☐ NOT DONE ☐ N/A ☐ LATE	
AT CASE REVIEW	These should be signed off (where applicable) by the nurse attending CR			
12. KW/Associate worker attends CR	…./…./…		☐ NOT DONE	
13. Carer/relative attends CR	…./…./…		☐ NOT DONE ☐ N/A	
14. • Review PARS objectives • Referral to PARS (if appropriate) • Review at risk register • Review drug risk register • Update open door register (if appropriate) • Review telephone & mail censorship lists	…./…./…		☐ NOT DONE ☐ N/A ☐ LATE	
SAME DAY AS CASE REVIEW				
15. Update nursing notes on Clinical Team outcome	…./…./…		☐ NOT DONE ☐ N/A ☐ LATE	
16. Updated registers e.g. at risk, drug risk, open door (as appropriate) and circulated	…./…./…		☐ NOT DONE ☐ N/A ☐ LATE	
17. Discuss Case Review with patient	…./…./…		☐ NOT DONE ☐ N/A ☐ LATE	
AFTER CASE REVIEW	**(within 3 weeks)**			
18. List details of referrals in PARS table (if appropriate)	…./…./…		☐ NOT DONE ☐ N/A ☐ LATE	
19. Discuss new treatment plan with patient (if appropriate)	…./…./…		☐ NOT DONE ☐ N/A ☐ LATE	

T & R ICP JULY 03   Patient Name:..................................... Patient ID……………………………………..

Appendix 7.2   (Continued)

MEDICAL				
INTERVENTIONS	Case Review Date :-			INTERIM/ANNUAL REVIEW (circle which review)
PRIOR TO ALL CASE REVIEWS	Date completed	Initials	Variance (✔ box if appropriate)	ENTER VARIANCE CODE – See Page 2 (if intervention is late or not done)
20. Mental State Review	..../..../...		☐ NOT DONE ☐ LATE	
21. Review Physical Health	..../..../...		☐ NOT DONE ☐ LATE	
22. Check results and investigations (to include: Lithium, high dose and anti-convulsant monitoring results)	..../..../...		☐ NOT DONE ☐ N/A ☐ LATE	
PRIOR TO ANNUAL CASE REVIEWS				
23. Summary report for Annual Review (if appropriate)	..../..../...		☐ NOT DONE ☐ N/A ☐ LATE	
AT CASE REVIEW				
24. Consultant attends case review	..../..../...		☐ NOT DONE	
25. Standard Case Review interventions				
• Review medication/ pharmacology • Review planned activities • Review at risk register • Review ground access • Review outings • Review of Previous Case Review objectives • Check consent to treatment (Form 9/10) • Review need for patient information and consider suitable format (e.g. written, visual, audio) • Re: change in medication • Info re: illness	..../..../...		☐ NOT DONE ☐ N/A ☐ LATE	
26. Review open door	..../..../...		☐ NOT DONE ☐ N/A ☐ LATE	
AFTER CASE REVIEW	(WITHIN 2 WEEKS)			
27. Check further results and investigations (if appropriate)	..../..../...		☐ NOT DONE ☐ N/A ☐ LATE	

Appendix 7.2   (Continued)

PSYCHOLOGY

INTERVENTIONS	Case Review Date :-			INTERIM/ANNUAL REVIEW *(circle which review)*
PRIOR TO CASE REVIEW	Date completed	Initials	Variance (✔ box if appropriate)	**ENTER VARIANCE CODE – See Page 2** *(if intervention is late or not done)*
28. Case review update – review notes and contact relevant members of psychological therapies staff	..../..../...		☐ NOT DONE ☐ LATE	
29. Meet patient to discuss progress	..../..../...		☐ NOT DONE ☐ LATE	
30. Interim treatment plan report *(If appropriate)*	..../..../...		☐ NOT DONE ☐ N/A ☐ LATE	
31. Write Annual Report *(if appropriate)*	..../..../...		☐ NOT DONE ☐ N/A ☐ LATE	
AT CASE REVIEW				
32. Psychology representative attends review *(psychologist or psychology associate)*	..../..../...		☐ NOT DONE	

SOCIAL WORK

INTERVENTIONS	Case Review Date :-			INTERIM/ANNUAL REVIEW *(circle which review)*
PRIOR TO CASE REVIEW	Date completed	Initials	Variance (✔ box if appropriate)	**ENTER VARIANCE CODE – See Page 2** *(if intervention is late or not done)*
33. SW to see client re: – preparation of report	..../..../...		☐ NOT DONE ☐ N/A ☐ LATE	
34. SW Interim Report prepared *(as required)*	..../..../...		☐ NOT DONE ☐ N/A ☐ LATE	
35. SW Annual Report *(as required)*	..../..../...		☐ NOT DONE ☐ N/A ☐ LATE	
36. Liaise with Hosp/Comm/ Prison/SW *(if appropriate)*	..../..../...		☐ NOT DONE ☐ N/A ☐ LATE	
AT CASE REVIEW				
37. Social Worker to attend Case Review	..../..../...		☐ NOT DONE	
38. Review child visit/child contact *(if appropriate)*	..../..../...		☐ NOT DONE ☐ N/A ☐ LATE	
AFTER CASE REVIEW	**(WITHIN 2 WEEKS)**			
39. See client post Case Review *(if appropriate)*	..../..../...		☐ NOT DONE ☐ N/A ☐ LATE	

Appendix 7.2   *(Continued)*

SECURITY				
INTERVENTIONS	**Case Review Date :-**		**INTERIM/ANNUAL REVIEW** *(circle which review)*	
PRIOR TO CASE REVIEW	**Date completed**	**Initials**	**Variance** (✔ box if appropriate)	**ENTER VARIANCE CODE – See Page 2** *(if intervention is late or not done)*
40. Security assessment	…./…./…		☐ NOT DONE ☐ LATE	
41. Ensure patient photo is up to date	…./…./…		☐ NOT DONE ☐ LATE	
AT CASE REVIEW				
42. Attend Case Review	…./…./…		☐ NOT DONE	

Pharmacy section for Alexandra, Forth & Clyde wards

PHARMACY				
INTERVENTIONS	**Case Review Date :-**		**INTERIM/ANNUAL REVIEW** *(circle which review)*	
PRIOR TO CASE REVIEW	**Date completed**	**Initials**	**Variance** (✔ box if appropriate)	**ENTER VARIANCE CODE – See Page 2** *(if intervention is late or not done)*
43. Check prescription complies with consent to treatment plan *(Form 9/10)*	…./…./…		☐ NOT DONE ☐ N/A ☐ LATE	
44. Report prepared *(if appropriate)*	…./…./…		☐ NOT DONE ☐ N/A ☐ LATE	
AT CASE REVIEW				
45. Attend Case Review	…./…./…		☐ NOT DONE	

T & R ICP JULY 03   Patient Name:……………………………… Patient ID……………………………

Appendix 7.2 *(Continued)*

OCCUPATIONAL THERAPY				
INTERVENTIONS		**Case Review Date :-**		**INTERIM/ANNUAL REVIEW** (circle which review)
PRIOR TO CASE REVIEW		**Date completed**	**Initials**	**Variance** (✔box if appropriate)	**ENTER VARIANCE CODE – See Page 2** (if intervention is late or not done)
46. Initial assessment/ screening is commenced using the Model of Human Occupation Screening Tool		…./…./…		☐ NOT DONE ☐ N/A ☐ LATE	
47. Patient's need for life skills is assessed/ reviewed	Formal assessment/ review completed (if appropriate)	…./…./…		☐ NOT DONE ☐ N/A ☐ LATE	
	Informal assessment/ review completed (if appropriate)	…./…./…		☐ NOT DONE ☐ N/A ☐ LATE	
48. Patient's need for social skills is assessed/ reviewed	Formal assessment/ review completed (if appropriate)	…./…./…		☐ NOT DONE ☐ N/A ☐ LATE	
	Informal assessment/ review completed (if appropriate)	…./…./…		☐ NOT DONE ☐ N/A ☐ LATE	
49. Liaise with KW re: recommendation for pattern of occupation (if appropriate)		…./…./…		☐ NOT DONE ☐ N/A ☐ LATE	
50. Results of OT assessments and interventions are documented in the Case Review report (if appropriate)		…./…./…		☐ NOT DONE ☐ N/A ☐ LATE	
51. Results of all OT assessments and interventions are fed back to patient.		…./…./…		☐ NOT DONE ☐ N/A ☐ LATE	
52. Patient is shown & given the opportunity to contribute to the Case Review report prior to the Case Review (if appropriate)		…./…./…		☐ NOT DONE ☐ N/A ☐ LATE	
AT CASE REVIEW					
53. Attend Case Review		…./…./…		☐ NOT DONE	

T & RICP JULY 03   Patient Name:………………………………… Patient ID…………………………………………..

Appendix 7.2   (Continued)

OFF WARD ACTIVITIES/ CLINICAL PROGRAMMES TABLE

Please update groups as appropriate

WARD BASED GROUPS – to be completed prior to each case review				
List of groups patient attends	Is patient attending?	Action	Is patient attending?	Action

PATIENT ACTIVITY AND RECREATIONAL SERVICES						
Department	Date referred	Session Referred AM/PM	Date Ward Contacted with Outcome	Rationale for Outcome E.g. non-participation, lack of attendance etc.	Start Date & Agreed Sessions	
					Date	Sessions
Laundry						
Gardens / Pet Therapy						
Woodwork						
Social Centre						
Craft & Design						
Recreation						
Education						
Community Centre						
Book Club						

T & R ICP JULY 03   Patient Name:... Patient ID...

Appendix 7.2   (Continued)

PSYCHOLOGICAL THERAPIES SERVICE						
Service		Date Referred	Assessed for Suitability	Approximate Start Date	Progress (stages)	Finish Date / Outcome
Anger Management Programme						
SVRR (Sexual Violence Risk Reduction) Service						
DBT (Dialectical Behavioural Therapy) for women						
DBT for men						
Offending behaviour programmes	PSST (programme, problem solving skills training)					
	MR (moral reasoning)					
	R&R (reasoning and rehabilitation)					
Psychosocial interventions	CBT (Individual)					
	Coping with mental illness					
Alcohol & Drugs Service	Relapse prevention					
	Education					
Wilful fire raising						

T & R ICP JULY 03   Patient Name:...................................... Patient ID...

Appendix 7.2   (*Continued*)

REFERENCES

Clinical Standards Board for Scotland 2001 Clinical standards for schizophrenia. Clinical Standards Board for Scotland, Edinburgh

Duncan AS, Moody KJ 2003 Integrated care pathways in mental health settings: an occupational therapy perspective. British Journal of Occupational Therapy 66:473-478

Dykes PC, Slye DA 1997 Data collection, outcomes, measurement, and variance analysis. In: Dykes PC, Wheeler K Planning, implementing and evaluating critical pathways, ch 4. Springer Publishing, New York

McQueen J, Milloy S 2001 Why clinical guidelines or care pathways in mental health? Journal of Integrated Care Pathways 5:44-53

Mental Welfare Commission for Scotland 2000 Report into the inquiry of the care and treatment of Noel Ruddle 2000. Mental Welfare Commission for Scotland

Middleton S, Roberts A 2000 Integrated care pathways: a practical approach to implementation. Butterworth Heinemann, London

National Health Service Health Scotland 1998 A smoking cessation policy for Scotland. National Health Service Health Scotland, Edinburgh

National Health Service Quality Improvement Scotland 2004 National overview – June 2004 – schizophrenia. National Health Service Quality Improvement Scotland, Edinburgh

Parkinson S, Forsyth K 2001 A user's manual for the Model of Human Occupation Screening Tool (MOHOST): version 1.0 (unpublished material). UKCORE, London South Bank University, London

Scottish Executive Health Department 2001 Services, care, support and accommodation for mentally disordered offenders in Scotland: care pathway document. Scottish Executive Health Department, Edinburgh

A care pathway for patients presenting at Accident and Emergency who have self-harmed

Carol Jackson

INTRODUCTION	**IMPLEMENTATION**
BACKGROUND	**OUTCOMES AND CONCLUSIONS**
PATHWAY DEVELOPMENT	**REFERENCES**

INTRODUCTION

Deliberate self-harm (DSH) can be defined as intentional self-poisoning or self-injury, irrespective of the apparent purpose of the act (Hawton & Catalan 1987). It remains one of the top five reasons for medical admission to hospital within the United Kingdom (UK), with approximately 150,000 presentations each year (Hawton & Fagg 1992). Patients who deliberately harm themselves have a risk of suicide 100 times greater than that of the general population (Greer & Bagley 1971, Hawton & Fagg 1988). DSH is the strongest associated risk factor for patients who commit suicide. The overall suicide rate in the general population in the UK is 12 people per 100 000, with approximately 6000 deaths occurring in 2002 (Samaritans 2004). Perhaps more alarmingly, between 20 and 25% of patients who die by suicide have presented to a general hospital following acts of deliberate self-harm in the year before their death (Foster et al 1997), and approximately 25% had been in contact with mental health services (Department of Health 2001). During 2003, in Northern Ireland more people died as a result of suicide or self-inflicted injury (n = 133) than in road traffic accidents (n = 123) (Northern Ireland Research and Statistics Agency 2003). These deaths also have an astounding impact on the concept of potential years of life lost. Although the numbers of deaths from suicide may be much smaller than from coronary heart disease, they account for approximately the same proportion of potential years of life lost (Department of Health and Social Services and Public Safety 2000). These figures provide momentum for the promotion of effective interventions for patients following any episode of DSH.

Suicide prevention is now incorporated into health-related policies and strategies on a global, national and regional scale. The World Health Organisation (1992) includes a reduction in suicidal behaviour as one of the 'Health for All' targets. This integral theme is evidenced in Standard 7 of the Mental Health National Service Framework (Department of Health 1999), Priorities and Planning Framework 2002/2003 (Department of Health 2002), Priorities for Action 2003/2004 (Department of Health and Social Services and Public Safety 2003a), Safety First (Department of Health 2001) and Promoting Mental Health (Department of Health and Social Services and Public Safety 2003b). A target for the reduction of suicide by 20% by 2010 was cited in 'Our Healthier Nation' (Department of Health 1998), and replaced an earlier target of a 15% reduction which was set in 1992 (Department of Health 1992). This is the policy context which has been a significant driver for the development of the integrated care pathway (ICP) discussed in this chapter.

In order to address these targets, the need for an integrated and collaborative approach is forefront in governmental policy (Department of Health and Social Services 1997a, Department of Health and Social Services and Public Safety 2001). Where the ICP is in use the trust's strategic mental health services plan advocates a comprehensive, coordinated approach in the promotion of mental health (Down Lisburn Trust 1999). In addition to 'partnership' working, the acquisition of education and training, the use of 'effective' interventions and the availability of 'research and information' to enhance practice and policy are seen as pivotal (Department of Health and Social Services 1997b).

BACKGROUND

Previous consensus on the care and interventions for people who self-harm is available from the Department of Health and Social Security (1984) and the Royal College of Psychiatrists (1994). More recently, the National Institute of Clinical Excellence (NICE) (2004) published 'The short-term physical and psychological management and secondary prevention of self-harm in primary and secondary care', which provides a comprehensive clinical guideline. Each of the documents recommends that anyone presenting at Accident and Emergency (A & E) having deliberately self-harmed should undergo a psychosocial assessment. NICE (2004) promotes the completion of:

1. a needs assessment, which includes social situation, personal relationships, recent life events, psychiatric history, mental state examination and motivation for the act and
2. a risk assessment, which includes characteristics of the act of self-harm such as intent, evidence of planning, characteristics of the person such as forensic history, hopelessness and circumstances of the person, for example physical illness, recent bereavement and social isolation.

Additional recommendations from NICE (2004) include training for staff who come in contact with people who self-harm, the completion of an initial assessment by healthcare staff who have first contact with patients, appropriate facilities in emergency departments for the care of people who have self-harmed and offering treatment for physical injuries even if the person declines a psychosocial assessment or psychiatric treatment. Despite the availability of guidelines, general and psychiatric treatment and service provision remain variable and frequently inadequate (Bennewith et al 2004, Hughes et al 1998).

Down Lisburn Trust lies within the Eastern Board in Northern Ireland and serves an urban and rural population of approximately 170,000, which covers a wide geographical area. The mental health services provide both inpatient and community facilities for patients aged 18 years and over. Eight consultant psychiatrists lead multidisciplinary teams who provide care and support 24 hours per day, 7 days a week. Inpatient units include acute psychiatry, addiction services, dementia assessment, intensive care and continuing care. The community mental health teams provide a 9 a.m. to 5 p.m. service, and more recently have developed an 'out of hours' emergency psychiatric service from 5 p.m. to 9 a.m. The reconfiguration of the '24 hour' services was promoted as a result of the following key issues. Firstly, a consultation report on a strategic framework for adult mental health services in Northern Ireland (Department of Health and Social Services and Public Safety 2004). This outlined the need for mental health services not to be confined to normal working hours. This document also highlighted the new contract for general practitioners (GPs) (National Health Service Confederation and British Medical Association 2003) which allows practices to remove themselves from the provision of 24 hour care, whilst prompting boards and trusts to develop integrated 'out of hours' mental health care. Secondly, the Royal College of Psychiatrists had instructed that specialist registrars should not be 'first on call' to assess patients with mental health problems in casualty. Thirdly, the European Working Time Directive specified the number of hours junior doctors were permitted to work, which in turn has a direct impact on ensuring a provision of care and treatment for patients by other mental health professionals (Department of Health and Social Services and Public Safety 2003c). The 24 hour service by mental health professionals is also of significant importance to staff working within the casualty departments and medical wards.

In the year 2000 there were 57 deaths from suicide and self-inflicted injury, 19 of which were within the Down Lisburn Trust population (Northern Ireland Statistics and Research Agency 2003). In the year 2002-3 the acute psychiatric units admitted a total of 809 patients, approximately 50% of whom had a history of self-harm. These data do not include patients who presented (but were not admitted) having self-harmed. Subsequently, the information technology department has been working on systems to improve data recording. Hence, in 2003 it was found that in total 667 patients attended casualty in 2003 having self-harmed (and this also included those that were not admitted). The difficulties in recording are not unique to this trust. Regional data are generally limited to the number of patients admitted to hospital following self-harm, and do not include those who present at casualty but are not admitted.

PATHWAY DEVELOPMENT

The development of an ICP to assess and manage people at risk and individuals who engage in deliberate self-harm was identified as a service priority in both mental health and acute medicine. The Royal College of Psychiatrists (2004) suggests care pathways may decrease the potential for misunderstanding between services. It also acknowledges, however, that ICPs must be known, used and understood by staff to guarantee their efficacy. The authoring team for this ICP comprised medical and nursing staff from psychiatry, A & E, medical wards, training and development. ICP development was facilitated by the ICP coordinator from mental health services (the author of this chapter). The consultants in psychiatry and A & E accepted joint responsibility as the 'clinical leads' for the pathway development team. This ICP would therefore cross the boundaries of the acute hospital and mental health services.

The scope of the ICP would address the needs of those aged 18 years and over, who presented at casualty having self-harmed. It was anticipated that the ICP would incorporate interventions and psychosocial assessments which would be completed by staff in A & E, medical wards and liaison psychiatry. The overall objectives were to:

- develop a tool which would ensure the delivery of evidence-based and best practice guidelines
- assist staff in their assessment and treatment of patients
- enhance communication between disciplines
- improve record keeping and documentation.

Thus the ICP would cover the entire patient journey, and provide guidance for discharge and follow-up.

Prior to pathway development in 2001 an audit was carried out which looked at various factors in relation to self-harm (Down Lisburn Trust 2001). The audit identified the number of patients who presented at A & E, the way in which patients had self-harmed and the completion of documentation. During a 3 monthly period, 26 patients presented at casualty having self-harmed, 25 of whom had taken an overdose. Of the original 26 patients who presented to A & E with DSH, one (4%) patient was not admitted and one (4%) refused to stay upon reaching the medical ward. Overall, 24 patients were admitted to the medical wards. Of these 24, two (8%) patients were not referred to Psychiatric Liaison and were discharged without psychiatric assessment. Four (17%) patients were referred but not seen, leaving hospital contrary to medical advice. Therefore, in total six (25%) patients received no risk assessment. The A & E record, medical inpatient charts and psychiatric liaison forms were audited by an audit facilitator.

It was found that risk assessments were generally very poorly recorded. For example, in A & E only 19% of patients had suicidal ideas documented, 23% had a previous psychiatric history recorded and only 15% were asked if they had attempted overdose previously. It would appear that no patients had documentary evidence recorded regarding any future propensity for self-harm attempts.

Assessment in medical wards was better, with 75% of patients having a record of suicidal ideas, 58% had a previous psychiatric history recorded, 54% were asked about previous overdoses and 21% were asked about future intent to self-harm. Psychiatric assessments highlighted areas for improvement as only 11% had a recording in relation to the seriousness of the attempt and 67% were assessed as having future self-harm intent.

Pathway development continued with mapping the process of the patient journey. This enabled each professional group the opportunity to re-examine their current practice and identify areas for improvement. Acute hospital and psychiatry staff reviewed their accident and emergency triage assessment against the NICE (2004) recommendations of using the Australian Mental Health Triage Scale (Pollard 1998). The ICP coordinator contacted the author of this scale, and obtained the most recent copy of the assessment. Following intense discussion and review of triage scales, local consensus arrived at a colour-coded assessment scale, which also has a section for documenting the response to each question. The triage nurse also records if a patient is in obvious severe distress and if they are likely to wait until seen by a casualty doctor, as recommended by guidelines (Royal College Psychiatrists 1994).

NICE (2004) outlines the physical management of patients who have self-harmed in both casualty and medical wards. The team utilised these guidelines to develop draft versions of the ICP. Interventions within the pathway include (where appropriate) the collection of blood and urine samples for analysis and guidance on treatment of patients who have taken an overdose. Appendices at the back of the ICP act as an aide memoire and provide information on paracetamol concentration levels, signs and symptoms of common poisons, and the detention process under the 1986 Mental Health Order (Northern Ireland) (Department of Health and Social Services 1986). The psychological treatment and assessment of patients are promoted by the use of a psychosocial assessment tool, which was devised by the team's consultant psychiatrist. This was based upon reference to guidelines from NICE (2004) and the Royal College of Psychiatrists (1994). This has resulted in an 'at a glance' tool whereby the assessment can be completed in either A & E or the medical ward. Therefore, if a patient is unable or unwilling to assist with the assessment in casualty, medical ward staff can identify this instantly and subsequently complete the assessment. Non-psychiatry staff were particularly interested in having a risk assessment scale with a scoring system. However, following debate, the team realised that a 'scoring' system did not always provide reliable and valid information. Considering this, some aspects of the assessment tool have been allocated a special '**' notation. Examples of indicators which have a notation are: suicide note left, attempt to end life at time of act, very serious previous self-harm, and hopelessness regarding the future. The notation '**' acts as an indicator that these are areas which should be given particular attention when assessing the patient.

The team utilised the available evidence to create sections of the pathway relevant to their department and discipline. The ICP coordinator combined the separate segments into a complete document. The team reviewed both the layout and content of the pathway until a final pilot version was agreed. It was established that a colour-coded document would help staff to recognise and access their section readily. The ICP coordinator formatted and supplied the pathway to the different departments.

IMPLEMENTATION

The pathway is commenced when a patient arrives at this department having committed DSH. When the patient is admitted to a medical ward, the document accompanies the patient on their journey. Liaison Psychiatry complete their section in either A & E or the medical ward. Upon discharge, the entire document is filed in the hospital records. Variance information is currently collected at the back of the ICP. Staff record the variance, the action taken and the outcome. The ICP coordinator collects the variances, compiles the results into specific groups, such as patient, staff, internal or external systems, and feeds back the results to the team for comment and action.

It was evident from the pre-pathway audit previously outlined and as a consequence of developing the ICP that paying attention to the training of staff in using the ICP and developing their practice would be crucial to success. Whilst the audit identified deficits in the recording of assessments, it also highlighted the necessity to provide education and training for acute hospital staff in mental health assessment and detention of patients if required. The ICP authoring team agreed this should be undertaken by the consultant psychiatrist, Liaison Psychiatry nurse and the Acute Services Training and Development nurse. Staff training about completion of the pathway document was undertaken by authoring team members. Medical staff in each of the areas made use of induction days and nursing staff devoted time as and when possible. The ICP coordinator was allocated time for training with the mental health 'emergency out of hours' staff. The number of staff that required information and training proved quite daunting, and the reasons for this are twofold: firstly, the crossing of services and boundaries, but also the fact that during development and implementation, the services involved with the ICP continued to change and evolve.

It was agreed initially that the pathway would be piloted for 20 patients. However, this was then extended to make the pilot longer to enable a more comprehensive review of the ICP. The benefits reported from the pilot by staff referred to the positive use of an evidence-based document, which is entirely multidisciplinary. It was agreed that when using the ICP, professionals have access to information which was previously not available, such as psychosocial assessment tools, mental state assessment tools, detention algorithms, mental health triage scales, and specific guidelines for discharging patients. The standardisation of documentation has encouraged equality of service for patients, and promotes a consistent approach from staff. The version of the pathway currently in use is shown in Appendix 8.1.

As with any ICP, the variance tracking enables any deviation from the pathway to be recorded. This promotes both autonomy for the clinician and individualises patient care. Attention to variance tracking will focus on key elements such as the completion of initial psychosocial assessments, early discharge, follow-up and liaison psychiatry documentation. These areas assist in ensuring the delivery of guidelines into practice, whilst enabling staff to obtain a more holistic overview of the patient, their needs and requirements. By concentrating on assessment, outcome and follow-up, the integrated care approach should assist the team in the delivery of effective and efficient interventions. Hence, the pathway encourages identification and management of risk throughout the patient's journey from presentation, admission and through to discharge.

This ICP is an initiative to ensure a more coordinated approach to care and improve the quality of care delivered to patients. These themes are outlined in the trust's Clinical and Social Care Governance Strategy (Down Lisburn Trust 2004a) and the Strategy for Mental Health 2004-2007 (Down Lisburn Trust 2004b). They suggest the 'building blocks' of effective practice include multi-professional audit, research and development, evidence-based practice, continuous professional development, risk management, user involvement and staff involvement. In addition, the mental health strategy advocates the implementation of ICPs in order to provide high-quality and ever improving services. The deliberate self-harm pathway is an instrument which will drive forward the expectations of patients, staff and the organisation, in order to ensure the patient's journey is timely and progressive with positive outcomes.

OUTCOMES AND CONCLUSIONS

Although this care pathway is in its infancy at the time of writing, it is clear that its introduction has promoted communication between staff, departments and services. Each area is now much more aware of the challenges and similarities professionals in acute and mental health fields have to face. Initial review of completed pathways indicates more comprehensive use and recording of triage scales and the psychosocial assessment tools. Our experience has been that staff training is highlighted as an area which requires constant input. Enthusiastic staff in all departments promote continuous pathway training for others at every opportunity. Full implementation of the ICP will follow a robust review of the extended pilot.

Integrated working across organisational boundaries has brought a variety of challenges and benefits. Even within one organisation, different 'sectors' have differences in processes, documentation and information technology. However, the staff in these organisations have taken on this project with commitment and enthusiasm. Using this ICP as a vehicle, they are persistent in their desire to deliver evidence-based care to every patient who has self-harmed with whom they come into contact.

An integrated care pathway for patients
presenting at A&E who have self-harmed

Surname: (Block Capitals)	Forenames:	Preferred Name:
Address: (including Postcode)		D.O.B: Age:
Telephone Number:	Admission Date and Time:	G.P. : Address & Telephone Number

Does patient have other professionals involved? if so please complete details below.

Tick appropriate box (☐√) to indicate professional involved and enter name

Community Psychiatric Nurse☐

Social Worker☐

Community Alcohol Team☐

Consultant Psychiatrist ☐

Other☐ . Please Specify ☐

Contact Numbers:

Liaison Psychiatry = 9am-5pm x3242 (under 65's) x3258 (over 65's)

Out of hours – via switchboard

Social Services – via switchboard

COLOUR CODING OF PAGES: White = All staff   Green = Nursing   Yellow = Medical

Pink = Psychiatry   Blue = Variance recording & Appendices

SELF HARM INTEGRATED CARE PATHWAY (ICP) (patients aged 18 +)

- This ICP has been developed by a multidisciplinary team from Mental Health and Acute Services.

- Patients MUST be removed from the pathway if complications requiring a specialist unit, e.g. intensive care unit, high dependency unit.

Signing the Care Pathway:

- You should use your signature to confirm that an intervention has been carried out, or an outcome achieved.

Variance:

- Whilst the ICP is based on 'Best practice' guidelines each patient is an individual and 'variances' may occur to that plan of care. In the event of a variance occurring, enter a 'V' at the signature section and then complete the variance section – page 35. Variances should be documented in numerical order, e.g. V1, V2, V3 etc.

Appendix 8.1
ICP in use

TRIAGE NURSING ASSESSMENT – Accident & Emergency

- **Is there obvious distress?**   Yes ☐ No ☐
- **Is he/she likely to wait until seen by Accident & Emergency Doctor?** Yes ☐ No ☐

Information about circumstances volunteered by patient

Information from/to relatives/others

Observations on admission:

GCS: _____Total. Temp _____ Pulse _____   BP ___/___ Respirations_____/min

Oxygen saturation: _____ %   BM:_____

Name: _____ Signature:_____

Date: _____ Time seen: _____

	RED	ORANGE	YELLOW	GREEN	BLUE
TRIAGE (Tick)					

Appendix 8.1   (*Continued*)

ATTACH TOXBASE PRINT OUT TO PATHWAY

Tick when done ☐

Mental Health/Deliberate Self-Harm Triage

		Yes	No
Red ▶ ▶ ▶	Airways compromised		
	Inadequate breathing		
	Shock		
	Currently fitting		
	Exsanguinating haemorrhage		
	▼ N		
Orange ▶ ▶ ▶	Altered level of consciousness		
	Significant incident history		
	Mechanism of injury		
	High lethality		
	Altered conscious level		
	Acutely short of breath		
	Uncontrollable major haemorrhage		
	Severe pain		
	High risk of further self-harm		
	▼ N		
Yellow ▶ ▶ ▶	Moderate lethality		
	Moderate pain		
	Moderate risk of further self-harm		
	Marked distress		
	Significant psychiatric history		
	Lacks insight into condition		
	Disruptive		
	Unwilling to stay for treatment		
	Inappropriate history		
	Uncontrollable minor haemorrhage		
	▼ N Green		

Appendix 8.1 *(Continued)*

ACCIDENT & EMERGENCY ASSESSMENT – Medical Staff

TOXIN:*

Type_____Time Ingested_____

Amount_____

Type_____Time Ingested_____

Amount_____

Type_____Time Ingested_____

Amount_____

ALCOHOL:

Amount_____Time Ingested_____

ILLICIT SUBSTANCES:

Amount_____Time Ingested_____

CIRCUMSTANCES SURROUNDING OVERDOSE:

_____

_____

_____

_____

*If the toxin is unknown;
see Appendix A for advice on diagnosis*

PHYSICAL EXAMINATION

Airway :   patent /compromised   **Breathing**_____

Circulation_____

Glasgow Coma Scale: E   V   M   Total_____

Physical Injuries_____

_____

_____

Other_____

_____

Appendix 8.1   (*Continued*)

ACCIDENT & EMERGENCY ASSESSMENT – Medical Staff

INVESTIGATIONS – as appropriate

Investigation	Done √ = yes x = no	Time 24 hour clock	Results	Signature
ABG		:		
ECG		:		
Glucose		:		
U/E (Istat)		:		
U/E		:		
LFT		:		
INR/PT		:		
FBP				
Paracetamol	4hrly	:		
Salicylates		:		
Urine tox		:		
		:		
		:		
		:		

TREATMENT GIVEN

Activated charcoal	No/Yes	Time	Notes
Repeat dose charcoal	No/Yes	Time started	Notes
Specific antidote	No/Yes	Time	Specify
Other e.g. sutures	No/Yes	Time	Specify

Appendix 8.1   (*Continued*)

PARACETAMOL TREATMENT

Tick the relevant box if any of the following factors are present. These put the patient at increased risk of hepatotoxicity and the high risk line should be used to decide the need for antidotal treatment. REFER TO APPENDIX B – GRAPH

- Chronic (not acute) excessive alcohol consumption   ☐

- Use of enzyme inducing drugs*   ☐

- Starvation/anorexia   ☐

*NB. Enzyme inducing drugs include carbamazepine, phenytoin, phenobarbitone, primidone, rifampicin and St John's wort

ACCIDENT AND EMERGENCY – MEDICAL STAFF

Key findings of Mental State Assessment: (page 11)				
Looks Depressed ☐	Hopeless ☐	Distressed ☐	Suicide Ideation ☐	Suicide Plan ☐

ONGOING CARE :

Admit: Yes/No Date Time	Hospital/Ward		
Discharge: Yes/No – if yes complete below	Yes/No	Date	Time
REFERRAL			
Community Psychiatric Nurse/Social Worker/Health Visitor			
Out of hours team			
Liaison Psychiatry			
G.P./Community Care			
Contrary to Medical Advice (CTMA)			
If patient leaves contrary to medical advice, staff MUST inform G.P. and Next of Kin within 24 hours.			
• G.P. informed			
• Next of Kin informed			
• Police informed (only if detained or major concerns)			

Appendix 8.1   (Continued)

Psychosocial Assessment of Risk Factors and Needs Assessment

Prior to discharge from hospital Sections A & B must be completed at some time during hospital attendance.
Please answer YES/NO or UTA (Unable to assess) or add comments.

Sections A & B need only be repeated by next department, if previously unable to assess or there is new information.

A Mental State Assessment (Section C) _MUST ALWAYS_ be completed just prior to a patient being discharged home by a department.

	Accident & Emergency (Dr.)	Medical/Surgical Ward (Dr.)	Liaison Psychiatry
Section A Deliberate Self Harm Act			
Give reason if Unable to Assess e.g. intoxicated, uncooperative, not medically fit			
What were the precipitating events?			
What were the motives of the act?			
What were the circumstances of the act?			
Have there been any signs/symptoms of depression?			
Evidence of planning **			
Precautions taken to prevent rescue **			
Suicide note left **			
Intent to end life at time of act **			
Violent method used e.g. hanging, shooting			
Medically serious act			
Any other comment			

Appendix 8.1   (_Continued_)

Section B Other Risk Factors and Needs Assessment	A & E	Medical	Liais Psych
Give reason if Unable to Assess e.g. intoxicated, uncooperative, not medically fit			
Previous deliberate self harm			
Very serious previous self harm **			
Past psychiatric illness			
Current psychiatric illness			
Currently attends psychiatric services (who are current professional contacts?)			
Alcohol misuse			
Drug misuse/Smoking			
Past/Present physical illness present e.g. chronic pain, terminal illness			
Recent life events e.g. bereavement			
Relationship difficulties and status			
Does the patient live alone?			
Does the patient live with dependent children?			
Work or unemployment difficulties			
Financial difficulties			
Other specific difficulties			
Any other comment **Insert:** Date, Time, Signature, Designation			

Appendix 8.1   (*Continued*)

Section C Current Mental State Assessment	A & E	Medical	Liais Psych
Appears distressed, agitated, restless			
Subjectively states feels depressed			
Objectively appears depressed			
Does patient's mood change during the day?			
Do they have impaired sleep pattern?			
Do they have feelings of guilt, unworthiness or self blame?			
Hopeless regarding the future **			
Regrets committing self-harm			
Regrets surviving self-harm **			
Still wants to die **			
Current suicidal ideas **			
Current suicidal plans **			
Psychotic features present e.g. delusions or hallucinations **			
Orientated to time, place & person			
Insight into problems			
Summary **Insert:** Date, Time, Signature, Designation			

Appendix 8.1   (*Continued*)

MEDICAL WARD ASSESSMENT: to be completed by JHO/SHO

THE FOLLOWING SECTION SHOULD BE COMPLETED WHEN THE PATIENT IS NOT DROWSY

****** PLEASE COMPLETE/REFER TO PSYCHOSOCIAL ASSESSMENT – PAGES 9, 10, 11*****

Presenting complaint
Social history
Systematic questioning

Past Medical History:
Family history

Drug history
Allergies
Physical examination

Appendix 8.1   (*Continued*)

MEDICAL WARD ASSESSMENT continued – JHO/SHO

MANAGEMENT

NURSING MANAGEMENT REQUIRED:

If concern that the patient is at RISK of further self-harm, discuss with senior staff nurse and SHO

*Consider factors in Psychosocial Assessment (Pages 9 – 11) – particular attention should be given to factors with ** beside them.*

Consider Detention – see appendix. Specify level of nursing observation here: Indicate with √ : General ☐   Constant ☐

IF CONSTANT OBSERVATION – NOTIFY SENIOR NURSE ON CALL

Post take ward round

Appendix 8.1   (*Continued*)

LIAISON PSYCHIATRY

Assessment Prompt List:

1. Brief History of DSH event

- What were the precipitating events?
- What were the motives for the act?
- What were the circumstances of the act?
- Were any precautions taken against discovery?
- Was the act impulsive or planned?
- How violent/lethal was the method?
- Have there been any signs/symptoms of depression?
- Is there any sign of the use or abuse of alcohol?

2. General Psychiatric and Medical History

- Have there been any previous acts of DSH?
- What was the nature of any previous psychiatric disorder?
- How was this treated? Who are the current professional contacts?
- Is there any family history of depression, psychiatric disorder, suicide or alcoholism?
- Is there any present or past physical illness?

3. Social Circumstances

- Housing – does the patient live alone?
- Does the patient live with dependent children?
- Does the patient have a job?
- What is the reaction of the family and friends to the act of DSH?
- Who will take the patient home and look after him/her?
- Family attitudes are important – are relatives sympathetic?
- The quality of family relations – is there evidence of abuse?
- Are conditions likely to change following DSH?

4. Background

- Is there any relevant family or personal history?
- Is there a pre-morbid personality problem or disorder?
- Is there any forensic history?
- Is there an extended history of alcohol/drug abuse?

5. Mental State (Points for particular attention)

- Consider whether the patient is of dejected appearance, agitated, restless or depressed.
- Ask does the patient's mood change during the day?
- Do they have impaired sleep?
- Do they have feelings of guilt, unworthiness or self-blame?
- Is there loss of appetite or unexplained weight loss?
- Is there a delusional system?
- Is the patient pessimistic about their ability to cope with and resume a normal life?
- Is there another psychiatric syndrome?

6. Formulation

- Why was the overdose taken or episode of DSH committed?
- Psychiatric diagnosis (illness and personality). There may be no psychiatric disorder.
- Assessment of risk of suicide or non-fatal repetition.
- Problem areas.
- Action to be taken.

Appendix 8.1   (*Continued*)

LIAISON PSYCHIATRY

Client Name _____ D.O.B. _____

Address _____

_____

1. Brief History of DSH Event

2. General Psychiatric and Medical History

3. Social Circumstances

4. Background

5. Mental State (Points for particular attention)

6. Clinical Impression/Formulation

Appendix 8.1   (*Continued*)

LIAISON PSYCHIATRY Continued

Senior Advice Sought: Yes ☐ No ☐ Whom _____

By Telephone ☐   Face to face ☐

Senior Assessed Patient   Yes ☐ No ☐

Risk Assessment for repeat

High ☐   Moderate ☐   Low ☐   Very Low ☐

Likely severity of repeat:

Severe ☐   Moderate ☐   Mild ☐

Are there risk factors amenable to interventions?

Management Plan

Admitted: Voluntary ☐   **Detained** ☐   **Hospital Ward.....**

Complete if Not Admitted	Yes/No	Routine/Urgent	Specify	Contact by Telephone/Letter
Offered admission but refused				
No requirement for admission				
Accepted follow up when offered with: • Out Patient Clinic • Community Psychiatric Nurse • Community Addictions Team • Community Social Worker • G.P. • Other				
Declined all follow up				
Action:				

Mental Health Professional

Name_____   Grade_____

Date_____Time_____   Signature_____

REFERENCES

Bennewith O, Gunnell D, Peters T et al 2004 Variations in the hospital management of self harm adults in England: an observational study. British Medical Journal 328:1108-1109

Department of Health 1992 The health of the nation. HMSO, London

Department of Health 1998 Our healthier nation. HMSO, London

Department of Health 1999 National service framework for mental health. Executive summary. HMSO, London

Department of Health 2001 Safety first: five year report of the national confidential inquiry into suicide and homicide by people with mental illness. Department of Health, London

Department of Health 2002 Priorities and planning framework 2002/2003. HMSO, London

Department of Health and Social Security 1984 The management of deliberate self-harm. HMSO, London

Department of Health and Social Services 1986 Mental health (Northern Ireland) order. HMSO, Belfast

Department of Health and Social Services 1997a Health and wellbeing: into the next millennium. Executive summary. DHSS, Belfast

Department of Health and Social Services 1997b Well into 2000. Positive agenda for health and wellbeing. DHSS, Belfast

Department of Health and Social Services and Public Safety 2000 The health of the public in Northern Ireland – report of the Chief Medical Officer. DHSSPS, Belfast

Department of Health and Social Services and Public Safety 2001 Best practice-best care: a framework for setting standards, delivering services and improving monitoring and regulation in the HPSS: a consultation paper. DHSSPS, Belfast

Department of Health and Social Services and Public Safety 2003a Priorities for action 2003/2004. DHSSPS, Belfast

Department of Health and Social Services and Public Safety 2003b Promoting mental health – strategy and action plan 2003-2008. DHSSPS, Belfast

Department of Health and Social Services and Public Safety 2003c Guidance on working patterns for junior doctors. Strategic Change Unit. DHSSPS, Belfast

Department of Health and Social Services and Public Safety 2004 A consultation report – the review of mental health and learning disability (Northern Ireland) – a strategic framework for adult mental health services. DHSSPS, Belfast

Down Lisburn Trust 1999 Mental health services strategic plan 1999-2002. Down Lisburn Trust, Downpatrick

Down Lisburn Trust 2001 Suicidal risk assessment in self-poisoning patients. Down Lisburn Trust, Downpatrick

Down Lisburn Trust 2004a Clinical and social care governance strategy: 2004/2006. Down Lisburn Trust, Downpatrick

Down Lisburn Trust 2004b A strategy for mental health 2004-2007. Down Lisburn Trust, Downpatrick

Foster T, Gillespie K, McClelland R 1997 Mental disorders and suicide in Northern Ireland. British Journal of Psychiatry 170:447-452

Greer S, Bagley C 1971 Effect of psychiatric intervention in attempted suicide: a controlled study. British Medical Journal 1:310-312

Hawton K, Catalan J 1987 Attempted suicide: a practical guide to its nature and management. Oxford University Press, Oxford

Hawton K, Fagg J 1988 Suicide, and other causes of death, following attempted suicide. British Journal of Psychiatry 152:359-366

Hawton K, Fagg J 1992 Trends in deliberate self poisoning and self injury in Oxford. British Medical Journal 304:1409-1411

Hughes T, Hampshaw S, Renvoize E et al 1998 General hospital services for those who carry out deliberate self-harm. Psychiatric Bulletin 22:88-91

National Health Service Confederation and British Medical Association 2003 New General Medical Services Contract 2003 – investing in general practice. NHS Confederation and BMA, London

National Institute for Clinical Excellence 2004 The short-term physical and psychological management and secondary prevention of self-harm in primary and secondary care. National Institute of Clinical Excellence, London.

Northern Ireland Statistics and Research Agency 2003 Statistics press notice births and deaths in Northern Ireland. Department of Finance and Personnel Northern Ireland, Belfast

Pollard C 1998 Mental health triage and assessment for emergency medicine. A guide for nurses. Department of Community and Health Services, Tasmania

Samaritans 2004 Information resource pack. Samaritans, London.

Royal College of Psychiatrists 1994 The general hospital management of adult deliberate self harm. Royal College of Psychiatrists, London

Royal College of Psychiatrists 2004 Psychiatric services in Accident and Emergency departments. Council Report CR118. Royal College of Psychiatrists, London

World Health Organisation 1992 Health-for-all targets. The health policy for Europe. Summary of the updated edition. World Health Organisation, Copenhagen

Implementing the Scottish schizophrenia guidelines through the use of integrated care pathways

Mark Fleming

INTRODUCTION	**CARE PATHWAY IMPLEMENTATION**
BACKGROUND	**OUTCOMES AND CONCLUSIONS**
PATHWAY DEVELOPMENT	**REFERENCES**

INTRODUCTION

Often in the development of new initiatives within health care there are key drivers for the purpose of any change. The key driver for the development of an integrated care pathway (ICP) for schizophrenia in NHS Ayrshire and Arran was the launch of a set of clinical standards for schizophrenia by the Clinical Standards Board for Scotland (now Quality Improvement Scotland). Table 9.1 shows a summary of the standard statements (Clinical Standards Board for Scotland 2001) and steps towards solutions for each of the 11 standards. Also influential were the evolving electronic health strategies and the developing joint working agenda across Scotland – the Joint Future Initiative (Scottish Executive 2000). A further driver was the formation of Community Health Partnerships (CHPs) in local areas who are tasked to plan, deliver and evaluate services to support the health needs of local populations (Scottish Executive 2004).

The local mental health services in Ayrshire and Arran have experienced joint working with social services and the voluntary sector for many years. The community mental health teams who play a significant role in this ICP are made up of staff from health, social services and housing. Joint management, information sharing and care recording protocols underpin integrated working. Many joint projects have involved the voluntary sector, including the securing

Table 9.1
Clinical standards for
schizophrenia (Clinical
Standards Board for
Scotland 2001)

Standard	Summary of standard statement	Electronic ICP solutions
Standard 1		
Information on populations and individuals	Recording the number of people who have a diagnosis of schizophrenia, and their met and unmet needs	The Reporting and Outcomes tools of the Electronic Patient Record (EPR) mean easy collation of assessment profiles of patient groups as defined by their diagnosis
Standard 2		
Initial diagnosis	Review by a psychiatrist and other disciplines to confirm or refute a considered diagnosis, actively involving the person and carer	Pathway monitoring of assessment process to confirm diagnosis. Diagnosis recorded in EPR using International Classification of Diseases diagnosis codes
Standard 3		
Initial assessment and care planning	Multidisciplinary assessment incorporating health and social needs, risk to self and others, and their need for information on their illness and related services/treatments	Introduction of Functional Analysis of Care Environments (FACE) assessment tools – health and social assessment, risk profile. Pathway monitoring of assessment process and provision of approved information
Standard 4		
Ongoing assessment and care planning	Providing coordinated access to services and regular review of needs	Pathway monitoring of reassessment and review process. Unique assessment flagging function to identify needs for care planning
Standard 5		
Transferring care – admission to hospital	Involving person in all aspects to assist early return to the community	Having a networked EPR and electronic integrated care pathway (e-ICP) ensures clinicians have appropriate access to up-to-date information on person's care needs

Table 9.1   *Continued*

Standard	Summary of standard statement	Electronic ICP solutions
Standard 6		
Transferring care – discharge from hospital	Involving person in all aspects to ensure coordination of discharge	Having a networked EPR and e-ICP ensures clinicians have appropriate access to up-to-date information on person's care needs
Standard 7		
Information and support for carers	Provision of practical support, accessible information and discussion opportunities regarding the person's illness and care	The e-ICP guides clinicians in assessment of the carer's needs and the provision of information on available treatment and services
Standard 8		
Prescribing anti-psychotic drugs – general principles	Provision and regular review of treatment with an appropriate anti-psychotic drug	The e-ICP monitors this review process and hosts the local drug algorithm
Standard 9		
Prescribing anti-psychotic drugs – special circumstances	Documenting rationale for dual prescription or any doses exceeding British National Formulary recommendations	The e-ICP monitors this documentation process and hosts the local drug algorithm
Standard 10		
Social and psychological approaches to care	Assessment of need for life and social skills training, and a person and their carer's need for psychological therapy	Development of local discipline specific assessments recorded in the EPR and monitored by the e-ICP
Standard 11		
Misuse of alcohol and illicit drugs	Review of a person's use of alcohol and illicit drugs, and provision of access to specialist addiction services where appropriate	Development of local assessment recorded in the EPR and monitored by the e-ICP

of transitional employment places for service users who were involved in a local mental health clubhouse. It was on the back of this joint working that a decision was made to apply for funds from the Mental Health and Wellbeing Fund at the Scottish Executive to develop an integrated care pathway and apply it within an electronic patient record framework. It is believed that this joint working approach helped to secure the £164,000 funding which allowed the project to develop. In the first few months following the award, the project team were recruited, with the author as project manager, and development began.

BACKGROUND

The 2001 Census showed that the population served by NHS Ayrshire and Arran stood at just over 368,000 (General Register Office for Scotland 2001). In terms of its make-up, the population profile is much like that of Scotland as a whole. North Ayrshire was however placed as the seventh lowest area of deprivation in Scotland with 13% of the population living in the 10% most deprived areas in Scotland. At the time, North Ayrshire had 1080 patients with severe mental illness and 380 of these had a diagnosis of schizophrenia or psychosis. Geographically, NHS Ayrshire covers a range of rural and urban areas including two islands. High deprivation falls across both rural and urban settings. Adult mental health services are offered from six community mental health teams, which are supported by two acute inpatient units, an intensive psychiatric care unit and two day hospitals. A recent addition has been an intensive community support service which supports the community teams in assertive outreach and crisis care for service users who are in the most need. Rehabilitation and long-stay beds are provided from hospital services based at Ailsa Hospital in Ayr.

Care pathway development, the pathway philosophy and framework were to offer multidisciplinary teams the opportunity to consider carefully and negotiate with service users and carers the most appropriate package of care; as well as assisting managers in identifying client needs and the service infrastructure required to support the processes and outcomes of the care offered. The ICP project team defined a set of aims and objectives for the project, which were signed off by a multidisciplinary project board. The NHS Ayrshire and Arran schizophrenia care pathway aims to:

- provide care for patients with schizophrenia/psychosis underpinned by evidence-based treatment, best practice and the support options available in Ayrshire and Arran
- apply the Quality Improvement Scotland standards for schizophrenia and monitor/audit these
- ensure the same level of care is provided to all patients across Ayrshire
- provide data to clinical governance teams to aid service planning, identify resource issues and improve patient care/journeys.

Implementing the pathway aspired to:

- provide key staff with appropriate training and support in implementing the pathway
- introduce an electronic patient record implementing computer-based assessment, care planning, care recording, outcome measurement and needs analysis tools
- develop networked communication between community services and agencies, inpatient services and primary care to aid the care process
- involve service providers, users and carers in the development process and ongoing evaluation of the pathway
- utilise the outcomes reporting tools to facilitate the clinical governance agenda within the local area.

In practice, the aim is to give users and carers greater choice and say in services planned for them and confidence that these services are efficient, effective and of a high quality. This requires the use of evidence-based practice, regular audit of the clinical outcomes and the quality of services providing these interventions. If best practice were to be offered, this must be cost effective as well as clinically proven. Achieving this is a complex task in mental health; however, the development of care pathways offers an inroad to achieving this. Integrated care pathways address these concerns, as they not only consider the outcome of individual care but they start to explore the overall performance of the care delivery process within the pathway. The key agenda is to streamline tasks and structure them in such a way that reduces repetition, minimises delay and simplifies the care process. Involvement ensures that the service user and carer can understand fully the care process, which will in turn facilitate inclusion in their care.

In order to identify the target group for the pathway, the project team decided upon key diagnostic criteria that would facilitate access to the pathway by service users. A decision had to be made whether this would be a process pathway or a diagnostic type pathway. The project board agreed that this would be a diagnostic pathway, as this would correspond with the structures and evidence base laid down in the national schizophrenia standards. It was agreed that one of four diagnoses would precipitate a service user's access to the pathway. These are the ICD10 (International Classification of Diseases) categories of:

- F20 schizophrenia
- F22 persistent delusional disorders
- F25 schizo-affective disorders
- F29 non specified psychosis (Royal College of Psychiatrists 1992).

A decision was also taken to include new referrals where psychotic symptoms were evident and an early intervention approach would benefit the service user and their family. The age of the service user group accessing the pathway was intended to be 16-65 years. However, it was evident that service users who continued to remain under the care of adult services over the age of 65 due to their specific needs would be included in components of the pathway. So the proposed upper age limit was removed. The local NHS board were involved in the initial development process. 'Buy in' from this group and the directors of the Trust was essential to support the development process and implement the change programme.

At the outset, the project board identified one of the critical success factors of the project as engagement with service users and carers in the development of the pathway and clinical information system. It was therefore essential that the chosen project team included staff who were respected, influential and from various backgrounds. Overseen by the project board was an initial project team made up of a nurse, an administration staff member and a social worker. This mix of experiences worked well in the development and implementation phases of the pathway. However, over the time of the project, the social worker moved to a senior position and was replaced by a nurse with beneficial IT (information technology) skills. This 'added value' during the IT implementation and evaluation phases. The selection of these particular individuals and their working relationships with others helped engagement with teams and groups, which has been one of the key success factors of the project. The project was managed by an ICP facilitator who utilised project management skills, having a grasp of effective change management in a complex organisation. The ICP facilitator acted as change agent, negotiator, supporter, politician, motivator, planner and time manager. These roles were accompanied by perseverance, diplomacy, confidence, credibility and self-motivation. The responsibilities of the project team were plentiful and changed as the project developed across the differing phases (Stephens 1997).

PATHWAY DEVELOPMENT

Firstly, the project team researched models of care pathway development. Implementation of the model was supervised by the project board, where key decisions were to be taken and direction given. The project board was multidisciplinary and involved people from different levels of the organisation; its aim was to give strategic direction as well as a realistic view of what could be achieved at the clinical interface.

The aims of the project board were to:

- provide strategic direction to the project and to help the project team understand the relationships of the project with other initiatives across the organisation
- develop the philosophy, model and methods of developing and introducing the integrated care pathway
- establish the desired outcomes and benefits of the project
- develop an effective communications strategy for the project
- promote the uptake of the pathway approach across the organisation
- monitor and support the development work of the project team
- support the project team in all aspects of its work
- sign off the pathways developed and support their implementation in clinical practice.

Previous experience had shown that where project boards function well, integrated care pathways flourish and develop quickly. Where there is no project board, pathways often do not succeed.

The care pathway development model agreed for use by the project board was an adaptation of a tool from NHS Wales (Welsh National Assembly 1999). This is a five-phase approach to the care pathway development and is structured as follows:

1. raising awareness and gaining commitment from all concerned
2. development of the integrated care pathway
3. development of documentation systems
4. implementation of the integrated care pathway systems
5. evaluation of the integrated care pathway.

The project team felt it was important to raise the awareness of the project across the Trust and develop working groups in order to gain the commitment of staff across all levels. Presentations were made to board members, managers and teams of clinicians to inform staff of the model and the process they would be involved in over the next 2 years. To provide this information, the project team had to complete initial research about how care pathways could be applied in mental health services. There was at that time limited published information relating to mental health ICPs, so the team developed information leaflets and presentations by adapting work from acute health care. The project team during this activity also raised awareness of the new national standards for schizophrenia and explored with staff how the standards could be implemented within an integrated care pathway framework. This collaborative work with clinicians was essential at the early stage of the project to secure staff involvement. One other key factor at this stage was developing the structure to support the eventual geographical roll-out of the integrated care pathway. NHS Ayrshire and Arran was divided into three sectors, which are coterminous with the local authorities and local healthcare cooperatives. The integrated care pathway was to be developed in one geographical area before wider roll-out. Still, it was essential to have as wide a 'buy in' as possible from the beginning. This was achieved by structuring the integrated care pathway development process around small working groups that had been set up in each area to support the development of care processes to sustain the new national schizophrenia standards. The project team therefore promoted the integrated care pathway approach in these forums and used the recommendations from these groups within the development phase.

The project team and project board identified at the outset the importance of involving service users and carers in the development, implementation and evaluation of the integrated care pathway. They wanted to do this in a meaningful way and enlisted the help of the North Ayrshire Advocacy Service to work with the project team. Advocates supported service users and carers to ensure they were given the opportunity to influence processes and explore with the project team potential solutions to issues that service users, carers and the wider public raised. The Advocacy Support Service held an 'open space' meeting to explore the pathways of care and present to service users and carers the approach being taken. This ensured that those service users and carers wishing to be involved fully understood the work that they were becoming engaged in. At this point, a number of issues were raised by service users and carers about their involvement in the project, and the project team were able to explore these issues and offer potential solutions. For example, a decision was made that service users and carers would be paid for attending meetings to cover their expenses and time.

When the project group and Advocacy Service began to work together, the first decision made was to use structured interviews with service users, carers and members of the public. The purpose of the interviews was to allow the development team to gain an understanding of the current care standards and secure the users' and carers' views on issues relating to care processes. Members of the Advocacy Service completed these interviews after initially supporting each other by role-playing the interviews. They interviewed service users, carers and the general public with whom they had routine contact and felt comfortable interviewing. After confidence grew, they used a factual approach to disseminate and collate information, seek out additional concerns and recruit new members to the group. The feedback from this was positive on all sides and the project team began to understand the key issues that were causing problems within the current pathways of care. Issues raised most frequently by the service users and carers interviewed related to the lack of structured information about the illness and the resources available locally to support people. It was identified that service users and carers were repeatedly reassessed, particularly by different medical locum staff. It was evident that information about service users' assessments or care was not readily available which led to staff repeatedly asking service users about the same issues over and over again (if they did not know the service user). It was suggested that inpatient care was chaotic, with little therapeutic intervention taking place. It was agreed with the project team that care pathway development would intervene in these issues.

As previously mentioned, there were a number of small groups established to work on aspects of both the pathway and the implementation of the changes required to support the new national schizophrenia standards. The groups explored the following aspects of the pathway:

- referral criteria to the pathway and the information required to support fast access to services for patients and carers
- the psychosocial assessment process and the assessments required for diagnostic purposes
- needs analysis and systems to identify and record diagnosis in a structured way
- care planning and specific psychological and occupational interventions
- transfer of care between services and the care/information processes around it
- care and treatment whilst in hospital.
- discharge planning
- provision of standardised information about services and illness (this involved users/carers deciding upon good material and assessing its quality)

- medication algorithms
- alcohol/drug assessment and joint working with alcohol/drug services.

The small working groups were made up of staff from all disciplines, service users, carers and representatives from the voluntary sector. They all provided reports on their findings and fed recommendations to the project team and the schizophrenia standards project board. When the small groups made recommendations, these were written in guideline form. These guidelines then formed the basis on which the integrated care pathway would be structured. Whilst this work was underway, the project team were procuring a software product which would support the implementation and evaluation of the integrated care pathway. The Trust had to go through the European procurement process to buy the product, as it exceeded the specified financial threshold. This was a new experience for the project team and presented a steep learning curve. This process took 9 months and after many visits, demonstrations and meetings the Trust decided to work with Intermation Limited to develop their FACE (Functional Analysis of Care Environments) software to manage the care pathway. Within the finances available, there was no product developed enough to serve on the Trust's IT network which had integrated care pathways as a core on their electronic patient record. Subsequently, a development approach had to be taken with the company concerned. The benefit of this was that the system would be developed as per the Trust's requirements. This development was a real challenge as the project team had only seen integrated care pathways in a paper format and had to think dynamically to structure all of the components within an information technology framework. The components that had to be built included:

- recording of demographic and personal information
- information collected by different services and centres of care
- keyworker and Responsible Medical Officer information
- referral information
- assessments and the ability to identify key needs/problems
- diagnosis
- key interventions within the pathway available for variance tracking
- guidelines on each aspect of the pathway
- person-centred plans of care based on needs assessments
- ability to record staff activity records with action type and outcome at its core.

Reporting tools needed to profile needs for groups and individuals; provide progress or deterioration views of clinical outcomes when compared with different intervention types; allow variance aggregation views from the defined pathway components; and analyse demographics, activity and assessment tools. These requirements were integral to the software development process. Consequently, the view of the pathway clinicians now have is very different from the traditional paper care pathway format. With this in mind, it was important to consider an evaluation framework, which would not only suffice for the integrated care pathway but would also assess the clinician's use of the new software. After 6 months of development an electronic integrated care pathway format became available. Figure 9.1 shows the structure of the pathway as it is currently seen on a computer screen. Guidance notes on the different sections of the pathway are available for viewing within the clinical information system. Clinicians can use these notes to guide them through each section of the pathway and give them support.

As part of the development phase, the project team developed the variance tool used on the clinical information system. The team initially felt a free text variance and action point system of collection would be useful to identify the key variances from the care pathway. This was then revised to coded variances identified within the clinical information system, with the action points structured within a free text/notes section. Figure 9.2 shows where clinicians select the coded variances from the software. Clinicians use the coded lists to record when they have been able to achieve a component of the pathway or when they have had difficulty in doing so. There is the facility to add a free text note to further describe variances. Feedback is ongoing from clinicians on how these coded variances are used and how they can be developed.

CARE PATHWAY IMPLEMENTATION

Initially it was agreed that there would be two-tier implementation, with North Ayrshire implementing the pathway using the new electronic clinical information system and the other two geographic areas initially implementing a paper pathway. The decision not to implement the IT system across all areas at once was due to the need to develop IT skills for staff and the resources required to do this on such a large scale. The implementation phase of the project required the project team to complete training as close to the 'going live' date as possible. However, the previous decision to limit the roll-out of the electronic system was reversed by the project board. It was decided to go straight for the IT solution in all areas and not to introduce the pathway in a paper format. This required large-scale IT skills training and support by the project team.

Following training, the electronic integrated care pathway went live on 1 July 2002. Going live was rather uneventful. In reality, it took at least a year to build up the patient information for the 380 service users who had existing contact with the service and met the criteria for accessing the care pathway. A decision was made to structure information inputting around the yearly review process that was included within the pathway. This spread out the initial data inputting for clinicians over a year, making it less of a burden.

The largest part of the project team's work at this stage was to provide support in using the clinical information system and guidance on different aspects of the care pathway. During the implementation phase the project team's balance of work changed from IT skills support to more clinical guidance (and less IT skills support) as the clinicians became more proficient with the system. The project

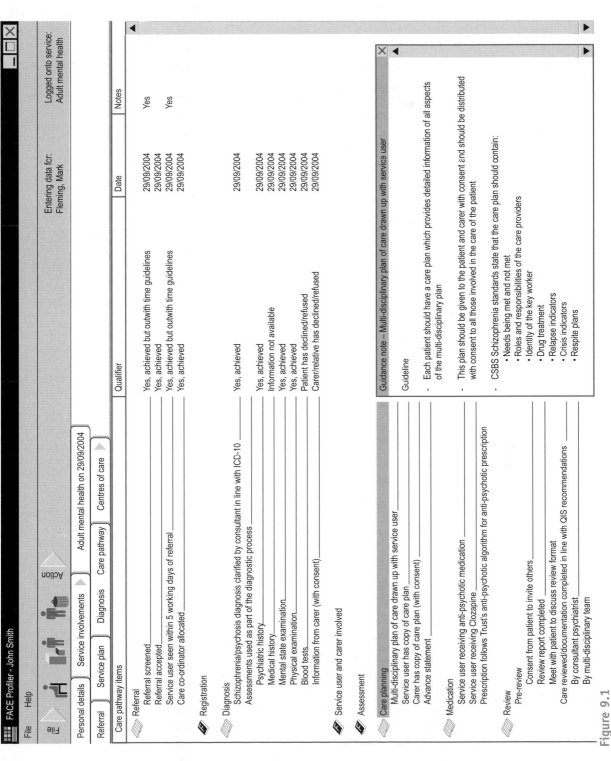

Figure 9.1

Screenshot showing the care pathway format

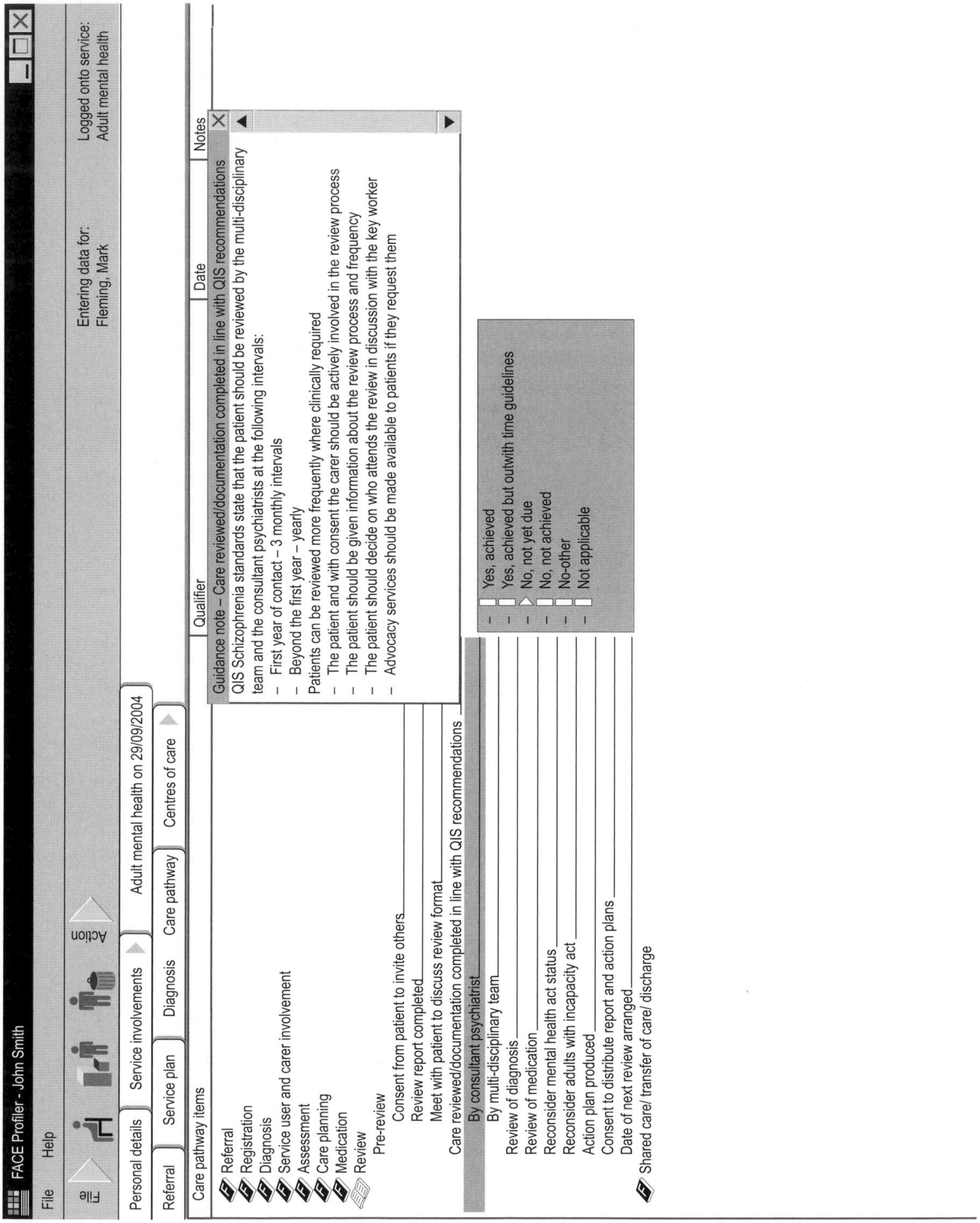

Figure 9.2
Screenshot of coded variance selection

board decided that the implementation phase would last for 1 year. At this point an evaluation would be made by clinicians and the service user/carer group. The service user and carer group, in conjunction with Advocacy Service, had developed a booklet about the integrated care pathway for use during the implementation phase. The booklet used simple language to describe the project and what service users and carers should expect from the pathway. A copy of this booklet can be requested via the Scottish Integrated Care Pathway Users website (www.icpus.org.uk). This resource was well received by users and carers and will be reviewed in 2005.

OUTCOMES AND CONCLUSIONS

Evaluation of the integrated care pathway is being undertaken in three phases:

1. The development of the integrated care pathway and quality of the tools developed.
2. The impact of the integrated care pathway upon the experience of care felt by service users and carers.
3. The use of the software to support the care pathway.

The project team intend to explore the quality of the integrated care pathway and adherence to the model of development used. This is to be undertaken using the Integrated Care Pathway Appraisal Tool developed at Birmingham University (Whittle et al 2004). The tool has been used to evaluate paper-based integrated care pathways and will be adapted by the project team to accommodate an electronic approach. The evaluation of impact upon the experience of service users and carers is being managed by a group of service users and carers with support from the advocacy group. The approach proposed is that interviews or focus groups will be held with new service users and carers who have accessed the service in the past 2 years. The groups or interviews will focus discussion around the key problems that were identified by the initial group (pre-pathway) to ascertain if there has been improvement. The third aspect (evaluation of the information system) has been completed using a series of questionnaires and focus groups with staff to identify the strengths and weaknesses of the product. Key issues raised were that staff found the support team essential in helping them to apply the integrated care pathway. There were a few problems with network/software speed, which needed to be rectified. Staff identified the need for remote access to the clinical information whilst they were in outlying clinics and the homes of service users.

To support clinical governance the project team currently produce clinical outcome reports as shown in Figure 9.3. The screenshot in this figure shows that an improvement or deterioration in the condition of a patient or a group of patients can be followed over a period of time. When coupled with the interventions associated with this patient group, this information allows clinicians to review their use of evidence-based practice. Over time, these reviews will help

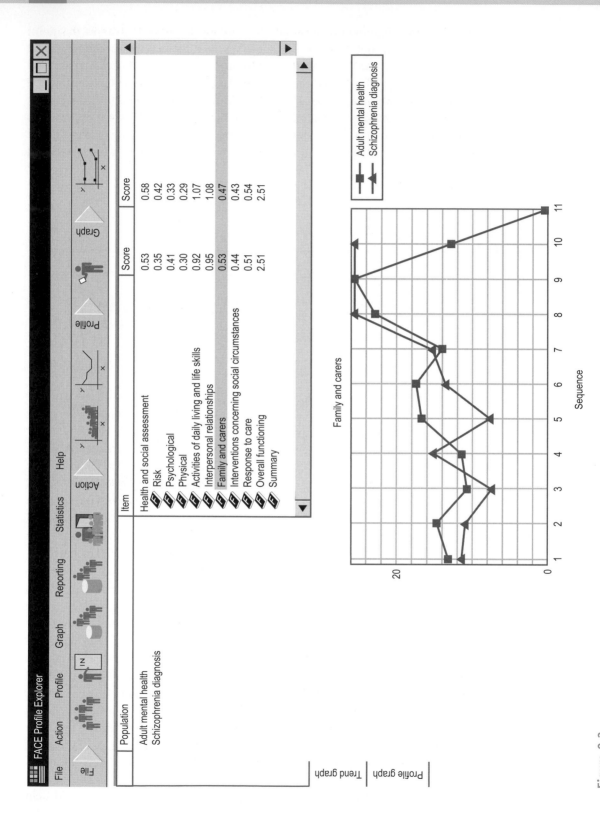

Figure 9.3
Screenshot of clinical outcomes report

ascertain whether the new structure of the care process has improved clinical outcomes for new service users entering the service. It is intended that these outcomes will be compared with the outcomes for a group of service users who accessed services 3 years ago (as the day hospital within the organisation was using the same outcome tools at that particular time). Completing this part of the evaluation has been delayed as the project team and project board believe that it will take some time for the change in culture and new ways of working to be fully embedded. This part of the evaluation will be completed in 2005/06. In the meantime, in order to review how change is progressing and how the pathway is being implemented the project team produce variance reports as shown in Figure 9.4. These highlight the areas of the pathway that are being adhered to and any variances. For example, the screenshot in the figure identifies that 32.88% of the time a multidisciplinary care plan has been drawn up with the service user. Obviously, this indicates that there is scope for improvement and reducing this variation. Clinical managers can focus on this and other areas that require improvement. The project team offers monthly reports of this nature to provide feedback to clinical governance groups. The clinical teams concerned then work on action plans to explore how improvements can be made within services. An example of such an action plan is shown in Figure 9.5. These reports can be used as the basis of new service developments, planning, developing staff skills and personal development plans.

One key development from this project has been the move towards becoming a learning organisation and securing the cultural changes required to move towards this. It will take some time to fully close the learning cycle, although there has been definite progress in the way that the organisation gathers information and promotes evidence-based practice by implementing clinical guidelines. Utilising integrated care pathways within an information management framework has been an essential step towards this. As a consequence of the work undertaken, the project team have learned a great deal from the development of the integrated care pathway for schizophrenia. There were a number of key critical success factors that the team would share with others developing a similar project. These include how valuable the project team approach was to embedding the processes into the patient journey, aiding compliance with the pathway. It was vital to ensure that there was support for ICPs at all levels of the organisation i.e. from directors to clinicians. It was essential to have a well supported user and carer reference group to sustain development, implementation and evaluation of the integrated care pathway. The use of an information technology system to support the care process and aid the development of variance reports to feed the audit/development loop has been fruitful. Particular benefits of this have been easy access to information and the use of reporting tools. The support of the clinicians working within this ever-changing environment has been a key to the success of the project. An appropriate model of integrated care pathway development and 'tried and tested' project management are required to ensure success and to realise the potential benefits.

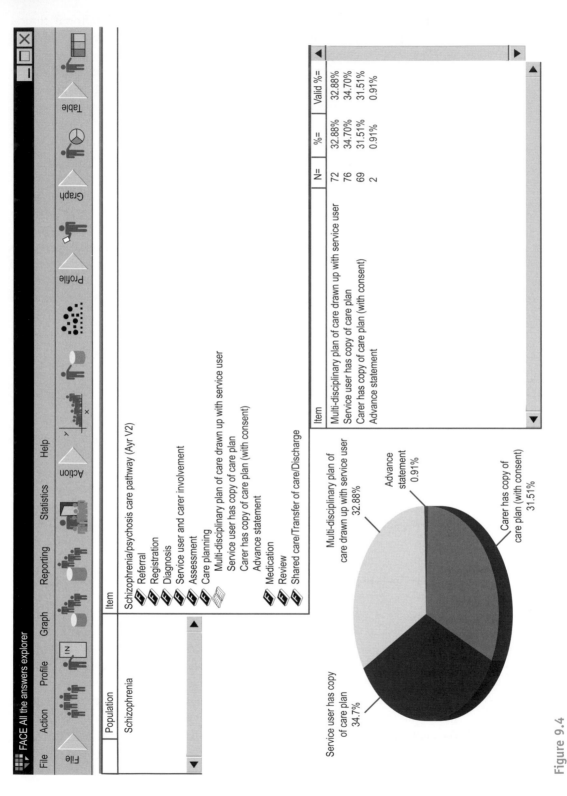

Figure 9.4

Screenshot of pathway variance report

Clinical governance action plans from FACE software information

Problem identified	Aim	Action	Responsibility	Timeframe	Outcome
22/8/04 Multidisciplinary care plan not being drawn up with patients. Only evidence of 32.88% success rate	To ensure 100% adherence to the care planning aspects of the pathway within 3 months	Team leaders and charge nurses build in importance of care planning into supervision with staff	Team leaders Charge nurse Clinical development manager	3 months from 22/08/04 New target 3 months from 22/11/04	22/9/04 Staff building aspects in to supervision. Improvement to 45% 24/10/04 Further improvement 77% 22/11/04 Now achieving 88% Continue action plan for a further 3 months
		Develop care planning documentation within software to make it more user friendly			

Action planning process

❖ From clinical governance reports the project leader will meet with team leader to identify problems.
❖ The project leader/team leader will explore:
   ▪ possible cause of problem
   ▪ aims
   ▪ possible actions/changes to clinical practice
   ▪ responsibility
   ▪ timeframe
   ▪ outcomes.
❖ Identify problem/achievement
❖ Reports will be fed back through the clinical governance forum
❖ Outcomes of these are also reported through the clinical governance framework

Figure 9.5
Example of a completed action plan

Acknowledgements   The screenshots were reproduced with the kind permission of Intermation Limited, 20 Fletcher Gate, Nottingham NG1 2FZ (www.facecode.com). Case details shown in the screen shots are fictitious.

REFERENCES

Clinical Standards Board for Scotland 2001 Clinical standards for schizophrenia. Clinical Standards Board for Scotland, Edinburgh

General Register Office for Scotland 2001 Scotland's census results online. www.scrol.gov.uk/scrol/common/home.jsp accessed 27.12.04, updated 21.10.2004, created

Royal College of Psychiatrists 1992 ICD-10: the ICD-10 classification of mental and behavioural disorders : clinical descriptions and diagnostic guidelines. Gaskell, London

Scottish Executive 2000 Joint Future Group report. Community care: a joint future. http://www.scotland.gov.uk/library3/social/rjfg-00.asp accessed 27.12.04, updated 24.12.04, created

Scottish Executive 2004 Community Health Partnerships statutory guidance. Scottish Executive Health Department, Edinburgh

Stephens R 1997 Setting up pathways in mental health. In: Wilson J (ed) Integrated care management: the path to success? Ch 9, pp 151-171. Butterworth Heinemann, Oxford

Welsh National Assembly 1999 Health: clinical pathways. www.wales.gov.uk/subihealth/content/keypubs/clinical/contents_e.htm accessed 27.12.04, updated, created

Whittle C, McDonald P, Dunn L et al 2004 Developing the integrated care pathway appraisal tool (ICPAT): a pilot study. Journal of Integrated Care Pathways 8(2):77-81

CHAPTER 10

Implementing care pathways for self-harm in acute inpatient care

Angus Forsyth

INTRODUCTION	**OUTCOMES AND CONCLUSIONS**
BACKGROUND	**APPENDIX**
CARE PATHWAY DEVELOPMENT	**REFERENCES**
PATHWAY IMPLEMENTATION	

INTRODUCTION

The Newcastle locality of the Newcastle, North Tyneside & Northumberland Mental Health Trust has six inpatient wards including 14 psychiatric intensive care beds providing a total of 100 inpatient beds to the city. With the development of specialist mental health teams there have been significant changes to the inpatient population, with the majority of service users having increasingly complex needs. More service users are admitted under a section of the Mental Health Act, have significant social difficulties, co-existing substance abuse problems and are severely at risk of suicide, self-harm and violence to others. Against this backdrop, the locality has been modernising adult acute care by reconfiguring services to reduce inpatient beds and reinvest further in community services. This has taken the form of home-based treatment to facilitate early discharge from hospital, development of acute day service provision and promoting a recovery model of service provision for community-based services. Integral to the success of these structural changes has been the development of care pathways to ensure that a high-quality service is delivered, that these are similar across the city and that service users are involved in developments. Integrated care pathways (ICPs) are being developed in tandem with the functions of adult acute inpatient care shown in Box 10.1.

Box 10.1 shows examples of process care pathways in accordance with the objectives of the adult acute wards. This provides a conceptual framework to make sense of the clinical work that needs to be undertaken in order to optimise expensive and scarce resources. The aim is reduce the likelihood of hospital admission and reduce length of stay whilst maintaining the quality of care for

Box 10.1   FUNCTIONS OF ADULT ACUTE WARD AND RELATED INTEGRATED CARE PATHWAYS

Engagement and stabilisation
- Assessment ICP
- Engagement ICP
- Safety and security ICP
- Mental Health Act ICP
- Reception ICP
- Medication concordance ICP

Conceptualisation and treatment planning
- Inpatient review meetings ICP
- Care coordination ICP
- Early discharge ICP

Coping and recovery
- Coping strategy development ICP
- Therapeutic activities: individual and group
- Relapse management ICP
- Transfer ICP (to other unit)

Sustaining recovery
- Transitional care plan ICP (community service)
- Family–carer networks
- Social and vocational support.

service users. Over the past 10 years there has been a greater focus upon service quality and improvement within the National Health Service (NHS) as a whole. Policy drivers are the Department of Health's (Department of Health 1998a) vision for the direction of the NHS as a modernised and dependable service better equipped to meet the needs of consumers. This was quickly followed by the publication of the *First class service* (Department of Health 1998b) that put forward a timetable to implement national standards to improve the quality of mental health services. Such standards were later described in the National Service Framework for Mental Health (Department of Health 1999).

Inherent within these documents is the need to improve patient experience with reference to evidence-based practice where it exists, to replicate similar standards of care irrespective of geography, reduce risk to service users and monitor performance and improvements in service delivery. Jones (1999) asserts that ICPs may be the vehicle for delivering such quality improvements. Following growing concerns about standards of care in adult acute inpatient settings, the Department of Health (2002) published the *Adult acute inpatient policy implementation guide* to improve the quality of care within these settings. A central tenet of the guidance was the establishment of acute care forums, which are multi-agency in nature. This engages a wide range of stakeholders to develop adult acute inpatient services across organisational boundaries. An important function of the forum is to define the therapeutic philosophy and overall service framework for adult acute care. Allied to this is the development of care pathways that engage multidisciplinary team members across the wide system of care. The policy guidance asserts that service planners need to concern themselves with the therapeutic approaches and interventions which are utilised to better meet the expectations of service users during the most vulnerable time of their illness. Thus the most recent guidance strengthens the need for ICPs and for inpatient mental health services to better define their role in the overall treatment process. Self-harm was selected as one target for an ICP due to the complexity of collaborating with service users, the proportion of service users that are unable to leave hospital because of the seriousness of their self-harm and the danger posed to others. Other factors included the range of responses to self-harm from care providers and the propensity for staff conflict in selecting appropriate treatment strategies.

BACKGROUND

According to NICE (National Institute for Clinical Excellence 2004, p 7), self-harm is defined as 'Intentional self-injury or poisoning, irrespective of the current purpose of the act'. It is estimated that approximately 1 in 10 people who engage in deliberate self-harm (DSH) will go on to commit suicide (Hawton 1997). Half of the suicides in England and Wales are committed by people with a history of self-harm, substance abuse or previous admission to hospital (Appleby et al 1999). Appleby (2000) states that approximately 4% of all suicides are psychiatric inpatients. A third of these occur during the first week of admission and another third during the period of planning discharge. Self-harm expressed by service users in acute psychiatric settings results in a range of interventions from 'high' observation to enabling clients to attend minor injury clinics on their own. The act of self-harm itself evokes a range of emotional reactions which can have a negative impact upon the service user and clinical teams (National Institute for Clinical Excellence 2004).

In an extensive review of the literature, Sharkey (2003) has likened self-harm to an addiction, in that service users can feel powerless to overcome their urges to self-harm which then results in release of emotions. This is seen as an important coping strategy. In keeping with this analogy, the author advocates that inpatient units adopt a harm reduction strategy for service users. This reduces potential for infection and reduction of subsequent scar tissue. Whilst acknowledging the importance of coping strategies for service users, this approach has been criticised by Forsyth (2003) as having the potential for inducing hopelessness in healthcare professionals and missing important opportunities to engage with service users. Additionally, this also fails to determine the individual meaning of the act of self-harm. Self-harm in a hospital setting is similar to that in community settings in that the act in itself cannot be viewed in isolation from other people. Whilst community practitioners can choose whether to intervene, this is difficult in a hospital setting due to the effect upon other service users. Feedback from service users is that they often feel frightened when another service user engages in self-harm.

The reality is that caring for service users who experience self-harm in an inpatient setting is extremely complex. A range of interventions are utilised by staff and these appear to be determined mainly by the culture of the caring team and become rule-bound procedures. For example, the philosophy of one unit in the locality was to enable service users to accept personal responsibility for self-harm and rarely explore the functional nature of the experience. This is in contrast to another unit with the maxim of keeping people safe and using observation until the risk has abated. Both approaches have their merits and drawbacks, and applied in blanket fashion neither reflects a collaborative relationship or the individual meaning of the act of self-harm. This variation of interventions between settings led to a project group in the Trust to explore this complex phenomenon, moving on to develop the ICP described in this chapter. When starting to develop the ICP, tools available from the NHS Modernisation Agency website were helpful. For example, *Developing protocol based care* offers a valuable guide to the development process and incorporates advice on service mapping, communication, training and auditing (NHS Modernisation Agency 2003).

CARE PATHWAY DEVELOPMENT

The first stage of ICP development was to set up a group to facilitate the development of the ICP. This acted as a steering group for ICP development and also provided an expert panel to judge the assumptions and issues posed by the phenomenon of self-harm. The group was established and led by the nurse consultant and included a range of stakeholders: service users, deliberate self-harm specialists, psychotherapists and cognitive therapists. Clinical nurse leaders and senior nurses from inpatient wards in the Trust were also part of the group. The aims of the group were to:

1. determine the impact of the problem of self-harm on the adult acute inpatient settings
2. identify the service responses to service users who engage in self-harm as inpatients
3. develop an evidence-based ICP to engage more effectively with service users who deliberately self-harm.

Before ICP development began, an audit of self-harm was undertaken using incident report forms (IR1) within the Trust during the previous 9 month period. The frequency of self-harm by gender is shown in Figure 10.1.

Figure 10.1

Frequency of self-harm by method and gender

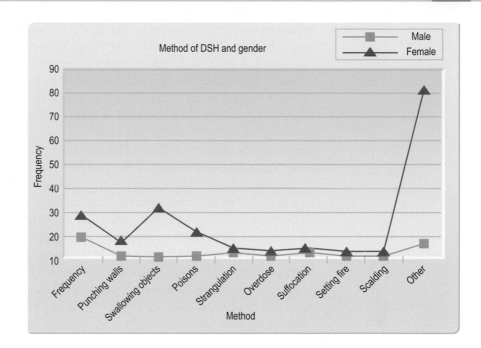

The main features of the findings showed during the previous 9 months:

- 36 acute inpatients expressed self-harm
- 161 episodes of self-harm were reported by IR1
- the age range of service users who self-harmed was 19-64 years
- the mean age of service users who engaged in self-harm is 34.7 years (men) and 37.2 years (women)
- the largest group of women who self-harmed were aged between 31 and 40
- the incidence of self-harm in men appeared to peak between 21 and 30 years of age
- the incidence of self-harm in females was greater than males
- cutting is the most frequent method; setting fire to self the least frequent
- men were more likely to engage in cutting and women more likely to swallow objects
- self-harm occurred most frequently in service users diagnosed with borderline personality disorder
- self-harm occurred less frequently in service users diagnosed with Huntington's chorea.

Three focus groups were used to collect data regarding nursing staff responses to service users who deliberately self-harmed whilst in adult acute inpatient wards. The focus groups comprised qualified mental health nurses and support workers. The findings revealed four main classes of response to service users who self-harm. The main strategies used were reducing access to means and high-level observation. These are related to clear goals of maintaining client safety and harm minimisation. However, it was viewed that these can result in negative outcomes for both staff and service users in that the interventions can be viewed as punitive, reducing client responsibility. This can result in further resentment and attributions of control which increase distance in the therapeutic relationship. Lack of confirmation to the service user about their experience stifles hope and optimism and is associated with further self-harm attempts (Lindgren et al 2004). This then results in resentment, conflict within the team, staff burn-out and a weakening effect upon the clinical team.

Nurses suggested that therapeutic engagement, one-to-one sessions, and giving responsibility back to the service user led to more positive feelings for staff. This is due to the focus upon collaboration and individual conceptualisation. This has an emphasis on developing alternative coping skills, whilst realising that service users would probably still self-harm. This leads to risk taking that contributes to anxiety within the practitioners and frustration when service users did not wish to receive care in this way. The major lessons learned from this exercise were that there appeared to be a hierarchy of interventions based upon the service user's level of complexity and understanding of the meaning of self-harm. However, generally, the clinical management strategy does not reflect the dynamic nature of this complexity and results in rule-bound interventions as previously highlighted. McAllister (2001) further infers that mental health nurses have uniform and inflexible responses to self-harming individuals. It is the author's view that there is a need to embrace new understanding of the service user's experience and ensure that service users are fully assessed with regard to their experience of self-harm. This was important for the development of the pathway, contributing to holistic assessment, security planning and engagement.

Service users were vital contributors to the development of the ICP. A focus group was undertaken with service users who had experienced adult acute inpatient care. Findings suggested that service users who have self-harmed feel misunderstood by staff but that developing helpful relationships is beneficial. Detachment has been found to be an antecedent for further self-harm and suicide attempts (Samuelson et al 2000). A large proportion of the group had not experienced self-harm prior to admission but had developed this strategy during their inpatient stay. This iatrogenesis raises an important issue with regard to the role and function of an acute ward.

Literature review

To support pathway development, a literature review was undertaken utilising the following keywords: deliberate self-harm, self-injury, self-inflicted wounds, self-wounding, parasuicide, acute mental health, and in-patient settings.

Studies of relevance to the ICP were selected using the following criteria:

- psychological approach
- psychosocial approach
- brief therapy

- outpatient
- inpatient
- adult population
- randomised control trials.

The following databases were accessed:

- Cochrane central register of controlled trials
- Cochrane database of systemic reviews
- Cochrane abstracts for reviews of effectiveness
- Psych-Info.

Table 10.1 shows the number of studies located that matched the above criteria. The systematic review matched several of the key words. Exploring the literature revealed studies that consisted of problem-solving therapy (Atha et al 1992), Manual Assisted Cognitive Therapy (MACT) (Evans et al 1999) and cognitive behaviour therapy (Raj et al 2001). Considered cumulatively, the literature indicates slight improvement after the use of problem solving and MACT. However, these findings were treated with caution due to small samples and the absence of outcome measures. The systemic review by Hawton et al (2002) compared the following treatments for DSH:

- problem-solving therapy versus standard aftercare
- intensive intervention outreach versus standard aftercare
- emergency card versus standard aftercare
- dialectical behaviour therapy versus standard aftercare
- inpatient behaviour therapy versus inpatient insight orientated therapy.

The limitations of most trials reviewed led to inconclusive results and failure to detect clinically meaningful differences between experimental and control groups. However, in overcoming this methodological criticism a large randomised controlled trial of MACT found similar attrition rates and no significant difference in repetition between the MACT and experimental groups. There were, though, significant differences in terms of cost effectiveness and subsequent use of services

Table 10.1
Results of the literature review

	Controlled trials	Systematic reviews	Review of effectiveness
Deliberate self-harm	14	9	3
Self-injury	27	4	2
Self-wounding	0	0	0
Parasuicide	16	2	1
Acute mental health	3	0	0
Inpatients	0	0	5

by service users with self-harm (Tyrer et al 2004). This raised the question on economic grounds that services should re-focus clinical efforts by switching to a lower cost but just as effective intervention. The NICE guidance concludes that the evidence base for the effective treatment of self-harm is extremely limited and that dialectical behaviour therapy is most effective for service users who repeatedly self-harm.

After presenting the literature review to the steering group, a 75 item ICP was developed to incorporate the following objectives in the care of service users who experienced self-harm:

1. to engage more effectively with service users who deliberately self-harm
2. to develop idiosyncratic case conceptualisations to guide team decision-making and interventions
3. to develop evidence-based interventions for service users
4. to provide a rationale for specific interventions depending on where the service user is on their journey to recovery.

PATHWAY IMPLEMENTATION

The pathway was developed to help those service users who are admitted to adult acute wards. These individuals are usually those who are:

- at moderate to severe risk of suicide, and
- have attempted self-harm, or
- at impending risk of serious self-harm and/or suicide
- detained under a section of the Mental Health Act
- working-age adults.

No formal criteria exist for diagnosis as this was felt to be too restrictive and excludes service users with complex needs that services hope to reach during the most vulnerable stage of their illness. Related to this was the function of reducing vulnerability, chronicity and minimising the duration of the service user's stay in hospital. The integrated care pathway standards and stages are briefly described.

An individual multidisciplinary assessment

According to the ICP each incidence of self-harm should be assessed to understand the individual meaning behind the act. This aims to enhance collaboration, understanding, engagement and prevent misinterpretations that are judgmental and dismissive. In order to develop this understanding, a range of methods have been used: self-report questionnaires, clinical interview and bibliotherapy. Risk assessment is also included within this part of the ICP. It is essential to complete the risk equation. This involves the immediate risk, long-term factors, coping resources and buffers. This may include accessibility of support and the service user's confidence in seeking help. It is important to explore the service user's previous experiences of self-harm, history of impulsivity and alcohol or substance misuse. Hazards in the form of access to means and the ward environment are also assessed and a risk management plan negotiated with the service user. Formal risk assessment models such as the validated Functional Assessment of Core Environments (FACE) risk assessment tool are used (Clifford 1995). This is in addition to a thorough mental state examination and medical assessment for hopelessness and suicide. The NICE guidance suggests that each individual act should be assessed to help the care team and service user understand the motivation and meaning behind each attempt. Then personalised care plans should be constructed.

An individual case conceptualisation

Models of understanding self-harm are related to deficits in problem solving, deficits in affect regulation, deficits in autobiographical memory, hopelessness, associations with early traumatic experiences, expression of dialectical tension, psychic distress turned inward on oneself, a demonstration of resistance against power and injustice, a way of expressing one's identity or as part of a psychiatric diagnosis such as borderline personality disorder. Developing a multidisciplinary formulation is essential to understanding and serves as an effective platform to deliver interventions. These are planned on this understanding rather than reactions to the service user's self-harm. An essential feature to enhance engagement is the joint understanding between professionals and service users. This aims to reduce conflict and malignant alienation towards service users. The cognitive model of Greenberger & Padesky (1995) is utilised to develop an individualised case conceptualisation for service users who experience self-harm. An example of the model applied to self-harm is illustrated in Figure 10.2.

Figure 10.2
Conceptualisation of self-harm from a cognitive behavioural perspective, adapted from Greenberger & Padesky (1995)

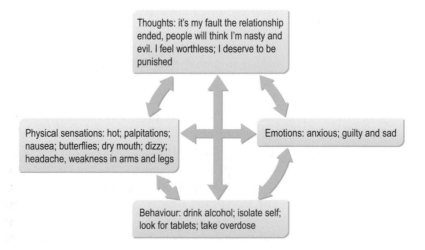

Thoughts: it's my fault the relationship ended, people will think I'm nasty and evil. I feel worthless; I deserve to be punished

Physical sensations: hot; palpitations; nausea; butterflies; dry mouth; dizzy; headache, weakness in arms and legs

Emotions: anxious; guilty and sad

Behaviour: drink alcohol; isolate self; look for tablets; take overdose

A clear framework for engagement and boundary setting

Shepherd & McAllister (2003) describe the CARE framework for responding therapeutically to service users who self-harm. This relates to Containment where the professional encourages the service user to seek help and responds in an empathic validating, non-judgmental manner. This works towards self-soothing and expression of emotion. Awareness is concerned with the analysis of the self-harm by developing an individual conceptualisation (as shown in Figure 10.2). Resilience is working together to develop strength and abilities, to connect with social networks and develop optimism for the future. Engagement relates to developing an empathic therapeutic relationship and working on problem issues. This promotes motivation and a new sense of meaning. By utilising this framework, nurses are able to develop more satisfaction in working and can complement existing multidisciplinary interventions. Strategies used include cognitive therapy sessions, use of the Trust's self-help guide and the development of collaborative security plans (Barker 2000).

A clear understanding of the process of therapeutic engagement and observation if required

Over the past 3 years the Newcastle Locality Acute Inpatient Service has embraced the Tidal model (Barker 2001, Stephenson et al 2002) to provide a conceptual framework for nursing practice. The model is based upon the fundamental principles of collaboration between the client and mental health nurse. This is built upon a therapeutic relationship whereby the two parties are able to empower each other to reach an increased understanding of current problems. The model identifies the risk posed by or to the client and provides guidance on a level of engagement. Together, a security plan and daily care plan are constructed and evaluated in order to help reduce risk. The inspiration of hope which is central to the process of caring is inherent within this paradigm.

Generally, observation is carried out by a range of professionals with differing understanding of the processes and interventions to facilitate inclusion. This can be characterised by nursing staff following clients wherever they go, sitting outside their room or lounge area and reduced capacity for a therapeutic relationship. With communication restricted to social 'chit chat' or helping clients with their physical needs, the practice can convey a lack of confirmation demonstrated by little personal contact. Staff perceptions are grounded in diagnosis or problem behaviour rather than individuality or functionality. This denies patients their feelings and does not offer hope in their given situation. Observation has been described as a low-skill activity, with junior support staff or students commonly being ascribed to the process (Barre & Evans 2002). The practice is often used to reduce organisational anxieties (Barker & Cutcliffe 1999) and contain staff angst (Reid & Long 1993). Close observation is a high-resource activity often directed by medical staff with nurses taking a passive role (Neilson & Brennan 2001) and, as Speedy (1999) describes, places the mental health nurse in the role of custodian. The therapeutic alliance is to convey meaning for the nurse and provide understanding of the client's current functioning. It is proposed that nurses who deliver observation without the clear involvement of the service user are further promoting custodial care. This benefits the organisation more than the consumer.

Providing clarity for practitioners, the ICP suggests that at times observation may be necessary, for example when the self-harm co-exists with acute suicidal ideation. This is used to maintain the safety of service users but with an increased emphasis on engaging with the service user to collaboratively reduce risk factors.

Understanding and planning to cope with urges to engage in self-harm

The NICE guidance suggests that individuals who self-harm and with a diagnosis of borderline personality disorder should be considered for treatment using Dialectical Behaviour Therapy (DBT). As other psychological interventions are not precluded and there are difficulties in local service provision for DBT, the following interventions identified in the literature review are included in the ICP:

- problem solving
- use of MACT self-help manual (Tyrer et al 2004)
- time-limited psychodynamic therapy
- medication
- contracting.

MACT was selected as this combines cognitive behaviour therapy approaches with problem solving and transferable aspects of DBT. This occurs in the form of a therapist-assisted self-help manual for service users. Outcomes are limited in terms of repetition of self-harm but beneficial in relation to increasing future positive thinking, reduced use of services and cost effectiveness. The structure and format of these sessions are shown in Box 10.2.

Box 10.2   STRUCTURE AND FORMAT OF MANUALISED COGNITIVE THERAPY (MACT) SESSIONS

The keyworker undertakes five sessions of 45 minutes' duration to facilitate the use of the manual. The main purposes of the sessions are to:

- consolidate self-help work
- problem-solve stuck points
- direct homework
- promote understanding and develop conceptualisation with the service user.

The sessions are collaborative in nature and underpinned by the values of cognitive behaviour therapy (Beck 1996). The daily engagement sessions will include the following elements:

1. development of problem list and targets
2. understanding self-harm
3. what to do in a crisis
4. learning to solve problems
5. learn to change your thinking
6. alcohol, drugs and pills: do you need to cut down or stop?
7. some further thoughts.

Awareness of the effects of self-harm upon other service users

Service users involved in the development of the ICP highlighted this issue. It was agreed that there needs to be a balance between the needs of the service user who engages in self-harm and service users who witness this. There are no recommendations in the literature although good sense suggests that all service users are treated within the bounds of safety, privacy and dignity. It is therefore suggested that when self-harm impacts upon others, the following arrangements are adopted:

- discussion of issues related to self-harm in community meetings/ward forums
- explore concerns regarding safety and possible contamination
- there is information about self-harm in ward orientation/reception information
- there is access to support for all service users
- there is a general awareness of imitation and escalation by other service users
- service user representatives raise awareness and explore concerns with service users.

Service users' treatment needs are explored in supervision with an experienced and expert practitioner

Acceptance of help by the client and their cooperation, enabling them to collaborate with treatment, is an important variable in determining how staff form an alliance with clients. There is a possibility that the mental health nurses make some form of causal attribution for the client's presentation (Weiner 1980). Hinshelwood (1999) states that professionals' attempts to reconcile their reactions or feelings towards clients are underpinned by an inability to understand the complex mental health needs that result in emotional discomfort. This is then attributed to an external source – the client. This in part may explain the difficulty of engaging with complex service users and professionals' poor adaptation to modern engagement interventions. Because of the complexities, it is therefore recommended that professionals caring for service users who self-harm:

- attend supervision sessions on a weekly basis
- develop multidisciplinary conceptualisation of case and platform for interventions
- facilitate team understanding
- troubleshoot effects of interventions
- re-evaluate personal and professional reactions to clients who self-harm
- reduce alienation to clients who self-harm
- shadow experienced specialist self-harm teams to develop skills and interest.

Multi-agency discharge and transitional arrangements in place prior to discharge

This ICP has been cross-referenced with the Department of Health's (2003) *Preventing suicide: a toolkit for mental health services*. The standards relate to joint planning of care with community agencies prior to discharge and include assessment of risk. The aftercare care plan has an engagement focus with appropriate 7 day follow-up and less toxic medication in limited supplies. Also included is the development of crisis plans and emergency cards with contact details of appropriate agencies. A copy of the full ICP is shown in the Appendix.

OUTCOMES AND CONCLUSIONS

At the time of writing, it has not been possible to fully evaluate the impact of the ICP due to the timeframe and integration of new clinical evidence into practice. However, a strategy for evaluation was used for piloting the individual standards within different clinical environments. This itself proved difficult due to shortages of staff and the competing demands of service reconfiguration. Also the service user lead obtained alternative employment before the service user monitoring of the new pathway was completed. Notwithstanding this, safety and security plans were compared pre- and post-ICP. Ten care plans were reviewed, and in the pre-pathway sample an average of four interventions for self-harm were found and these were very general in nature, for example one-to-one sessions and approach nurse for support. In the post-pathway sample, interventions increased to an average of 10 per case. These included more specific interventions, for instance identifying the advantages and disadvantages of harm and suicide, experiencing and expressing feelings, being assertive with others, use of distraction techniques and ignoring voices. Post-pathway service users who were cared for on formal observations had their situation reviewed more regularly. They were also more likely to progress to general observation within 2 to 3 days compared with an average of 7 days pre-pathway.

Currently, the author is evaluating part of the ICP by randomised control trial with 30 service users receiving interventions and 30 service users receiving standard treatment as usual. The main evaluation measures are Beck's Suicide Ideation Scale, duration of observation and length of hospital stay. The hypothesis is that the service users who receive the ICP and manualised approach to cognitive therapy will improve faster than those who receive the non-ICP standard treatment. The focus groups described pre-pathway for professionals' responses to service users who self-harm will be repeated after a year to identify whether their responses have altered in light of the ICP. The assertion is that there will be more evidence of engagement and collaboration with service users; and that this occurs whether formal observation is utilised or not. There should also be greater knowledge of underpinning practice, with this being reinforced through supervision sessions. Finally, qualitative data will be obtained to consider service user experiences, using the methodology of patient stories which capture the lived experience, and used to further service improvement. Service user representatives plan to undertake this work.

Staff reflections upon the ICP have been mixed. These ranged from enthusiasm to dismissal, that it would be ineffective and generate more work. The latter responses are consistent with barriers to new models of working and were expected. Interestingly, resistance to change was less where the Tidal model had been implemented and also where the author was primarily based. A group of senior and charge nurses fed-back anecdotal improved collaboration and effectiveness. The ICP is now featured in the training plan for adult acute inpatient staff within the locality. The training incorporates the Trust's suicide risk assessment and minimisation training, and cognitive behaviour therapy. Individuals who have self-harmed are also involved in the planning and delivery of training for staff.

This chapter has focused upon the development of an integrated care pathway for service users who self-harm. Implementation has been difficult within an ever-changing and complex environment. Staff in these environments work with some of the most complex service users, with very little investment in terms of specialist workers (i.e. psychologists and psychotherapists). This chapter has focused on the development of the ICP with a strong emphasis upon therapeutic engagement with a group of service users who can experience negative attitudes from health professionals. The ICP, rather than a checklist of interventions, provides multidisciplinary teams with a process for individual case formulations to better understand the experience of service users who self-harm. This leads to the development of collaborative relationships and interventions which have meaning for service users and professionals alike.

Care Pathway for Self-Harm (SH)

This integrated care pathway is for individuals admitted to acute inpatient services and who experience self-harm (SH). It is intended to guide assessment and intervention ensuring that a service user's journey is negotiated, managed and agreed. As inpatient care is implicitly a request for urgent/intensive intervention, there needs to be clarity regarding inputs and interventions required and how they will be delivered. Wherever possible interventions are based upon evidence and best practice. It is essential that the expectations of the individual service user are addressed as part of the overall care plan. This care plan will complement other process approaches undertaken during the inpatient journey, i.e. Mental Health Act obligations, reception best practice, care coordination.

Overall objectives of this care pathway are to:

1. engage more effectively with service users who deliberately self-harm
2. develop idiosyncratic case conceptualisations to guide team decision-making and interventions
3. develop evidence-based interventions for service users
4. provide a rationale for specific interventions depending on where the service user is on their journey to recovery.

Sources and evidence which inform the content of this pathway are:

- Barker, P (2000) The Tidal Model: Theory & Practice

- Department of Health (2003) Preventing Suicide: a Toolkit for Mental Health Services. London, DOH

- National Institute for Clinical Excellence (2003) Self-Harm: Short term physical and psychological management and secondary prevention of intentional self harm in primary and secondary care, 1st Draft

- Shepherd, C & McAllister, M (2003) CARE; A framework for responding therapeutically to the client who self-harms. Journal of Psychiatric & Mental Health Nursing, 10, 442-447

- Tyrer, P et al (2004) Differential effects of manual assisted cognitive behaviour therapy in the treatment of recurrent deliberate self harm and personality disturbance: The POPMACT Study. Journal of Personality Disorders. 18(1) pp 102-116

Appendix 10.1
Integrated Care Pathway to Self Harm

Following each episode of *Self Harm* the service user will have:-

1. An individual multi-disciplinary assessment comprising:-
(day 1)

Code	Intervention	Date & Sign	VARIANCE: Please tick box as appropriate, write reason for variance, action taken and final outcome
1.1	FACE risk assessment undertaken	../../..	☐ LATE ☐ NOT DONE ☐ N/A
1.2	Medical assessment for hopelessness and suicide completed	../../..	☐ LATE ☐ NOT DONE ☐ N/A
1.3	Mental state examination completed	../../..	☐ LATE ☐ NOT DONE ☐ N/A
1.4	Ascertain meaning of expression of self-harm: relief of distress; validate experience; kill self; communicate to others etc.	../../..	☐ LATE ☐ NOT DONE ☐ N/A
1.5	Identify any access to means and steps taken to minimise risk	../../..	☐ LATE ☐ NOT DONE ☐ N/A
1.6	Ward environment risk assessment undertaken and potential hazards identified and communicated to others in the care team	../../..	☐ LATE ☐ NOT DONE ☐ N/A
1.7	Determine alcohol and substance misuse	../../..	☐ LATE ☐ NOT DONE ☐ N/A
1.8	Use of DSH Risk Equation to determine observation & engagement level	../../..	☐ LATE ☐ NOT DONE ☐ N/A
1.9	History of previous impulsivity identified	../../..	☐ LATE ☐ NOT DONE ☐ N/A

Appendix 10.1   (*Continued*)

1.10	Beck Scale for Suicidal Ideation is administered	../../..	☐ LATE ☐ NOT DONE ☐ N/A
1.11	Measures of distress disruption & control are obtained	../../..	☐ LATE ☐ NOT DONE ☐ N/A
1.12	Beck Depression Inventory is administered	../../..	☐ LATE ☐ NOT DONE ☐ N/A
1.13	Brief Reason for Living Inventory Scale is administered	../../..	☐ LATE ☐ NOT DONE ☐ N/A
1.14	The Nurses' Global Assessment of Suicide Risk (NGASR) is obtained	../../..	☐ LATE ☐ NOT DONE ☐ N/A

2. An individual case conceptualisation completed and include:-
(day 1-2)

Code	Intervention	Date & Sign	VARIANCE: Please tick box as appropriate, write reason for variance, action taken and final outcome
2.1	A current description of the Deliberate Self Harm	../../..	☐ LATE ☐ NOT DONE ☐ N/A
2.2	Meaning of DSH is ascertained	../../..	☐ LATE ☐ NOT DONE ☐ N/A
2.3	Relationships between cognitive, emotional, physical and behavioural components of ? are represented	../../..	☐ LATE ☐ NOT DONE ☐ N/A
2.4	Short term risk factors are identified	../../..	☐ LATE ☐ NOT DONE ☐ N/A
2.5	Hazards are identified	../../..	☐ LATE ☐ NOT DONE ☐ N/A

Appendix 10.1   *(Continued)*

2.6	Protective factors are identified	../../..	☐ LATE ☐ NOT DONE ☐ N/A
2.7	A theoretical model(s) is used to understand the DSH	../../..	☐ LATE ☐ NOT DONE ☐ N/A
2.8	The service user has contributed to the conceptualisation	../../..	☐ LATE ☐ NOT DONE ☐ N/A
2.9	The multi-disciplinary team agree on the conceptualisation	../../..	☐ LATE ☐ NOT DONE ☐ N/A
2.10	The conceptualisation shows clear intervention points	../../..	☐ LATE ☐ NOT DONE ☐ N/A
2.11	Each professional is aware of his or her role in the treatment plan	../../..	☐ LATE ☐ NOT DONE ☐ N/A
2.12	The service user is aware of and contributed to the treatment plan	../../..	☐ LATE ☐ NOT DONE ☐ N/A
2.13	The carer (s) is (are) aware of and contributed to the treatment plan	../../..	☐ LATE ☐ NOT DONE ☐ N/A

3. A clear framework for engagement and boundary setting (day 1)

Code	Intervention	Date & Sign	VARIANCE: Please tick box as appropriate, write reason for variance, action taken and final outcome
3.1	Encourage client to participate in first aid/self management of injury where appropriate, for example lacerations	../../..	☐ LATE ☐ NOT DONE ☐ N/A
3.2	Reduce access to means for DSH & assign level of therapeutic engagement & observation if required, based on risk equation & risk assessment and suicidal intent and conceptualisation: Level 1 Level 2 Level 3	../../..	☐ LATE ☐ NOT DONE ☐ N/A

Appendix 10.1   (*Continued*)

3.3	Explain safety measures to service user	../../..	☐ LATE ☐ NOT DONE ☐ N/A
3.4	Service user and professional expectations are identified in terms of therapeutic goals and tasks	../../..	☐ LATE ☐ NOT DONE ☐ N/A
3.5	Service user is given Trust's self help guide & questionnaire to complete	../../..	☐ LATE ☐ NOT DONE ☐ N/A
3.6	Information is given to service user on regular engagement sessions with key worker or associate nurse	../../..	☐ LATE ☐ NOT DONE ☐ N/A
3.7	First engagement session appointment is made with service user	../../..	☐ LATE ☐ NOT DONE ☐ N/A
3.8	Single room accommodation is considered to promote safety, privacy and dignity of service user/s	../../..	☐ LATE ☐ NOT DONE ☐ N/A

4. A clear understanding of the process of therapeutic engagement and observation (Level 1)

Code	Intervention	Date & Sign	VARIANCE: Please tick box as appropriate, write reason for variance, action taken and final outcome
4.1	The service user will be given a file to help understand the process of therapeutic engagement and observation containing:-	../../..	
	▪ Information booklet	../../..	☐ LATE ☐ NOT DONE ☐ N/A
	▪ Self help guide	../../..	☐ LATE ☐ NOT DONE ☐ N/A
	▪ Security plans	../../..	☐ LATE ☐ NOT DONE ☐ N/A

Appendix 10.1   (*Continued*)

4.2	The service user and allocated nurse will complete a monitoring assessment of distress and control on a (minimum) 4 hourly basis:- ▪ Morning	../../..	☐ LATE ☐ NOT DONE ☐ N/A
	▪ Afternoon	../../..	☐ LATE ☐ NOT DONE ☐ N/A
	▪ Evening	../../..	☐ LATE ☐ NOT DONE ☐ N/A
4.3	The allocated nurse and service user will explore any divergence in ratings	../../..	☐ LATE ☐ NOT DONE ☐ N/A
4.4	The service user and allocated nurse will evaluate the security plan and examine ways of developing it	../../..	☐ LATE ☐ NOT DONE ☐ N/A
4.5	The service user and allocated nurse will evaluate the impact of the period of therapeutic engagement and observation	../../..	☐ LATE ☐ NOT DONE ☐ N/A

5. Understanding, and developing plans to cope with, urges to engage in DSH (days 2-7)

Code	Intervention	Date & Sign	VARIANCE: Please tick box as appropriate, write reason for variance, action taken and final outcome
5.1	The service user receives a minimum of 7 structured engagement sessions to understand their deliberate self harm	../../..	☐ LATE ☐ NOT DONE ☐ N/A
5.2	The service user is orientated to the structure of the sessions:- ▪ Homework review ▪ Main area of discussion ▪ Homework negotiation ▪ Session review	../../..	☐ LATE ☐ NOT DONE ☐ N/A

Appendix 10.1 (*Continued*)

5.3	The purpose of the sessions are explored with the service user:- • Consolidate self help work • Problem-solve stuck points • Direct homework • Promote understanding and develop collaborative conceptualisation with the service user	../../..	☐ LATE ☐ NOT DONE ☐ N/A
5.4	Daily engagement sessions using MACT are undertaken along the following themes:-	../../..	☐ LATE ☐ NOT DONE ☐ N/A
5.4.1	Development of problem list and targets in service user's own language	../../..	☐ LATE ☐ NOT DONE ☐ N/A
5.4.2	Understanding DSH	../../..	☐ LATE ☐ NOT DONE ☐ N/A
5.4.3	What to do in a crisis	../../..	☐ LATE ☐ NOT DONE ☐ N/A
5.4.4	Learning to solve problems	../../..	☐ LATE ☐ NOT DONE ☐ N/A
5.4.5	Learn to change your thinking	../../..	☐ LATE ☐ NOT DONE ☐ N/A
5.4.6	Alcohol, Drugs & Pills: do you need to cut down or stop?	../../..	☐ LATE ☐ NOT DONE ☐ N/A
5.4.7	Some further thoughts/relapse prevention	../../..	☐ LATE ☐ NOT DONE ☐ N/A
5.4.8	The DSH is understood by the service user	../../..	☐ LATE ☐ NOT DONE ☐ N/A

Appendix 10.1   (*Continued*)

6. An awareness of the effects of DSH on other service users

Code	Intervention	Date & Sign	VARIANCE: Please tick box as appropriate, write reason for variance, action taken and final outcome
6.1	The service user and allocated nurse have formulated a plan to cope with the impact of DSH on other service users.	../../..	☐ LATE ☐ NOT DONE ☐ N/A
6.2	Information about DSH in ward orientation/reception information	../../..	☐ LATE ☐ NOT DONE ☐ N/A
6.3	Discussion of issues related to DSH in community meetings/ward forums.	../../..	☐ LATE ☐ NOT DONE ☐ N/A
6.4	Explore concerns regarding safety and possible contamination	../../..	☐ LATE ☐ NOT DONE ☐ N/A
6.5	Information about accessing support is given to other service users	../../..	☐ LATE ☐ NOT DONE ☐ N/A
6.6	The service user is aware of the impact	../../..	☐ LATE ☐ NOT DONE ☐ N/A

7. Their treatment needs explored in supervision with an experienced and expert practitioner
(day 7 onwards)

Code	Intervention	Date & Sign	VARIANCE: Please tick box as appropriate, write reason for variance, action taken and final outcome
7.1	The key worker has obtained consent from the service user to explore their needs in regular supervision	../../..	☐ LATE ☐ NOT DONE ☐ N/A
7.2	The key worker attends supervision with the nurse consultant on a weekly basis	../../..	☐ LATE ☐ NOT DONE ☐ N/A

Appendix 10.1   *(Continued)*

7.3	The team have supervision with the nurse consultant on at least two occasions	../../..	☐ LATE ☐ NOT DONE ☐ N/A
7.4	The team and key worker have a clear case conceptualisation and platform for interventions	../../..	☐ LATE ☐ NOT DONE ☐ N/A
7.5	Personal and professional reactions to clients with DSH are explored and evaluated	../../..	☐ LATE ☐ NOT DONE ☐ N/A
7.6	The key worker and team members have shadowing experiences with specialist DSH teams to develop skills	../../..	☐ LATE ☐ NOT DONE ☐ N/A

8. Multi agency discharge and transitional arrangements in place prior to discharge
(day 7 onwards)

Code	Intervention	Date & Sign	VARIANCE– Please tick box as appropriate, write reason for variance, action taken and final outcome
8.1	Prior to discharge in-patient & community teams carry out a case review, including assessment of risk	../../..	☐ LATE ☐ NOT DONE ☐ N/A
8.2	All discharge care plans specify arrangements for promoting compliance/engagement with treatment	../../..	☐ LATE ☐ NOT DONE ☐ N/A
8.3	Service users who are treated with anti-depressants or antipsychotic medication receive newer less toxic drugs	../../..	☐ LATE ☐ NOT DONE ☐ N/A
8.4	Discharge prescription is for less than 14 days	../../..	☐ LATE ☐ NOT DONE ☐ N/A
8.5	Care plan and/or discharge letter includes explicit advice to the GP about appropriate prescribing quantities	../../..	☐ LATE ☐ NOT DONE ☐ N/A

Appendix 10.1   *(Continued)*

8.6	Crisis plan is constructed with service user	../../..	☐LATE ☐NOT DONE ☐N/A
8.7	An agreed member of the clinical team follows up service users at high risk of suicide during the period of admission within 48 hours of discharge.	../../..	☐LATE ☐NOT DONE ☐N/A
8.8	All service users with severe mental illness, or a history of self harm or illness, or a history of self harm of less than 3 months, including those who discharge themselves, are followed up within one week by an agreed member of the clinical team.	../../..	☐LATE ☐NOT DONE ☐N/A
8.9	Service users are given an emergency card with the contact numbers of key personnel to be contacted in case of crisis.	../../..	☐LATE ☐NOT DONE ☐N/A

Appendix 10.1 *(Continued)*

REFERENCES

Appleby L 2000 Prevention of suicide in psychiatric patients. In: Hawton K, Van Heerigen K (eds) The international handbook of attempted suicide, ch 35, pp 617-630. Wiley, New York

Appleby L, Shaw J, Amos T et al 1999 Safer services: national confidential inquiry into suicide and homicide by people with mental illness. Department of Health, London

Atha C, Salkovskis PMG, Storer D 1992 CBT problem solving in the treatment of patients attending a medical emergency department: a controlled trial. Journal of Psychosomatic Research 36(4):299-307

Barker P 2000 The Tidal model: from theory to practice. University of Newcastle, Newcastle

Barker P 2001 The Tidal model: developing an empowering, person-centred approach to recovery within psychiatric and mental health nursing. Journal of Psychiatric and Mental Health Nursing 8(3):233-240

Barker P, Cutcliffe JR 1999 Clinical risk: a need for engagement not observation. Mental Health Care 2(8):8-12

Barre T, Evans R 2002 Nursing observations in the acute in-patient setting: a contribution to the debate. Mental Health Practice 5(10):10-14

Beck J 1996 Cognitive therapy: basics and beyond. Guilford, New York

Clifford PI 1995 The FACE outcomes programme: validation of the approach. Report to the Department of Health, London. University College London Centre for Outcomes Research and Effectiveness

Department of Health 1998a The new NHS – modern and dependable. HMSO, London

Department of Health 1998b A first class service. Quality in the new NHS. HMSO, London

Department of Health 1999 The National Service Framework for mental health. Department of Health, London

Department of Health 2002 Mental health policy implementation guide: adult acute inpatient care provision. Crown Publications, London

Department of Health 2003 Preventing suicide: a toolkit for mental health services. Department of Health, London

Evans K, Tyrer P, Catalan J et al 1999 Manual assisted cognitive behaviour therapy (MACT): a randomized control trial of a brief intervention with bibliotherapy in the treatment of recurrent deliberate self harm. Psychological Medicine 29(1):19-25

Forsyth AS 2003 Cutting through hopelessness. Mental Health Practice 6(8):8

Greenberger D, Padesky C 1995 Mind over mood: change how you feel by changing the way you think. Guilford Press, New York

Hawton K 1997 Attempted suicide. In Clark CM, Fairburn CG (eds) Science and practice of cognitive behaviour therapy, ch 12, pp 285-312. Oxford University Press, Oxford

Hawton K, Townsend E, Arensman E et al 2002 Psychosocial and pharmacological treatments for deliberate self harm. [Review] Volume (issue 4) The Cochrane Database of Systematic Reviews. The Cochrane Library, The Cochrane Collaboration

Hinshelwood RD 1999 The difficult patient. British Journal of Psychiatry 174:187-199

Jones A 1999 A modernized mental health service: the role of care pathways. Journal of Nursing Management 7(6):331-338

Lindgren BM, Wilstrand C, Gilje F et al 2004 Struggling for hopefulness: a qualitative study of Swedish women who self harm. Acta Psychiatrica Scandinavica 11(3):284-291

McAllister M 2001 In harm's way; hidden aspects of deliberate self harm. Journal of Psychiatric and Mental Health Nursing 8:391-398

NHS Modernisation Agency 2002 A step-by-step guide to developing protocols. NHS Modernisation Agency, London

National Institute for Clinical Excellence (2004) Self-harm: short term physical and psychological management and secondary prevention of intentional self harm in primary and secondary care. National Institute for Clinical Excellence, London

Neilson P, Brennan W 2001 The use of special observations: an audit within a psychiatric unit. Journal of Psychiatric and Mental Health Nursing 8:147-155

Raj MSJ, Kumaraiah V, Bhide AV 2001 Cognitive behavioural intervention in deliberate self harm. Acta Psychiatrica Scandinavica 104(5):340-345

Reid W, Long A 1993 The role of the nurse providing therapeutic care for the suicidal patient. Journal of Advanced Nursing 18:1369-1376

Samuelson M, Wilklander M, Asberg M et al 2000 Psychiatric care as seen by the attempted suicide patient. Acta Psychiatrica Scandinavica 32(3):635-643

Sharkey V 2003 Self-wounding: a literature review. Mental Health Practice 6(7):35-37

Shepherd C, McAllister M 2003 CARE: a framework for responding therapeutically to the client who self-harms. Journal of Psychiatric and Mental Health Nursing 10:442-447

Speedy S 1999 The therapeutic alliance. In: Clinton M, Nelson S (eds) Advanced practice in mental health nursing. Blackwell Science, Oxford

Stephenson C, Barker P, Fletcher E 2002 Judgment days: developing and evaluation of an innovative nursing model. Journal of Psychiatric and Mental Health Nursing 9(3):271-276

Tyrer P, Tom B, Byford S et al 2004 Differential effects of manual assisted cognitive behaviour therapy in the treatment of recurrent deliberate self harm and personality disturbance: the POPMACT study. Journal of Personality Disorders 18(1):102-116

Weiner B 1980 A cognitive (attribution) – emotion-action model of motivated behaviour: an analysis of judgments of help giving. Journal of Personality and Social Psychology 39:186-200

Using an eating disorders integrated care pathway for child and adolescent mental health services

Marie Rawdon, Richard Oldham and Julie Lambert

INTRODUCTION	**IMPLEMENTATION**
BACKGROUND	**OUTCOMES AND CONCLUSIONS**
PATHWAY DEVELOPMENT	**REFERENCES**

INTRODUCTION

The purpose of this chapter is to share our experiences of integrated care pathway (ICP) development in this specialist service. In order to do this adequately, we will first clarify the core target client group who access the pathway. Throughout this chapter we will make reference to eating disorders. Whilst we recognise that this description generally encompasses four classifications, we ask readers to be aware that the ICP discussed in this chapter has been specifically developed for those experiencing anorexia nervosa and bulimia nervosa. To access the pathway in this service the young person would have been previously diagnosed under the following International Classification for Disease (ICD) classifications:

ICD 10 (F50.0) Anorexia nervosa: A disorder characterised by deliberate weight loss, induced and sustained by the patient. There is usually under-nutrition of varying severity, with secondary endocrine and metabolic changes and disturbances of bodily function. The symptoms include restricted dietary choice, excessive exercise, induced vomiting and purgation, and use of appetite suppressants and diuretics (World Health Organisation 1994, p 197).

ICD 10 (F50.2) Bulimia nervosa: A syndrome characterised by repeated bouts of overeating and an excessive preoccupation with the control of body weight, leading to a pattern of overeating followed by vomiting or use of purgatives. This disorder shares many psychological features with anorexia nervosa. Repeated vomiting is likely to give rise to disturbances of body electrolytes and physical complications (World Health Organisation 1994, p 199).

Eating disorders experienced by children and adolescents continue to be a serious problem and can result in premature death or long-term medical conditions (Sigman 1995). Caring for or living with the young person therefore creates many concerns and anxiety for professionals, individuals and families/carers. For example, in our clinical setting, such concerns were highlighted when a newly qualified nurse discussed these feelings within a clinical supervision situation. The newly qualified nurse expressed feelings of anxiety related to lack of skills and experience when working with young people with an eating disorder. After discussion, these perceptions were shared with colleagues who themselves expressed similar concerns. In turn this led to a decision to commence a proactive multidisciplinary approach towards the care of adolescents with eating disorders in our clinical setting, the aim being to improve the experience of receiving care, relieve these feelings and improve knowledge and skills. By using a reflective approach we entered into the process of learning through experience. This in turn empowered us to develop a focus for change. From this point the clinical team agreed to the concept of developing and implementing an ICP to work with young people admitted to the inpatient setting who were experiencing an eating disorder (Honig & Sharman 2000).

The rationale for choosing an ICP approach came from the concerns experienced and the desire of the team to have the right people doing the right things during the process of care. We had the collective intention that the right outcome would be achieved with the entire focus being on the young person's experience (National Health Service (NHS) Information Authority 2003). The team were aware that on occasions the care received by young people and their families was previously inconsistent. The staff team wanted to work in a positive way with young people and avoid negative conceptualisation, which resorted to labelling individuals as divisive or difficult. It was felt the development of an ICP would offer guidelines and direction; it would increase skills, knowledge and thus increase morale and confidence.

BACKGROUND

Within our locality, the patient journey for young people experiencing an eating disorder often begins with consultation with a general practitioner (GP). The GP then completes a referral to the Child and Adolescent Mental Health Services (CAMHS). Whether initiated by a parent, school nurse, teacher or social/health worker, often by the time GP consultation is sought, the young person has reached a point where symptoms match the criteria set within the ICD 10 (World Health Organisation 1994). A crisis point has probably already been reached. Delay in seeking advice may be prolonged due to the young person's ambivalence about whether they have a problem and the feeling of being out of control (Paterson 2002). Carers may struggle to recognise that there is a problem until this stage as weight loss is often gradual (Lask & Bryant-Waugh 2000). In addition, baggy clothing may be used to hide the weight loss. Consequently, due to the young person's entrenched thought processes, they are usually reluctant to visit the doctor (Paterson 2002). For the specialist mental health services, information from the GP referral is important, as assessment of the young person's health begins at this point. Height and weight are obviously pertinent to the initial assessment as to whether or not the young person is in any physical danger (Rome et al 2003). This in turn affects how quickly the individual is seen and what services are offered.

If it is required, admission to the child and adolescent inpatient service can be planned. In which case this follows the route shown in Figure 11.1, or an alternative emergency admission is triggered. The action taken in an emergency is very much dependent on the clinical judgment of the consultant psychiatrist at that time. Admission is used as a last resort where there is high risk of physical complications as a consequence of weight loss. As with any admission process consent to treatment needs to be ascertained. Prior to the development of the care pathway, parents and young people would consent to 'generalised treatment'. We believe that promoting informed consent enables the young person to understand fully what is being proposed (Christensen & Kockrow 1999), whilst promoting independence is key to working with children and families. Developing and maintaining trust are paramount in working with anyone experiencing a mental health problem (Graham 1999). However, it is known that the ongoing conflicts associated with the psychology of eating disorders can significantly influence levels

Figure 11.1
High-level process map showing access to the Child and Adolescent Mental Health Service for those experiencing an eating disorder

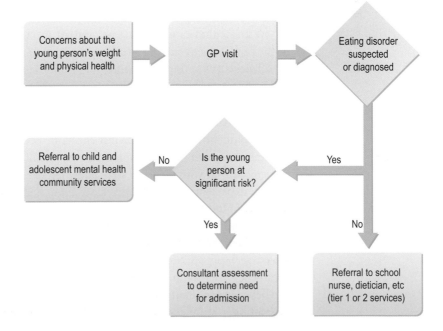

of trust (Paterson 2002). We feel that one of the most important and helpful tools in guiding the young person through their difficulties and strengthening trust is honesty. This needs to start right from admission at the beginning of the pathway and involves consent. Prior to beginning ICP development we reflected on how we could be honest with the young person, if we had no clear treatment plan (Cochrane 1998). Young people and their parents were signing consent to treatment whilst we questioned what they were signing for. What does 'treatment' mean? These are some of the questions that needed to be answered by care pathway development if possible.

To clarify our care process or treatment, we felt we needed to embark on a process involving young people, their families and multidisciplinary team members. The team consisted of nursing staff, consultant psychiatrists, a staff grade doctor, social worker, art therapist, psychologist, psychotherapist, dietician and housekeeping staff. This also meant becoming familiar with research and literature appertaining to management of an eating disorder. Our philosophy was to combine this information with clinical experience and the views of young people and their families. This would attempt to not only answer the questions about the care process, but enable an outcome that could be put into practice, and make a difference. Previously we had used 'generalised' consent to treatment and no specific nursing care plans. This left individual nurses to devise plans of care with the young person. Whilst we do not dispute the use of individualised care or care plans, our discussions and experiences told us that in cases there had been inconsistencies that directly affected the effectiveness of interventions and the progress of recovery. Prior to the ICP this was borne out in inequality, variation and inconsistencies in our approach to care. We recognised that different nursing staff planned care differently, and different shifts delivered care differently. This was not always intentional but could clearly impact upon the experience of receiving care.

We know that care plans are recognised and used amongst the broad spectrum of the care services and are a fundamental element to the nursing process (Schultz & Videbeck 1998). But we wanted to go one step further, with an ICP that would bring theory and practice experience together. This would then offer a sound guideline that encompasses the needs of young people who are experiencing an eating disorder whilst ensuring that professionals are offering a consistent service and 'singing from the same hymn sheet'. In preparation for developing the ICP we examined with young people and their families typical patient journeys. It was recognised that young people were admitted to the inpatient unit, perhaps having already experienced community care. They had received treatment for physical health problems or received interventions focusing on psychological well-being. Young people described the value of becoming gradually reintegrated to home and mainstream school during an inpatient stay. It was described how, following discharge, appropriate arrangements needed to be made to either continue or commence follow-up at home. It was agreed that the ICP needed to bridge the gap between inpatient and community services, offering a consistent approach and promoting a 'seamless service' (Department of Health 2005, p 1).

Young people told us that the fact they spend a good proportion of their day at school needed to be factored in to the ICP. For the young person experiencing an eating disorder, school is often a 'prime time' to skip breaks/snacks or throw lunch away. Schools involved with our service wanted to collaborate to promote the best interests of the young person, but often considered themselves to be lacking an adequate knowledge base and the relevant skills to manage situations during school time. This is also highlighted in the National Service Framework for Children, Young People and Maternity Services (Department of Health 2004). During preparation for pathway development, discussion clearly identified that transitions between inpatient and community care should be considered to offer a more cohesive approach. This is considered at various stages in the pathway although particularly evident in the green (latter) stage of the care pathway, which specifically prepares for the transition period between inpatient care and the involvement of the community mental health team. The experiences of young people and their families highlighted the need for communication between services across the tiers of the service (see Figure 11.2). Tier 1, in most cases (with the exception of an emergency), would be the first services encountered by a young person experiencing mental health related concerns. Tier 2 bridges the gap between Tiers 1 and 3 and is where many specialist assessments occur. An example of a professional working within Tier 2 is a primary mental health worker. Within Tier 3, there are services provided by multidisciplinary teams, who offer specialist community support to young people and their families. Tier 4 is the provision of more intensive support within an inpatient setting. In developing a comprehensive care pathway we needed to ensure continuity across the tiers of the service where this is needed.

Figure 11.2
The structure of Child and Adolescent Mental Health Services – the four-tier service. The mental health needs of children are described using a four-tier service model. Tier 4 describes the most intensive interventions offered by child and adolescent mental health services for those experiencing more severe or complex problems, whilst Tier 1 describes services providing brief interventions offered by a range of services

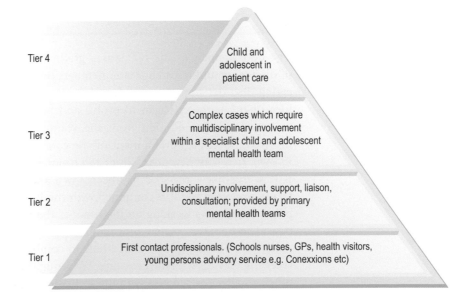

Tier 4 — Child and adolescent in patient care

Tier 3 — Complex cases which require multidisciplinary involvement within a specialist child and adolescent mental health team

Tier 2 — Unidisciplinary involvement, support, liaison, consultation; provided by primary mental health teams

Tier 1 — First contact professionals. (Schools nurses, GPs, health visitors, young persons advisory service e.g. Conexxions etc)

Previous clinical experience and discussions with young people and their families clarified that anorexia nervosa and bulimia nervosa hugely impact on the family unit. The experience can place much strain on family members and carers. Family therapy, therefore, was indicated as an essential component of the care pathway by all stakeholders and the literature (Atkins & Warner 2000). Family therapy sessions are based on psychological principles (National Institute of Clinical Excellence (NICE) 2004). Guidelines suggest that individuals experiencing an eating disorder may experience a degree of developmental conflict; between the need to individuate and the need to conform to the professed expectations of families (Steinberg-Nye & Johnson 1999). Prior to the implementation of the care pathway, the forms of interventions offered were somewhat arbitrary and very much depended on the skills and judgment of individual clinicians. By delivering a research-based ICP we hoped to ensure that families are offered the therapeutic interventions that are the most effective. The NICE guidelines for the management of eating disorders, although not published at the time of development, later confirmed that 'you should be admitted to a unit that is skilled in increasing people's levels of nutrients, you should be closely monitored in the first few days whilst this is happening' (National Institute for Clinical Excellence 2004, p. 4). Inpatient treatment for anorexia nervosa should also consist of a structured psychological treatment to help gain weight; this should focus upon eating habits, attitudes to weight and shape, and feelings about gaining weight. Physical weight should be closely monitored (National Institute for Clinical Excellence 2004). The general crux of our motivation for the development of the care pathway clearly revolved around the consistency, equality and effectiveness of care. Motivated by deficiencies in our current practice and armed with the determination that all young people, families, carers and professionals could work together to change this, we set out to develop the ICP.

PATHWAY DEVELOPMENT

The development of the ICP was a gradual process which took many months of discussion and research. Team members took the opportunity to visit specialist eating disorder units to consider the approaches offered by other services. The idea of the pathway began to evolve and became underpinned by enthusiasm, motivation and dedication from the young people, families and professionals involved. Soon the development of the care pathway began to take on a life of its own, rich with new possibilities and room for growth. We began to think of the ICP as tree-like – the seed had been sown and brought about hope for change. Development of the ICP continued with the ICP interest group, including young people and carers working on the roots of the pathway – this being the evidence base. The literature review process formally began and this was shared amongst the group. The group considered how to combine experiences from practice and receiving services with the literature. We brought into this the lessons learned from others during our contacts with the specialist services we had visited.

Essentially, this became both a reflective and proactive process, whereby elements of practice from all these sources were discussed and adapted to embrace the philosophy of care of the unit.

We believe in supporting the well-being of young people and their families, building on their courage, knowledge and strengths.

We related this to the research, working within the parameters of local Trust policy and professional codes of conduct. As suggested previously at the time of ICP development, the NICE guidelines for the management of eating disorders (National Institute for Clinical Excellence 2004) had not been published. Undoubtedly this would have made the task of reviewing the literature and incorporating theoretical evidence much easier. Indeed, when these guidelines did become available, the ICP content was reviewed to ensure concordance and to see if any changes were needed.

Having gathered all of this knowledge, the next stage was to consider where to apply the evidence in the patient journey. What would be beneficial to the care process and what would work in practice, for the young person, their family and the team? We felt the only way to do this was to continue to involve all stakeholders, our philosophy being that this is a young person focused care pathway and its content needed to reflect their individual thoughts and needs relating to their recovery. Young people and their carers continued to volunteer and were involved in structured discussions about the ICP content. Collaboratively we identified areas for practice change or practice based upon previous positive outcomes. It was at this point we had a new care pathway in map form and we began to consider a format that would make it accessible to colleagues.

Continuing our tree-like model of ICP development, we considered this as the move from the root to the trunk, the trunk then resembling the content of the patient journey, and particularly modelling what interventions would happen at what stage. It was at this point we devised the three stages of the ICP, now more commonly recognised as the red, amber and green stages of the ICP. These three stages enabled us to conceptualise stages of the patient journey and allowed us to map activities on a continuum. The red stage represents the part of the process where young people are most physically unwell. They have a low body mass index and require intensive psychological stabilisation and interventions to prevent severe physical deterioration. The need to establish a therapeutic relationship is critical. The red stage interventions begin to reduce the symptoms of the eating disorder and include monitoring physical health, regular observations, recording dietary intake and output, establishing a base weight and assessing and maintaining skin integrity. Decreasing the obsessive preoccupations with food is important, as is being mindful of the re-feeding syndrome and the need to relieve tiredness and depression.

The amber stage corresponds with a stage where young people are less physically at risk and more able to focus upon their psychological self and assume more gradual autonomy. Interventions at this stage start to encompass psychological treatments, as well as continuing to monitor physical health and well-being throughout the care journey. The green stage represents a period of increased independence, skills development and decision-making. The young person is now able to demonstrate independence and autonomy towards their care package, working towards extended leave and discharge. Psychological interventions and physical health monitoring continue through this stage. Here we also note that the young person may proceed to the next stage of the ICP and then, due to circumstances, return to a previous stage in the journey. The green, amber and red stages can been seen in the process map shown in Figure 11.3. Pooling together the feedback of all stakeholders was key to the development of these stages.

Once the pathway content had been formulated, we began to work within the multidisciplinary team, raising awareness, promoting knowledge and improving skills. We used this time to gain feedback from the team about the pathway so that full cooperation for implementation was secured by this preparation. Example extracts of the 29-page paper pathway in use are shown in Appendix 11.1. At the time of writing, we have moved on to the branches of the tree in our model of development. From undertaking this process there has been evidence of growth, both personal and professional. Since implementing the ICP we have considered how it can be further developed. We are extending the boundaries of the ICP. Early intervention and prevention are of vital importance, and evidence suggests that early recognition of eating disorders can prevent full development of the illness and the subsequent need for inpatient treatment (Rome et al 2003). Although prevention was considered at the initial stage of developing the ICP, we did not pursue it any further at that time. We have now begun to develop closer links with the primary mental health team, extending education about eating disorders into this service and their involvement in the green stage of the ICP. In time, we may see this early intervention initiative grow to schools and GPs. Additionally we have begun liaising and improving communication with local paediatric wards. The aim of this is to promote good practice between services. We have facilitated learning sessions, sharing knowledge and skills, and gained feedback as to how best to support each other in promoting the mental well-being of young people and their families. Also, families using the pathway have made us aware of a lack of local parent/support groups. We feel that this is yet another branch of the ICP to be developed in the future. Our overall 'tree-like' model of ICP development is shown in Figure 11.4.

IMPLEMENTATION

We feel that implementation of the ICP is appropriately illustrated by outlining a case study. The details used are purely fictitious but describe how a young person can progress along the ICP. Alice is a 14-year-old girl who presents on the surface as a confident, bubbly, young adolescent. However, during the assessment with her parents it transpires that although Alice previously had a good network of friends she has become more socially withdrawn and isolated. Alice's mother states

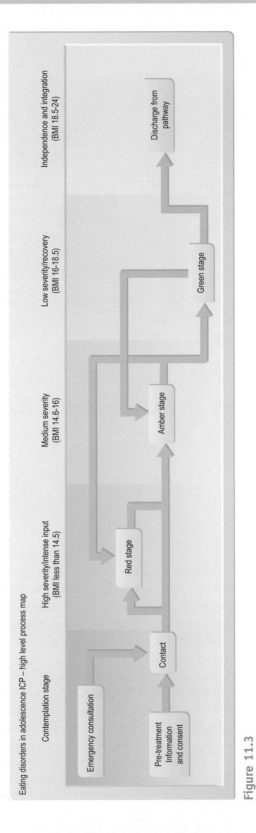

Figure 11.3
High-level map of the red, amber and green stages

Figure 11.4
The 'tree-like' model of
ICP development

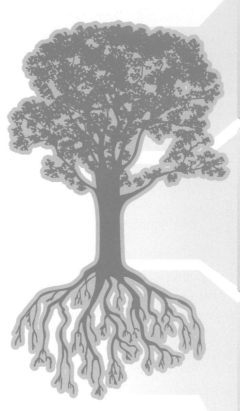

The branches – review, evaluation and
future development
• Audit/review
• Development of steering group
  (teachers, school nurses)
• Liaison with other professionals
• Involvement of primary mental health workers
• Education of different stakeholders
• Contribution of user groups
• Development of a parenting/support group

The trunk – patient journey, process and content
• Development of the process map
• Production of the ICP document
• Preparation for practice change
• Piloting
• Presentations to different stakeholders
• Continued regular meetings with core
  ICP developers
• Training to ICP users
• Evaluation via team, family and
  service user feedback
• Internal and external review of the content

Roots – the concept, background
and evidence base
• Literature searches
• Review of evidence
• Reflection on practice
• Clinical experience
• Clinical supervision
• Courses/training specifically related to
  eating disorders
• Special interest groups (professions and
  service users – gaining views and ideas)
• Visits to other services

that Alice spends the majority of her time in her bedroom and she is not mixing with her siblings. Alice refuses to join the family at mealtimes. Her mother said that Alice makes excuses like she has already eaten, etc. Her mother and father amicably separated 2 years ago. Alice and her siblings still have regular contact with their father. He has a new partner with whom he now lives.

Alice had a planned admission to the inpatient child and adolescent unit. The school had contacted her mother when Alice's friend had approached the school nurse and reported that Alice was vomiting every lunchtime. The school advised her mother that Alice was undertaking extra exercise activities every lunch time and attending several after-school exercise activities. They also informed her mother that over the last 6 months Alice had become more socially withdrawn, choosing to spend the majority of her time with just one close friend. Her mother then took Alice to the doctor who made the referral to the child and adolescent mental health team. At this time, Alice's BMI (body mass index) was 14. Alice had a slow irregular pulse, low blood pressure, secondary amenorrhoea and severe malnutrition.

Alice's mother states that Alice is academically a high achiever but over the last couple of months she has been finding the pressure of academic work too much. During the admission process Alice talked about being fat, ugly and that she has no friends. Her mother suggests that Alice only sleeps for a couple of hours each night and that previously Alice used to enjoy going to the cinema with her friends but now lacks any enthusiasm and finds it difficult to concentrate on tasks. Alice refuses to go out unless she is taken in the car and her mother feels that this is due to Alice having low self-esteem and that she is lacking in confidence. Her mother and father are very supportive of Alice, but unaware of the implications of Alice having an eating disorder.

Alice was assessed by the team, who took an in-depth holistic view of the situation. Pre-admission information was given to the family relating to the integrated care pathway and the various stages involved. The philosophy of care, possible therapies and information about eating disorders were also given at this time. Consent for treatment was obtained and the family discussed the contract of care and what this would entail. Alice and her family began on the pathway at the red stage. The integrated care pathway is a structured intervention ensuring that Alice and her family's journey is negotiated, managed and agreed. It remained the responsibility of the professionals to ensure that the journey is flexible enough to take into consideration Alice's individual needs.

Once admitted, it was agreed that Alice would benefit from intensive individual one-to-one support as described in the red stage. Three main factors contributed to this decision: a low BMI, physical symptoms of malnutrition and poor psychological well-being. Due to Alice's intense fear of food, an inability to control her impulse to exercise, vomiting and her poor physical health, it was advised that Alice take bed rest, with physical health monitoring. Initially, meals were taken away from peers alongside staff, so as to provide monitoring and support. Food and eating around peers increased Alice's anxiety; therefore a process of desensitisation and intensive one-to-one support began to promote Alice's privacy and dignity during this difficult time. Alice was weighed twice per week, once on a regular day and once randomly. This continued throughout all stages of the ICP. Alice was able to omit five foods from her diet after discussion with her dietician and named nurse. Various assessments were implemented throughout the stages to monitor Alice's mood and attitude towards eating.

As suggested by the progress described in the ICP, Alice began to gain around 1 kg per week until she progressed to the amber stage of the ICP. Alice accessed and benefited from ongoing family therapy, individual therapy with her named nurse and art therapy (as well as other interventions from varying members of the team). Alice began to increase her independence during the amber stage and began having meals in the dining room with staff and peers, as well as taking weekend leave. Once Alice achieved the weight gain that indicated progression to the green stage, she continued to access the therapeutic interventions offered before. However, her autonomy increased to the point where Alice went back into mainstream school and had extended leave once her target weight had been reached. At this point Tier 3 services commenced more contacts with Alice and her family with a view to continuing support following discharge.

OUTCOMES AND CONCLUSIONS

We have begun to consider the outcomes of the implementation of this ICP. To date, there has been anecdotal feedback which supports continued efforts towards further development and evaluation. One of the main benefits has been the use of a process that enables the team to involve the young person and family from the start of their journey towards recovery. We have a live guideline which we can use pre-admission, on admission and throughout the inpatient stay. This helps us to discuss the pathway of care, empowering the young person and their family with knowledge of what to expect and, most importantly, to incorporate what they expect. We agree that evaluation is integral to the implementation of change in healthcare provision and this ICP warrants such attention (Pollit et al 2001). Our formative means of evaluating the ICP were to observe and discuss its use with team members, asking how they viewed the changes of practice involved in the ICP. Discussion occurred on an individual basis and within multidisciplinary staff meetings. This helped us to gauge the professional response to the ICP and practice changes. After time other techniques were used to consider the progress of the ICP.

Further individual and multidisciplinary discussions and use of questionnaires centred upon how the team felt the ICP document performed and whether they found it usable, i.e. the ease of interpretation. Some queries were raised and answered, and impressions were generally favourable. Time was taken to observe whether the practice changes anticipated were incorporated into day-to-day care. It was most notable that this had occurred by reflecting on how the individual young person's care is being negotiated and importantly whether the interventions described in the ICP are being offered. Examples of interventions introduced since the development of the ICP are: formal family therapy, family meals and parenting sessions. There is post-ICP an all-round clarity of care and expectations and increased promotion of young people's autonomy, especially regarding dietary requirements and care. Although these observations may be considered as subjective it is our impression that there have been observed changes in practice since using the pathway. A noticeable change is that staff informally report feeling more autonomous and empowered working with young people and their families. What is noticeable is that there is collaboration beyond the named nurse; the young person's relationship and continuity and understanding moves beyond this to wider relationships. Feedback from the team and young people confirm that the environment in general has become more productive and supportive towards the needs of the young person. This perhaps cannot be directly attributed solely to using the ICP, although the development process has certainly impacted upon collaboration and teamworking.

We have had discussions with young people in regard to their impressions of care whist the ICP has been used. This has been investigated on an individual face-to-face basis and during a user/carer feedback day where the ICP was presented in full and feedback was given by young people and their families. The parents and young people involved stated that they liked the structure that the ICP offered and felt it empowered them to work alongside professionals. It was also suggested that they had clarity in knowing what to expect, which relieved their anxieties. Parents also added that it gave them some guidance as how to help the young person at home. The young people reported that they valued the level of honesty and ability to mark their progress along a journey. We have been able to consult several young people involved in the ICP development about the content of this account who agreed that it does truly reflect a young person's feelings on the experience of developing the ICP. We intend to add a more substantial evaluation to our plans and further assess the use of the ICP. Most importantly, we believe that this will help us to determine any future ICP developments.

PART 1 – PRE ADMISSION RED STAGE (INPATIENT) CONTRACT

To be completed and copied as required prior to commencing the Red Stage

When the young person's Body Mass Index is below 14.5 he or she can be admitted to this inpatient unit and cared for as described in the "red" stage of this care pathway. Later the young person can proceed to the "amber" and "green" stages as he or she progresses. Occasionally due to circumstances the young person may return back to a previous stage in the pathway. Information about the "red" "amber" and "green" stages are contained in the accompanying information leaflet.

If the care offered becomes compromised for any reason, a review of the contract will be arranged at the earliest opportunity.

Specific aims of the "red" stage are for the young person to:

- Achieve adequate nutrition, hydration, elimination resulting in adequate electrolyte and fluid balance
- Eliminate signs and symptoms of malnutrition
- Gain weight as appropriate
- Attain an appropriate state of physical health
- Begin to reduce the symptoms of the eating disorder and desire an appropriate state of physical health
- Maintain skin integrity
- Decrease obsessive preoccupations with food
- Reduce the urge to binge eat/purge
- Relieve tiredness and depression
- Improve sleep and ability to meet self care needs
- Approach carers for help and support

Long-term aims are for the young person to:

- Maintain appropriate food and fluid intake habits
- Demonstrate the beginning of ability to meet basic needs or ask for help
- Experience decreased symptoms of an Eating Disorder.
- Verbalize anxieties and concerns

I/we agree to work within the above contract.
I/we have got a copy of the following information; "stages" leaflet, families' philosophy
of care, information on possible therapies and the information leaflet for parents and families.
I have had this explained by a health care professional.

Signed:

Date:

Appendix 11.1

PART 3 – RED STAGE INITIAL INTERVENTIONS

3. PRACTICE GUIDE
It is expected that these activities have been completed unless they are recorded as a variance

Code	Activity completed by the Nursing Staff at the beginning of the RED Stage
1.1	The young person and family have received and had explained the information detailed in the red stage contract
1.2	The client and family have completed the red stage contract
1.3	Weight at the beginning of the red stage is _____
1.4	The current body mass index is _____ (date & sign)
1.5	The plateau weight is _____ for progression onto the next (amber) stage; this weight is suggested to be 1/3 of the overall target weight for discharge
1.6	The scheme for exercise and progression are recorded below
	Activity completed by the Medical Staff at the beginning of the RED Stage
1.7	Assessment of Capacity, Consent, Mental and Physical State
1.8	Review prescribing & initial plan and case review process explained
1.9	Investigations requested HB ☐ ESR ☐ FBC ☐ Other (please state) U&Es ☐ LFTs ☐ ECG ☐
1.10	State as required: Continued monitoring of physical state (i.e. TPR, Bloods etc)

Coordinated by: (date, time & sign)

4. MEAL GUIDE
Discussed with the client and completed by the Named Nurse/Nominated other

WARNING: Regarding re-feeding; avoid overloading the system prematurely

MEAL	PLANNED DURATION
Breakfast	Maximum 45 minutes working towards 30 minutes Or state otherwise:
Lunch & Tea	Maximum I hour working towards 35 minutes Or state otherwise:
Breaks & Supper	Maximum 30 minutes working towards 15 minutes Or state otherwise:

Appendix 11.1   (Continued)

5. PROGRESS PLAN   Discussed with the client and completed by the Named Nurse/Nominated other

Exercise, Mealtimes, Privacy & Self Care:

Progress and Contingencies:

Recorded by: (date, time & sign)

Appendix 11.1   (*Continued*)

PART 16 – GREEN STAGE INITIAL INTERVENTIONS

21. PRACTICE GUIDE   It is expected that these activities have been completed unless they are recorded as a variance

Code	Activity completed by Named Nurse or Nominated other	
5.1	The young person and family have received and had explained the information detailed in the green stage contract	
5.2	The young person and family have completed the green stage contract	
5.3	Weight at the beginning of the green stage is _____	
5.4	The current body mass index is _____	
5.5	The plateau weight _____ at the point of discharge	(date & sign)

PART 17 – GREEN STAGE INTERVENTIONS

22. PRACTICE GUIDE   It is expected that these activities have been completed unless they are recorded as a variance

Code	Activity maintained by all Nursing Staff
5.6	The young person has complete autonomy to exercise
5.7	Meals are taken with peers and without supervision
5.8	No supervision is required after meals
5.9	The young person can make and receive phone calls as per the unit policy
5.10	Visiting times are not restricted apart from those guidelines already set by the unit
5.11	The overall target weight is achieved and maintained for 2 weeks prior to discharge
5.12	The Individual Therapy Plan and school activity continues
5.13	The young person accepts full individual responsibility for day to day care
5.14	The young person orders meals without supervision
5.15	Dietary intake no longer needs to be recorded
5.16	The young person is weighed once a month at random
5.17	Supervision is on normal unit terms, i.e. minimal supervision to encourage independence
	Activity by the Multidisciplinary Team
5.19	Weekly review of progress and interventions
	Individualised Interventions (activities offered and not described above) (date, time, sign)
	Coordinated by: (date, time & sign)

23. VARIANCE RECORDING   Only complete when recommended & individualised interventions do not occur as suggested

Code	Date, Time & Sign	Code	Date, Time & Sign

Appendix 11.1   (*Continued*)

PART 18 – GREEN STAGE PREPARATION FOR DISCHARGE

24. RELAPSE INDICATORS

25. CONTINGENCY PLAN

Detailing the arrangements to be used at key points after discharge

Nature of response to a crisis/out of hours

26. PRACTICE GUIDE   It is expected that these activities have been completed unless they are recorded as a variance

Code	Activity maintained by all Nursing Staff
6.1	Weekend leave progresses towards extended leave with an overall aim of discharge.
6.2	To attend the unit as an day-patient
6.3	The young person actively participates in discharge planning, including community workers/services/family
6.4	The young person and family are aware of help-line and contingency arrangements
6.5	The young person has an outpatients appointment prior to discharge
6.6	The young person and family have met on occasions prior to discharge the person who is responsible for their aftercare
	Activity by the Multidisciplinary Team
6.7	Review of progress and interventions
Individualised Interventions (activities offered and not described above)	

Coordinated by: (date, time & sign)

27. VARIANCE RECORDING   Only complete when recommended & individualised interventions do not occur as suggested

Code	Date, Time & Sign		Code	Date, Time & Sign

28. PROGRESS

Discharge Return to Amber Stage Agreed	(date, time & sign)

Appendix 11.1   *(Continued)*

Acknowledgements   We would like to take this opportunity to thank all the young people, their families and other team members involved in developing this ICP. Our thanks also to Sarah Cimgioula for her inspiration and support in the early stages of development.

REFERENCES

Atkins L, Warner B 2000 Systemic family therapy in the treatment of eating disorders. In: Hindmarsh T (ed) Eating disorders: a multiprofessional approach, ch 7, pp 107-134. Whurr, London & Philadelphia

Christensen, B, Kockrow E 1999 Foundations of nursing, 3rd edn. Mosby, USA

Cochrane C 1998 Eating regulation responses and eating disorders. In: Stuart G, Laraia M (eds) Principles and Practices of Psychiatric Nursing 6th edn, ch 25, pp 523-543 Mosby, USA

Department of Health 2004 National service framework for children and maternity services: executive summary. Department of Health, London

Department of Health 2005 Care services efficiency delivery programme. www.dh.gov.uk/policyandguidance/healthandsocialcare/healthandsocialcarearticle/fs/en?CONTENTUNDERSCOREID=4089166&mIxVT8. Accessed 11/01/05

Graham P 1999 Ethics and child psychiatry. In: Bloch S, Chodoff P, Green SA (eds) Psychiatric ethics 3rd edn. Oxford University Press, Oxford

Honig P, Sharman W 2000 Inpatient management. In: Lask B, Bryant-Waugh R (eds) Anorexia nervosa and related eating disorders in childhood and adolescence 2nd edn, ch 13, pp 265-303. Psychology Press, UK

Lask B, Bryant-Waugh R 2000 Anorexia nervosa and related eating disorders in childhood and adolescence 2nd edn. Psychology Press, New York

National Health Service Information Authority 2003 Care pathways know-how zone: about integrated care pathways (ICPs). http://www.nelh.nhs.uk/carepathways/icp Accessed 21.12.2004. Last updated on: 16.01.2003

National Institute for Clinical Excellence 2004 Eating disorders: anorexia nervosa, bulimia nervosa and related eating disorders. understanding NICE guidance; a guide for people with eating disorders, their advocates and carers, and the public. NHS, London

Paterson A 2002 Diet of despair, a book about eating disorders for young people and their families. Lucky Duck Publishing, Bristol

Pollit D, Beck C, Hungler B 2001 Essentials of nursing research: methods, appraisal and utilization 5th edn. Lippincott, New York

Rome E, Ammerman S, Rosen D et al 2003 Children and adolescents with eating disorders: the state of the art. Paediatrics 111(1):98-108

Schultz J, Videbeck S 1998 Lippincott's manual of psychiatric nursing care plans 5th edn. Lippincotts/Raven Publishers, Philadelphia

Sigman G 1995 How has the care of eating disorder patients been altered and upset by payment and insurance issues? Let me count the ways. Journal Adolescent Health 16:415

Steinberg-Nye S, Johnson CL 1999 Eating disorders. In: Netherton S, Holmes D, Walker C (eds) Child and adolescent psychological disorders; a comprehensive textbook, ch 19, pp 397-414. Oxford University Press, Oxford

World Health Organisation 1994 The pocket guide to the ICD 10 classification of mental and behavioural disorders. Churchill Livingstone, London

Using an integrated care pathway to deliver a nurse-led clozapine clinic

Susan Wakefield, Jon Painter, Malcolm Peet and Joanna Chave

INTRODUCTION

Clozapine is an antipsychotic drug which is used in the management of treatment-resistant schizophrenia. Because clozapine is associated with the potentially fatal side effect of agranulocytosis, this drug can be prescribed only with careful monitoring procedures. Therefore, the use of clozapine lends itself to being managed by an integrated care pathway (ICP). This chapter outlines our rationale for, and experiences of, developing an ICP for our locally run nurse-led clozapine clinic.

The use of ICPs is still relatively uncommon in mental health services. In Rotherham we have been fortunate in obtaining funding for a full-time, dedicated ICP coordinator since October 2000. ICPs are an integral part of our care planning and delivery process and, for some patients, the ICP replaces the Care Programme Approach (CPA) care plan (Department of Health 1990). We have developed ICPs in several clinical areas, including the management of electroconvulsive therapy (ECT), an inpatient rehabilitation unit, an assertive outreach team and treatment with atypical antipsychotics. The aim of this chapter is to share the process of developing an ICP for use in our clozapine clinic. We will use this account to illustrate the main challenges and benefits of implementing an ICP, and we hope to 'bring alive' the process of developing and implementing an ICP and to offer insights to other mental health practitioners who are planning to undertake such an endeavour.

BACKGROUND

ICPs are particularly useful in situations where numerous professionals are involved in the care-giving process, and where breakdowns in communication could lead to adverse patient care (De Luc, 2001). In addition, any situation where there is an inherent potential for risk, requiring management and reduction, can also benefit. Both phenomena are evident in the prescribing and administration of the antipsychotic medication clozapine. The defined administration and monitoring procedures for clozapine readily lend themselves to an ICP. The well written manufacturer's guidelines also support these processes. We believed, therefore, that turning these into a usable ICP would be a realistic task. This chapter therefore outlines how we developed and implemented the ICP to be used with all patients who are prescribed and receiving clozapine. The ICP starts at the pre-commencement phase of the process (before the patient has actually taken clozapine) and therefore includes such interventions as a record of the decision to prescribe clozapine (which conforms to current National Institute for Clinical Excellence (NICE) guidance on the use of clozapine). NICE advises that trials with two different antipsychotics, including one atypical, must have failed before clozapine is prescribed (National Institute for Clinical Excellence 2002). The ICP also directs clinicians towards undertaking education sessions with the service user in order to gain informed consent, and records details of the initiation and titration of clozapine through to maintenance therapy (see Appendix 12.1).

Clozapine and treatment issues

Clozapine is often effective where other antipsychotic drugs have failed (National Institute for Clinical Excellence 2002). Recent guidance recommends that clozapine should be introduced at the earliest opportunity to treat the 30% of people who suffer from schizophrenia that do not respond to treatment with other antipsychotic drugs (National Institute for Clinical Excellence 2002). Clozapine treatment requires careful monitoring because it can cause agranulocytosis and other significant side effects (British Medical Association 2004). In our experience, through talking with clinicians within our own Trust and those in other organisations, it is acknowledged that arrangements for monitoring vary widely between, and even within, NHS trusts. One increasingly popular tool to address this varition is via a specialised clozapine clinic (Camprubi et al 1996). This approach was adopted by our Trust in 2000; however, variations remained and the clinic model did not fully address the issue of consistency.

The clozapine clinic was initially set up in 2000 in order to provide a more structured service to clients, essentially 'a one-stop shop' for all clozapine-related interventions including blood sampling, side-effect monitoring and administration. Following the appointment of one of the authors as day hospital manager, and lead clinician for the clinic, the clinic was evaluated and a number of issues were highlighted which indicated that the system used required development:

- Historically, two members of nursing staff had run the clinic, one qualified, one unqualified. Over-reliance on the expertise of these two members of staff had made the clinic vulnerable. The processes that were essential for safe monitoring were only fully understood by the clinic practitioners and were, at times, unclear to the larger staff group.
- Outside of the clinic, particularly in the inpatient areas, staff awareness of, and involvement in, the clozapine treatment process was poor. Disjointed care was a particular concern to the clinic staff as it meant that even the smallest issues were diverted back to the clinic rather than being dealt with as they occurred on the wards, thereby preventing the delivery of a 'seamless service'.
- Initiation of clozapine in the inpatient area and routine monitoring at the clinic were seen as two separate entities, not as interlinked stages of the patient journey.

Having considered these issues, we believed that an ICP would be the most useful tool to improve the situation.

The rationale for using an ICP

Having identified many of the problems with our current clozapine care, and having established that an integrated care pathway was a potential solution, we began considering the benefits of ICPs in relation to each issue identified and quickly made many satisfactory links:

- ICPs fulfil clients' desire for more information about their treatment (Lovell 1995, Quirk & Lelliot 2001, Wallace et al 1999) as they provide a tangible outline of the care process (De Luc 2001).
- The development and use of ICPs enhance inter-professional communication (De Luc 2001) which, in itself, improves client satisfaction (Ricketts 1996, Wallace et al 1999).
- The development process provides an opportunity to highlight bottlenecks, address unwanted gaps/disjointed care (e.g. between ward and clinic), and avoid duplication (De Luc 2001).
- ICPs have been found to be an effective educational tool (Chan & Wong 1999) and provide the structure and guidance required to increase the competence of less experienced staff when delivering complex, evidence-based interventions.
- One benefit of using ICPs to coordinate care delivery is their ability to schedule interventions over a prolonged period of time without any being forgotten (De Luc 2001). Hunt (1991) warns that with a treatment-resistant, 'difficult to engage' client group, excessive form filling and other bureaucratic demands can significantly damage the therapeutic relationship. Whilst accurate record keeping is essential, the ICP format can minimise the impact this has on the client experience, ultimately ensuring continued engagement with the service.

An ICP for the care of patients receiving clozapine therefore seemed to provide potential solutions to the majority of the problems identified (see Table 12.1).

Table 12.1
Issues arising from evaluation of current clozapine care and potential solutions offered by an ICP

Clinical issue	Benefits derived from the process of developing integrated care pathways	Benefits derived from the operation or use of integrated care pathways
Teamwork Wider staff group not 'owning' the process or consistently following best practice guidelines	Encourages multidisciplinary and multi-agency team development Clarification of roles and responsibilities within the team Identification and agreement on standards or practice guidelines	They encourage the development of multidisciplinary clinical documentation
User involvement/ perspective Poor inter-professional communication, potential for patient dissatisfaction	The process involves a review of patient/user information and education The process ensures care is developed from a patient/user perspective	Facilitation of communication between staff and between patients/ users and staff
Evidence-based practice Wider staff group not aware of best practice guidelines, leading to an over-reliance on clinic staff expertise	A consensus is reached which ensures consistency in practice	Integration of the latest evidence-based practice and guidelines within it Structuring of the clinical documentation and information collected so that it assists in retrospective review Identification of areas for further research Provision of a dynamic tool, which can be continually reviewed and refined
Process and practice issues Disjointed process of care	Streamlining of the patient/user path or journey Highlighting of bottlenecks and unnecessary duplications	Provision of an outline of the anticipated course of treatment (template/ prompt) Provision of an aid to the day-to-day management of the individual patient/user

PATHWAY DEVELOPMENT

We were in a fortunate position as we had an enthusiastic staff team and a dedicated, full-time ICP coordinator. In our view, it is essential if a trust wishes to develop ICPs that there is a worker with time dedicated to the development and monitoring of ICPs. This is a critical success factor and ensures ICPs reflect practice and are sustainable (Wakefield & Peet 2003). Once it had been decided to develop an ICP, the first step in the process was to form a working group in order to analyse the clinic processes and take practice forward. Initially this group comprised solely of the clinic staff and the ICP coordinator who undertook a service mapping exercise. The exercise was aimed at identifying all the disciplines integral to the administration of clozapine (Peet & Wakefield 2002).

The final membership of the working group was agreed once all staff who were involved in the prescribing, administration and monitoring of clozapine had been identified. The final working group comprised:

- the ward manager (to cover the pre-commencement, initiation and transition phase)
- the day hospital manager and nursing assistant (to cover the maintenance phase and clinic-based care)
- the ICP coordinator (to ensure consistency of approach and project management)
- the mental health pharmacist (to consider the dispensing of clozapine and offer specialist advice)
- the local clozapine advisor (to ensure the ICP encompassed manufacturer's recommended guidelines and contemporary best practice).

This process was aided by the fact that the clozapine clinic and day hospital were run from the same site as the inpatient ward, and were all overseen by one psychiatrist. Medical involvement was therefore consistent, uncomplicated and supportive of both ICPs and a nurse-led initiative.

Having established the full working group, our first task was to undertake a process mapping exercise whereby the existing systems were reviewed and incorporated into an all-encompassing flow chart, allowing us to identify particularly complex areas. This ensured that vital activities/interventions would not be missed from the final care delivery process (see Figure 12.1). More importantly, it also allowed us to consider objectively and discuss the quality as well as the mere content of care; in our experience an integral part of the development of an ICP. For example, within the clinic regular blood sampling is undertaken by a member of the clinic staff, a familiar member of staff, as opposed to an impersonal phlebotomy department. This has the added benefit of allowing frank dialogue around, and monitoring of, the service user's mental state. This is important because a well designed ICP must be far more than a checklist of interventions; it must holistically address the entire service user experience (Peet & Wakefield 2002).

Figure 12.1

Process mapping exercise for proposed clozapine care

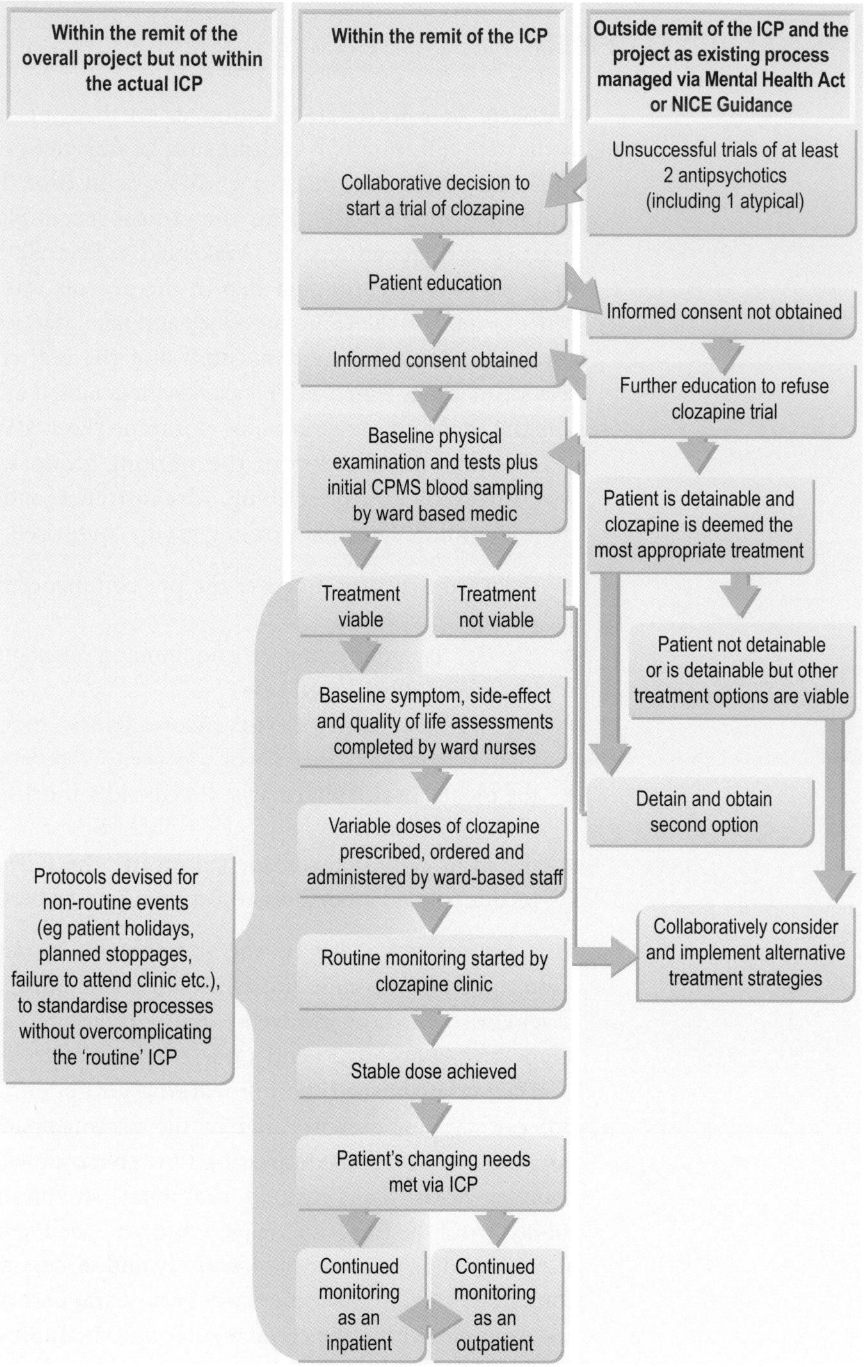

Within the remit of the overall project but not within the actual ICP	Within the remit of the ICP	Outside remit of the ICP and the project as existing process managed via Mental Health Act or NICE Guidance

The working group met on a number of occasions, using the meetings to share ideas about the evidence base, as well as current local practice that the members had found to be effective. On this occasion, gathering the relevant evidence was relatively straightforward as, in addition to the British National Formulary (British Medical Association 2004), the drug company itself had produced numerous leaflets relating to best practice. Also, by having their local advisor on the authoring group, we were able to access easily many other pertinent articles. This was checked against our own review of the published literature using Medline, as well as published national guidelines for the treatment of schizophrenia (National Institute for Clinical Excellence 2002). The available evidence thus covered all aspects of clozapine treatment, including such issues as physical health checks and side-effect monitoring. The exercise then continued by identifying each individual task performed in relation to clozapine, from the decision to commence, through cross-titration, full handover to the clinic for continued monitoring, to planned and unplanned discontinuation. Once we had identified the tasks and arranged them in sequential order, we began to allocate them to specific timeframes and to the discipline/clinician responsible. Considering the process in this analytical manner gave us the chance to identify both existing and potential problems with care provision. In our experience, the opportunity for a full range of professionals to stand back from care and consider it philosophically, as a group of equally valued practitioners, is rare within today's pressured healthcare arena. Un-surprisingly, we found this to be a liberating educational experience which encouraged teamworking, as experienced by De Luc (2001).

Having agreed on the content and qualitative aspects of a patient's clozapine experience, it was relatively straightforward to transfer this to an ICP format (Wakefield & Peet 2003). Certain non-routine situations, e.g. planning for service users' holidays, were then given special consideration. For each situation a decision was taken as to whether the issue was a rarity or the norm. If it occurred for the majority of service users it was fully integrated into the body of the ICP. If not, it was included as a clear and simple protocol in a separate file, effectively signposted from the ICP (as shown in the examples in Figures 12.2 and 12.3). This ensured safety was maintained for all eventualities without over-complicating the tool. It is crucial when developing an ICP that it is not designed to account for every eventuality, however rare and infrequent, as this will lead to a cumbersome document which is unwieldy and would result in excessive variance recording. However, an ICP that is vague and non-specific will be meaningless and staff will continue to use existing systems and paperwork which more closely meet their needs. An ICP needs to reflect reality and the clinical situation; it needs to take account of interventions which should occur most of the time. Anomalies can then be dealt with via protocols and variance tracking, both of which should be embedded within the process without over-complicating the ICP itself. Involving staff from the area in which the ICP will be used will increase the likelihood of an ICP being developed which truly meets the needs of patients and that will actually be used by staff.

Figure 12.2
Example of a protocol
embedded in the ICP

Doncaster & South Humber NHS
Healthcare NHS Trust

ROTHERHAM MENTAL HEALTH SERVICES

ROTHERHAM CLOZAPINE CLINICS

PROTOCOL FOR PATIENTS GOING ON HOLIDAY WHILST ON CLOZAPINE
(Note: This protocol does not need to be followed if the holiday does not exceed the normal sampling time)

Patients may holiday for a maximum of 2 weeks if established on fortnightly monitoring or a maximum of four weeks if established on 4 weekly monitoring.

HOLIDAY IN THE UK:

The RMO (or Clozapine Clinic staff) will need to liaise with a psychiatrist at the holiday destination to arrange:

- Routine blood sample
- Send a sample to CPMS laboratory
- Confirm a satisfactory blood result has been obtained
- Authorise supply of Clozapine
- Be emergency contact for patient and CPMS.

HOLIDAY ABROAD:

The following must have occurred prior to the holiday:

- The consultant has assessed the likely effect of the trip on the patient's health
- Emergency contact between the medical team and patient is possible at all times
- Patient had a satisfactory blood result prior to leaving the country. If necessary a sample should be taken and analysed locally just prior to departure and the result phoned through to CPMS.
- No more than 14 days' (or 28 days' for 4 weekly monitoring) supply of Clozapine is taken on holiday with patient, unless special arrangements have been made in advance with CPMS.
- Patient and carers aware what action to follow if the patient develops an infection. If an infection does develop an emergency white blood count with differential should be performed immediately and the results transmitted urgently to the patient's consultant.

If you are unsure of contact details in any destination contact CPMS for information.

The experience of developing an ICP was interesting and informative, raising issues of current practice, the evidence base and highlighting areas where interventions were being duplicated. Development alone also improved communication (De Luc 2001) between the ward, day hospital and pharmacy. Further benefits were then derived from using the ICP in practice.

Figure 12.3
Further example of a protocol embedded in the ICP

> **Doncaster & South Humber** NHS
> Healthcare NHS Trust
>
> ROTHERHAM MENTAL HEALTH SERVICES
>
> ROTHERHAM CLOZAPINE CLINICS
>
> PROTOCOL FOR PLANNED DISCONTINUATION OF CLOZAPINE
>
> This protocol should be used following the decision by the multidisciplinary team to discontinue Clozapine.
>
> 1. As with all antipsychotic medication, discontinuation from Clozapine should be done gradually. Patients should gradually discontinue over a period of one to two weeks.
>
> 2. The patient should be carefully monitored for symptoms of psychosis during this period.
>
> 3. The 'discontinuation card' should be returned to CMPS when treatment stops.
>
> 4. Blood monitoring should be continued for a further 4 weeks at the established frequency from the day the last dose was taken.
>
> 5. Sudden withdrawal from Clozapine may give rise to physical symptoms such as confusion, sweating, restlessness, nausea, dyskinesia, headache, insomnia and vomiting. If necessary treatment with an anticholinergic agent may be helpful.

IMPLEMENTATION

We were in the fortunate position that staff were already familiar with the basic principles of ICPs and their use. This had been achieved through taught, small group sessions when previously launching another ICP. In our experience, we have found thorough staff training to be vital for the success of any ICP as, without it, resistance will be incurred through negative preconceptions regarding excessive demands on practitioners' time, formulaic practice and the perceived removal of their ability to apply professional judgments. Despite this existing knowledge base, we still felt a staggered implementation would be prudent. This began with the transfer, by clinic staff, of all existing clozapine patients' records onto the maintenance section of the ICP (this section is only completed by clinic staff but acts as a point of reference to others). During this phase, the ward manager and the ICP coordinator trained qualified ward staff and associated medical staff in the use of the initiation section of the ICP. Once both phases were complete, any patients being considered for a trial of clozapine had care delivered via the whole ICP. As the number of patients involved was small and sporadic, it was possible for the ward manager and the ICP coordinator to supervise closely use of the ICPs, in addition to problems being picked up at clinic visits. The arduous and time-consuming nature of this part of the implementation phase should not be underestimated, especially if the ICP is to be widely used or is acute/high volume in nature.

Once the ICP had been piloted for several months, it was evaluated by the original working party. At this stage, this involved qualitative feedback from practitioners about their experiences of using the ICP as well as more quantitative evaluation through variance tracking. Minor amendments were then made (e.g. agreement that drug cards would be sent to clinic with the patient and their ICP), staff informed and the new version launched. It is vital that when a new version is introduced all blank supplies of earlier versions are removed from the clinical area. The ICP shown in Appendix 12.1 is now used for all patients who are prescribed clozapine; it is their plan, and record of clozapine-related care and, as such, sits in and forms part of the patient record.

OUTCOMES AND CONCLUSIONS

Since implementing the clozapine ICP in our nurse-led clinic we are confident that the quality of the service has improved. Box 12.1 describes what we view as the outcomes of implementation. For those patients who are commencing on clozapine we have observed a smoother pathway with greater involvement from the wider staff team.

Box 12.1   OUTCOMES OF THE CLOZAPINE ICP

- Clearly defined processes for commencement and ongoing treatment
- Simple protocols for all eventualities
- Improved communication between ward and clinic
- Easy to access record of care
- Auditable record of care
- Improved knowledge base, and greater involvement from the wider staff team
- Seamless transition from commencement to monitoring
- Positive patient feedback
- A staff-owned process
- A detailed, holistic package of care incorporating interpersonal relationships as opposed to pure task performance.

Generally, staff feedback has been positive; they find the ICP easy to use as it clearly outlines the tasks required and who is responsible for them. The ICP is not only useful for outlining and recording the structured, pre-defined care but, in addition, by using the supplementary protocols (which are referred to in the ICP) it also takes into account the specific action required in unexpected and unusual situations (see Figures 12.2 and 12.3). This being the case, in terms of risk management, our clozapine ICP is a powerful tool in that it can direct even the most inexperienced staff should the unexpected occur.

Early feedback from patients and staff has been positive; however, a more structured evaluation of the re-launched version will be undertaken, giving further consideration to the following:

- staff experiences of using the ICP
- staff knowledge of, and involvement in, the clozapine process
- variance analysis
- auditing practice against the standards outlined in the ICP (this would strengthen the validity and reliability of the variance analysis)
- patient and carer experiences of receiving care via the ICP.

Given the early indications of success, we have also developed an ICP for community initiation of clozapine and have begun using an ICP for the administration and monitoring of other atypical antipsychotic medication (which fell outside the remit of this project during the process mapping exercise). The initiation and monitoring of clozapine need to be standardised and organised in order to deliver safe, effective care and ensure a positive service user experience. Our experience has led us to believe the ICP tool lends itself perfectly to this process.

Doncaster & South Humber NHS
Healthcare NHS Trust

Patient Label

INTEGRATED CARE PATHWAY: CLOZAPINE

Information on Integrated Care Pathways:

This Integrated Care Pathway is for all patients who are commencing on Clozapine and attending the Clozapine Clinic.

It covers the period from staff decision to start Clozapine therapy and includes all clinic appointments. There are a number of protocols which accompany this ICP, and these should be referred to and followed where indicated in the ICP. Wherever possible, the interventions are based on evidence and best practice.

Instructions for use:

Before writing in this Integrated Care Pathway, please ensure you have signed the signature sheet in the patient's notes. Please ensure you date, time and sign against each activity when it has been completed.

It is important to remember that the aim of the Integrated Care Pathway (ICP) is to ensure the most appropriate care is given at the correct time. If an activity outlined in the ICP has not, for whatever reason, been completed then this must be shown as a variance. A 'V' should therefore be placed in the sign box next to the intervention. The variance record sheet should then be completed.

To view an example of a completed ICP please read the ICP file, which is in your ward/area.

If you require further information please contact the Integrated Care Pathway Co-ordinator on xxxxxxx.

Endorsed by: LOCAL CLINICAL GOVERNANCE

Date Endorsed: 13 FEBRUARY 2003

List of abbreviations:

ICP: Integrated Care Pathway
SE: Side effects
RMO: Responsible Medical Officer
LUNSERS: Liverpool University Neuroleptic Side Effect Rating Scale
BPRS: Brief Pyschiatric Rating Scale
SQLS: Schizophrenia Quality Life Scale
CPMS: Clozapine Patient Monitoring System
BP: Blood pressure
ECG: Electrocardiogram
KGV: Krawiecka Goldbergh & Vaughan

Appendix 12.1

Doncaster & South Humber NHS
Healthcare NHS Trust

INTEGRATED CARE PATHWAY: CLOZAPINE

SIGNATURE SHEET

Would all disciplines please sign below prior to writing in this ICP.

Patient Label

Full name (print)	Designation	Signature	Initials	Date of Entry

Appendix 12.1   (*Continued*)

Doncaster & South Humber NHS
Healthcare NHS Trust

INTEGRATED CARE PATHWAY: CLOZAPINE

Patient Label

Patient Information Sheet
CPMS number:

Date commenced on Clozapine / /		
Frequency of bloods	Date changed	Signed

Current dose: ....Date commenced on current dose   /   /
....Date commenced on current dose   /   /
....Date commenced on current dose   /   /
....Date commenced on current dose   /   /

Use this space to record other relevant patient information:

Appendix 12.1   (*Continued*)

Doncaster & South Humber NHS
Healthcare NHS Trust

	Patient Label

INTEGRATED CARE PATHWAY: CLOZAPINE

Prior to Commencement of Clozapine					
MDT Responsibilities					
Date	Time	Intervention Code	Intervention	Comments	Sign
		MDT1	MDT decision to start Clozapine therapy has been made.		
Nursing Responsibilities					
		N1	First education session carried out by named nurse covering: Clozapine booklet on Schizophrenia ☐ Clozapine patient handbook ☐		
		N2	Second education session carried out by named nurse covering: Clozapine booklet on Schizophrenia ☐ Clozapine patient handbook ☐		
		N3	Baseline LUNSERS completed: Score:		
		N4	Baseline SQLS completed: Score:		

		N5	Baseline
			        BPRS ☐
			        KGV ☐ completed:
			Score:		

		N6	Date of next assessment placed in Clozapine Clinic diary.		
Medical Responsibilities					
		M1	Informed consent obtained from patient (if unable to obtain consent follow protocol in Clozapine file).		
		M2	Baseline physical examination as per Clozapine check list completed: Weight: BP: Temp: Pulse: Bloods Glucose: ECG:		
		M3	Blood sample taken and sent to CPMS.		

Appendix 12.1   *(Continued)*

Doncaster & South Humber NHS
Healthcare NHS Trust

INTEGRATED CARE PATHWAY: CLOZAPINE

			Prior to Commencement of Clozapine Cont.		
			Medical Responsibilities		
		M4	Blood result review: Green result Red result Amber result If red/amber result further blood sample must be taken. NB: (If second red result is received discuss with RMO)		
		M5	Blood glucose level reviewed		
		M6	Register patient with CPMS		
		M7	Consultant registered with CPMS		

			Friday Prior to Commencement of Clozapine		
			Nursing Responsibilities		
		N7	Above results and assessments discussed with medical staff.		
		N8	Medication ordered from pharmacy (ensure arrival for Friday before commencement date)		
		N9	Clozapine medication received from pharmacy and checked.		
		N10	Book in for medic.		
			Medical Responsibilities		
		M8	First 9 doses of variable dose regime of Clozapine prescribed. First dose to commence on Monday morning and within 10 days of initial blood test.		
		M9	ECG results reviewed (if abnormal discuss with consultant)		

Appendix 12.1   (*Continued*)

Doncaster & South Humber NHS
Healthcare NHS Trust

PATIENT LABEL

INTEGRATED CARE PATHWAY: CLOZAPINE

Day One Clozapine Therapy			(Monday)	Date: / /		
Nursing Responsibilities						
Date	Time	Intervention Code	Intervention	Comments		Sign
		N11	Immediately prior to first dose, following physical assessments carried out: BP: Temp: Pulse: (if any abnormalities/concerns discuss with medical staff before administering Clozapine)			
		N12	First dose of Clozapine administered (ensure this falls within 10 days of initial blood test)			
		N13	Appointment made to attend Clozapine clinic in 10 days and clinic staff informed. (Clinic Appt: Thursday / /)			
		N14	Following to be taken and recorded every 2 hours: BP: Temp: Pulse: (Follow protocol)			
		N15	Following to be taken and recorded every 2 hours: BP: Temp: Pulse: (Follow protocol)			
		N16	Following to be taken and recorded every 2 hours: BP: Temp: Pulse: (Follow protocol)			
		N17	Administer further doses of Clozapine as per variable dose on drug card.			

Appendix 12.1   *(Continued)*

Doncaster & South Humber NHS
Healthcare NHS Trust

INTEGRATED CARE PATHWAY: CLOZAPINE

Patient Label

On 3rd day of commencement of Clozapine therapy (Wednesday)				Date: / /	
Date	Time	Intervention Code	Intervention	Comments	Sign
Medical Responsibilities					
		M10	Blood sample taken and sent to CPMS		

First Friday after commencement of Clozapine therapy				Date: / /	
Date	Time	Intervention Code	Intervention	Comments	Sign
Nursing Responsibilities					
		N18	Clozapine ordered from Pharmacy.		
		N19	Clozapine received by Friday pm.		
Medical Responsibilities					
		M11	Previous blood result reviewed by medic. Green: [ ] Red: [ ] **NB: If red withhold further doses of Clozapine and discuss immediately with medical staff**		
		M12	Friday am: Six doses of Clozapine prescribed (Ensure this will last over the weekend) Friday am:		

Monday prior to attending first Clozapine Clinic				Date: / /	
Date	Time	Intervention Code	Intervention	Comments	Sign
Nursing Responsibilities					
		N20	Clozapine ordered from pharmacy ordered before noon.		
Medical Responsibilities					
		M13	Variable doses of Clozapine prescribed. (Up to and including Thursday am)		
		M14	Blood result reviewed: Green: [ ] Red: [ ] **NB: If red withhold further doses of Clozapine and discuss immediately with medical staff**		

Appendix 12.1   *(Continued)*

Doncaster & South Humber NHS
Healthcare NHS Trust

INTEGRATED CARE PATHWAY: CLOZAPINE

Patient Label

First appointment at Clozapine Clinic — Date: / /

Date	Time	Intervention Code	Intervention	Comments	Sign
Nursing Responsibilities					
		N21	Patient attended at first appointment at Clozapine clinic.		
		N22	Role of Clozapine clinic explained to patient and copy of leaflet given.		
		N23	Clozapine ordered from pharmacy.		
Medical Responsibilities					
		M15	Further variable doses of Clozapine prescribed.		

Second Clozapine Clinic appointment — Date: / /

Date	Time	Intervention Code	Intervention	Comments	Sign
Nursing Responsibilities					
		N24	Patient attended at Clozapine Clinic.		
		N25	Clozapine ordered from pharmacy.		
Medical Responsibilities					
		M16	Further variable doses of Clozapine prescribed.		

Third Clozapine Clinic appointment — Date: / /

Date	Time	Intervention Code	Intervention	Comments	Sign
Nursing Responsibilities					
		N26	Patient attended at Clozapine Clinic.		
		N27	Clozapine ordered from pharmacy.		
Medical Responsibilities					
		M17	Further variable doses of Clozapine prescribed.		

Appendix 12.1   (*Continued*)

Doncaster & South Humber NHS
Healthcare NHS Trust

Patient Label

INTEGRATED CARE PATHWAY: CLOZAPINE

Interventions to be carried out at each subsequent Clozapine Clinic appointment				Date: / /	
Date	Time	Intervention Code	Intervention	Comments	Sign
		N28	**Patient attended clinic:** **Yes** [ ] **No** [ ] *If no, complete variance record and follow DNA protocol. Complete date patient does attend in date/time column.*		
		N29	<u>**Inpatients only:**</u> Telephone call to ward to remind them of appointment.		
		N30	<u>**Outpatients only:**</u> Telephone call to patient's home to remind them of appointment.		
		N31	Blood sample obtained: Local: [ ] CPMS: [ ] *If unable to obtain a sample, record as a variance. (Indicate date and time sample was then sucessfully obtained).* Date obtained: Time obtained:		
		N32	Observations completed: Pulse: BP: Temp: Weight:		
		N33	Side effects questionnaire completed. **NB: medic must be informed if an increase in side effects.**		
		N34	Brief assessment of current mental state completed. Including mood, thinking, behaviour.		
		N35	Clinic appointment made and date recorded in: ICP: [ ] Clinic Diary: [ ] Patient's name placed on list to fax to pharmacy.		

Continued on next sheet

Appendix 12.1   *(Continued)*

Doncaster & South Humber NHS
Healthcare NHS Trust

INTEGRATED CARE PATHWAY: CLOZAPINE

Patient Label

		N36	Inpatients only: Ward informed of next clinic date and of any local samples (if required). Medication dispensed by: Ward ☐ Day Services ☐ Pharmacy ☐ Hostel ☐		

Appendix 12.1 *(Continued)*

Doncaster & South Humber NHS
Healthcare NHS Trust

INTEGRATED CARE PATHWAY: CLOZAPINE

Affix Patient Label Here

Variance Record Sheet for Clozapine ICP

Date	Time	Intervention Code	Reason for Variance Code	Action to be Taken	Sign

User/carer codes

1.1 User unavailable
1.2 Carer unavailable
1.3 User refused
1.4 Carer refused
1.5 Intervention inappropriate
1.6 Deterioration of mental state: intervention inappropriate
1.7 Improvement of mental state: intervention inappropriate
1.8 User refused due to poor motivation
1.9 Intervention repeated due to lack of understanding and/or skills
1.10 Drug/alcohol intoxification

Ward codes

2.1 Date and time of appointment changed
2.2 Awaiting feedback from others
2.3 Staff unavailable
2.4 Lack of time
2.5 Meeting postponed/cancelled

Agencies

3.1 Accommodation not available
3.2 Community support not available
3.3 Day services not available

Appendix 12.1   *(Continued)*

REFERENCES

British Medical Association 2004 British national formulary. Pharmaceutical Press, London

Camprubi M, Bagary M, Riccio M 1996 The clozapine clinic. The Lancet 347(8994):124

Chan S, Wong K 1999 The use of critical pathways in caring for schizophrenic patients in a mental hospital. Archives of Psychiatric Nursing 13:145-153

De Luc K 2001 Developing care pathways: the handbook. Radcliffe Medical Press, Oxford

Department of Health 1990 The Care Programme Approach. HC(90) 23/LASSL (90) 11. Department of Health, London

Hunt A 1991 The admission process. Nursing Times 87(20):30-32

Lovell K 1995 User satisfaction with in-patient mental health services. Journal of Psychiatric and Mental Health Nursing 2:143-150

National Institute for Clinical Excellence 2002 Guidance on the use of newer (atypical) antipsychotic drugs for the treatment of schizophrenia. NICE Technology Appraisal Guidance No.43 National Institute for Clinical Excellence, London

Peet M, Wakefield S 2002 Integrated care pathways in mental health: the need for the human touch. Journal of Integrated Care Pathways 6:108-114

Quirk A, Lelliot P 2001 What do we know about life on acute psychiatric wards in the UK? A review of the research evidence. Social Science and Medicine 53:1565-1574

Ricketts T 1996 General satisfaction and satisfaction with nursing communication on an adult psychiatric ward. Journal of Advanced Nursing 24:479-487

Wakefield S, Peet M 2003 Developing integrated care pathways in mental health: the critical success factors. Journal of Integrated Care Pathways 7:47-49

Wallace T, Robertson E, Frisch S 1999 Perceptions of care and services by the clients and families: a personal experience. Journal of Advanced Nursing 29(5):1144-1153

CHAPTER

13

Care pathways for older people's mental health care

Adrian Roberts

INTRODUCTION	**IMPLEMENTATION**
BACKGROUND	**OUTCOMES AND CONCLUSIONS**
PATHWAY DEVELOPMENT	**REFERENCES**

INTRODUCTION

Integrated care pathways (ICPs) are now routinely used across modern healthcare systems. From their initial development within the United States they have spread widely via Australia and Canada to Western Europe and beyond. Wherever they have been applied, understanding about the concept of pathways has been refined. Within the United Kingdom (UK), the development of care pathways has been given added impetus by the concept of clinical governance, the need to apply the service models outlined in the various UK National Service Frameworks and further develop information for health. Consistent drivers for adopting ICPs are the need for a proactive approach to 'quality' rather than reacting as and when new problems arise, the need to focus care around the needs of patients and to encourage active patient participation in care. Whilst a successful programme is dependent on a number of factors, carefully planned and reflective care pathways can certainly help to address some of these issues, whilst also meeting the professional duties of health and social care staff – that of maintaining standards of practice and legally defensible levels of documentation. The care pathways described in this chapter span a variety of older people's mental health settings. Examples specifically focus upon a falls care pathway and an inpatient assessment care pathway which considers the requirements of the Single Assessment Process (Department of Health 2004) and the Care Programme Approach (Department of Health 1999).

In simple terms, the care pathways described in this chapter are multi-disciplinary, interdisciplinary or multi-agency documents that both define and record the care given, including interventions, milestones and outcomes. The care pathways are robust in that they:

- Are based on what is expected to happen for a group of patients or for a particular process (e.g. admission) with a focus on improving care coordination and communication
- Include patient goals and outcomes which support monitoring of progress and incorporate available evidence and/or a consensus of best practice, subject to regular review
- Focus on the patient (and carers) and the way care is delivered to them, rather than upon organisational structures. The intention is to view the 'patient journey' from a different perspective and identify how it can be improved – tying in with the developing principle of clinical networks
- Help to make sure we do the right things at the right time, for the right person.

BACKGROUND

It is the author's view that care pathways are much more than the pieces of paper (or indeed data on a screen) which they first appear to be; that they are in fact a care delivery model that can be used to drive service design and delivery. The care pathway and development model described in this chapter represents a deceptively powerful cycle of change, which is familiar across all types of business from private industry to public sector services. It is embedded within virtually all quality improvement frameworks and is, in essence, applied common sense:

1. If we are trying to improve something, then we first must establish what we are trying to achieve (i.e. establish what success will look like)
2. Once we know what we are trying to achieve we can plan how we intend to achieve it
3. With a plan in place we can then try it out
4. Once implementation is underway, we need to understand the impact it has – this is done by review, to see whether success has been achieved. We can then use the results to guide our next steps – we can alter our targets and therefore our idea of what success will look like. Alternatively, we can alter our plan or we may wish to try a combination of the two approaches
5. The cycle continues.

ICP development and use are practical applications of this quality improvement framework, as demonstrated by the model in Box 13.1.

It is, of course, the concept of variance that helps to make care pathways so powerful – and, at a basic level – anything that does not have a facility to record and monitor variance is not really a care pathway. In simple terms, a variation ('variance') as explained in Chapter 2 occurs when an activity or outcome set out in the pathway does not happen as planned. In my experience, recording variance

Box 13.1   CARE PATHWAYS MODEL: A PRACTICAL APPLICATION OF THE CONTINUOUS IMPROVEMENT CYCLE

1. Agree patient outcomes and key milestones (indicators of progress)
2. Agree the clinical processes/procedures and treatment designed to achieve the defined indicators and milestones
3. Design and implement the care pathway
4. Review the care pathway through variance analysis, with a focus on outcomes and key milestones.

is an effective way of completing the 'patient's story' in terms of a comprehensive record of care, whilst monitoring variance helps us to understand why different patients follow different paths. Experience has shown that in mental health less predictable patient journeys mean that the care process may be more complex and the number of variations greater overall. However, defining an expected route of care within a care pathway helps us to focus on (patient) progress and also means that when progress varies, potential problems may be picked up much earlier than they would have been otherwise. By acknowledging problems sooner we can hopefully implement solutions earlier, which benefits everybody – patients, staff and service providers.

There are two points to note here. Firstly, it is my view that care pathways, in keeping with the idea of a continuous improvement cycle, try to demonstrate a link between cause and effect. Secondly, they are also an ideal basis for a programme of clinical benchmarking, i.e. comparisons between different health-care service providers (Middleton & Roberts 2000). In many ways, benchmarking based on a comparison of numbers and performance indicators is beset by difficulties due to arguments over different service configurations, local populations and different levels of skill. Care pathways help in this situation because they break contexts down to the level of processes (i.e. the work that is actually done) and as a result this allows organisations to learn from the successes and failures of others, regardless of the service environment in which they operate.

With regard to the pathways discussed in this chapter, the National Service Framework (NSF) for Older People (Department of Health 2001) now provides the context for service delivery for older people, in keeping with the NHS Plan and its central aims of improving overall standards, and rebuilding the NHS around the needs of patients. The NSF is made up of a number of key themes including the development of person-centred care and coordinated and integrated service provision. The eight standards within the NSF for Older People are outlined in Box 13.2. These standards recognise the complex health needs of this patient group and that there is often the need for coordination of a greater number and range of services than for other groups. Coordinating this obviously represents a considerable challenge. The main principles and activities involved in the design and use of care pathways, however, offer a considerable advantage in meeting

Box 13.2   THE NATIONAL SERVICE FRAMEWORK FOR OLDER PEOPLE

The NSF for older people is based on eight standards (Department of Health 2001):

1. rooting out age discrimination
2. person-centred care
3. intermediate care
4. general hospital care
5. stroke
6. falls
7. mental health in older people
8. promoting an active healthy life in older age.

Box 13.3   THE RATIONALE FOR USING ICPS IN OLDER PEOPLE'S MENTAL HEALTH SERVICES

Reasons for introducing ICPs for older people using mental health services include:

- developing a 'roadmap' to support clarity and equity of care
- to help form relationships and develop care networks – the development of connections across different providers and sectors of care
- improving communication between those responsible for offering care and services
- quality assurance; information from pathways can be used as the basis for audit, to monitor and improve service delivery
- improving standards, access to services and equity
- identifying and reducing gaps in service provision
- targeting resources for improvement.

this challenge if they are carefully applied. The rationale for using ICPs in older people's mental health services is summarised in Box 13.3.

PATHWAY DEVELOPMENT

Firstly, by bringing together all stakeholders (including service users and carers) care pathway development allows stakeholders from different perspectives the time to understand their role within the care process and any areas of overlap. In the author's experience, what is interesting about these development sessions is that groups and individuals who may have worked together for some considerable time have never been given the opportunity to consider how their activities fit with the input of colleagues – and, if we are honest, we will all be aware of times when we look at situations solely from our own 'uniprofessional box'. The very act of developing a pathway breaks down such barriers and aids understanding of those times when duplication is necessary and when it is merely collecting the same information or repeating an intervention.

An important part of bringing people together to develop a care pathway is to establish clarity of purpose. Service delivery involves many different professionals across different parts of the National Health Service (NHS) and local government and reaches into the community including the voluntary, independent and business sectors. This often means that aims and objectives of care delivery are not necessarily shared although they may well be similar. In some instances, the aims and objectives of different agencies may conflict, particularly when taking into account resources or responsibility of payment for services. Unless these conflicts are explored and managed then it is unlikely that any processes deployed will meet with success, and partnership working will be undermined. When developing any pathway, it is therefore important to examine and define what it seeks to achieve as a starting point. This supports the ability to communicate shared aims and objectives to all those who will use the pathway. As an important guiding principle, any professional who will be expected to use a pathway should have the opportunity to influence the content rather than it being thrust upon them. In this context, the care pathway can help to establish a common language and a set of rules of engagement for all partners. This is particularly important at a time when older people's services are continually being encouraged to develop networks that work across traditional organisational boundaries in order to present a seamless service to patients and carers.

The next stage in the development of the pathway requires baseline assessment of what happens currently; which in turn leads to a focus on resolving problems and inconsistencies with local service delivery. If this assessment does not happen, then it is more likely that the pathway will fail on implementation. The most common way of undertaking a baseline assessment to inform pathway development is to develop a series of process maps or flow charts. Analysis of the completed flow charts allows pathway development teams to make a judgment on those things that are done well and those practices that require improvement. An example of an initial high-level process map is shown in Figure 13.1. Without such information, the temptation is to introduce solutions to the wrong problems or to assume that services are good when they may not be.

The ICPs shown later in this chapter (and indeed in other chapters) require interdisciplinary coordination and effective teamworking. Putting together process maps will quickly help to establish how effectively groups work together in teams and any barriers to teamworking that may exist. It is important not to merely assume that high levels of teamworking exist without further investigation. Process mapping enables teams to examine the patient journey across services and examine examples of blockages and ambiguity. For example, the value of a highly

Figure 13.1
Example of a high-level
process map

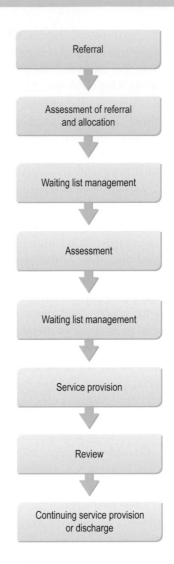

professional service may well be diminished if potential service users are referred to the service via routes that make it difficult to access. In the care pathway examples discussed in this chapter process mapping has been a crucial component in ensuring success. In the author's view it is difficult to envisage how any care pathway can be introduced in the absence of process mapping. If this stage is not completed, the resulting pathways are often disjointed and do not reflect the process of care for service users, carers or staff.

Process mapping has certainly become more common within health and social care in recent years. The activity has benefits beyond establishing the steps and activities that underpin successful services. These include:

■ developing an understanding of things as they happen, which can be quite different to expectations

- involving all stakeholders or their representatives is crucial to developing understanding as the experience of service users and carers can be dramatically different to that intended
- helping to identify roles and responsibilities – and helping everybody to understand how they work with others
- identifying problem areas, duplication, delays and 'waste' and focusing improvement efforts; process maps will also indicate where best to measure performance
- promoting trust and ownership to solve problems; as a result, even if the pathway ultimately fails, it still should be a positive experience for all involved.

Process mapping is probably best undertaken as a series of iterations, as it is unlikely that first attempts will accurately capture the information required for analysis and building robust care pathway documentation. Seeing process mapping as a series of steps allows groups to start off relatively simply (by producing an overview or high-level map, as shown in Figure 13.1) before becoming progressively more detailed (as shown in Figure 13.2).

Using process mapping within the ICP development process involves completing a number of steps (Bullivant 1997):

1. Define the scope of activity (for example, where does the single assessment process begin and end? Which departments and organisations impact upon it? How do patients enter into the assessment process?)
2. Define the desired outcome (for example, what objectives are we trying to achieve through the single assessment process? Are there any key principles we wish to work to?)
3. Map the processes undertaken now (this will probably result in a number of process maps) and define roles and responsibilities for each activity and the outcomes identified
4. Identify problem areas and opportunities for improvement; test processes against the evidence base, current research and good practice guidance. This work can be devolved to a series of multi-professional working groups
5. Define new processes taking account of all information collected and use as the basis for training and the development of care pathways.

Given the requirement for the ICP development team to review relevant health policy and research to ensure pathways are 'modernised' and based on contemporary evidence, recent policy developments within older people's mental health care are, of course, highly influential. For example, the eight standards outlined in the NSF for Older People (Department of Health 2001) provide a number of natural areas where the potential use of pathways can be explored. Given the number of competing priorities services face at any given moment (and also given the ever-increasing range of services on offer) it is difficult to imagine a time when fully functioning multi-agency care pathways will be in place to cover every activity. Given the time and resources involved, it would be necessary to question whether such a situation would be desirable! However, in terms of

Figure 13.2
Mental health
assessment ICP process
map

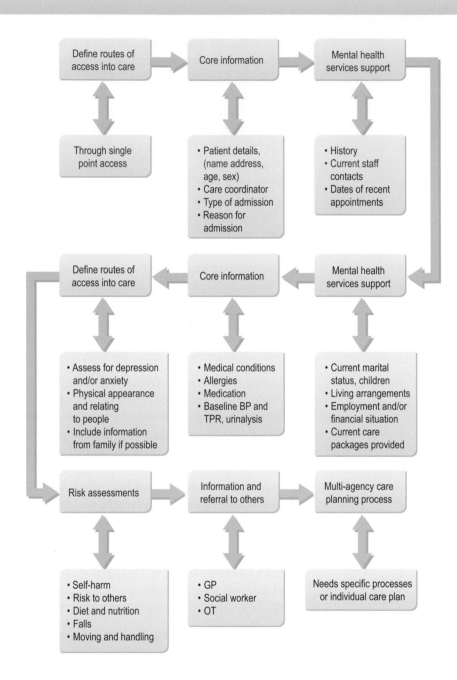

gaining value from care pathways it would seem sensible to suggest that services focus on those areas that present the biggest problems and tie in with important components of organisational strategy.

The NSF for Older People standard 6 (Department of Health 2001), which focuses upon falls, can be taken as an example here. Standard 6 proposes that the NHS, working in partnership with councils, takes action to prevent falls and reduce resultant fractures or other injuries in their populations of older people.

Older people who have fallen need to receive effective treatment and rehabilitation and, with their carers, receive advice on prevention through a specialised falls service. Many trusts have responded to this with care pathways for falls, specifically targeted for older people (White 2004). Strategies to reduce the likelihood of in-hospital falls are also being incorporated into care pathways by defining a falls assessment process. These pathways impact upon the provision of falls prevention information for those who have either fallen or are assessed as at risk of falling (see the example in Figure 13.3). The prevalence of falls increases with age, and the subsequent disability and mortality that arise indicate that this is a serious issue in the care of older adults. The example in figure 13.3 is intended to guide the prevention of falls and management of risk, and aims to close the gap between

Figure 13.3
Falls risk assessment (care pathway component)
Adapted from Morse (1997)

FALLS RISK ASSESSMENT			Score
1. History of falling. *Immediate or within 3 months*	No ☐		0
	Yes ☐		25
2. Secondary diagnosis. *Does the patient have more than one ongoing diagnosis documented in the patient record?*	No ☐		0
	Yes ☐		15
3. Ambulatory aid	None, bed rest, wheelchair, nurse ☐		0
	Crutches, cane, walker ☐		15
	Does not use walking aids but grasps furniture ☐		30
4. Equipment. *Is the patient attached to a syringe driver, IV fluids or have a catheter bag that has a stand*	No ☐		0
	Yes ☐		20
5. Gait/Transferring	Normal, bed rest, immobile ☐		0
	Weak ☐		10
	Impaired ☐		20
6. Mental status. *Ask the patient if they are able to go to the bathroom alone?*	Orientated to own ability (their answer is the same as your assessment of their capabilities) ☐		0
	Forgets limitations (they overestimate their abilities or seem unclear) ☐		15
Total Score =	Low risk 0-24; ☐		
	High risk > 50 ☐		
	Moderate risk 24-50; ☐		

Figure 13.3   (*Cont'd*)

	Time	Initial	VC
Falls Assessment completed			
Falls low risk			

FALLS ACTON PLAN	
Low Risk	• Document score in patient record • Communicate score to team • Keep bed on low setting unless performing procedures • Ensure required items in reach • Check footwear and ensure appropriate • Assess environment for safety hazards, avoid clutter and remove spillage • Ensure patient instructed in the use of call bell
Moderate Risk	Plus • Frequently re-orientate confused patients to facilities • Educate patient/carers in safe movement practices • Educate patient to request assistance when mobilising
High Risk	Plus • Place patient in an observable room where possible • Consider patient sensor alarm • Discuss interventions with team, document in patient record

	Time	Initial
Additional Notes		
Please continue overleaf		

Adapted from Morse (1997).

suggested good practice, research evidence and what happens in actual practice on a day-to-day basis. The overall objectives of this falls assessment are to:

■ reduce the likelihood of falling and subsequent injury
■ establish effective interdisciplinary working and ensure that appropriate and necessary treatments are part of post-fall care
■ determine a measure of risk by prompt and expert assessment
■ provide an effective and evidence-based treatment plan to manage the level of identified risk.

As soon as a particular assessment tool or care process has been introduced into a care pathway it is used as the actual record of care. If the assessment (as part of the ICP) is not used, the recording of variance should give the reason why; which, in turn, helps to monitor the implementation of the NSF standard. Within this context, the use of ICPs in older people's mental health services has helped to avoid a problem that is often perceived by healthcare staff – that, in a time of almost constant change, there appears little time to learn the lessons from one initiative before another replaces it. In the author's experience, another powerful advantage of pathways as a model of care delivery is that any new initiative (like the falls assessment) can be absorbed into the care pathways themselves and thereby provide some support and consistency for the staff who use them. The types of initiatives that have been absorbed by care pathways for older people with mental health problems include not only the various standards of the National Service Frameworks but also:

- the Care Programme Approach (Department of Health 1999) and/or Single Assessment Process (Department of Health 2004)
- local/national audit programmes
- clinical governance requirements (e.g. the need for continuing education and training)
- utilisation of evidence-based approaches e.g. information from Scottish Intercollegiate Guidelines Network and the National Institute of Clinical Excellence
- national and/or locally required risk assessments.

Another area where the application of ICPs for older people's services has been particularly helpful relates to the development of the Single Assessment Process (SAP) (Department of Health 2004) for older people and its relationship with the Care Programme Approach (CPA) (Department of Health 1999). SAP was introduced in the NSF for Older People as part of standard 2 – person-centred care. The SAP concept is intended to ensure that older people's needs are accurately assessed without needless duplication across different agencies. The key aims of SAP are defined as: older people should receive appropriate, effective, and timely responses to their health and social care needs and that older people and their carers will be involved in this process and a unified and standard process should be used to avoid duplication and waste (Department of Health 2004). A clear rationale for these aims can, of course, be established on the basis of providing more choice to patients; confirming roles and responsibilities of professionals and reducing the number of times decisions are deferred from one professional to another. At a basic level, the powerful advantage of any single assessment is also reported as an advantage of care pathways – that patients (and carers) do not have to continually answer the same questions asked by different health and social care professionals, unless there is a valid reason for asking questions again.

SAP (Department of Health 2004) is made up of a number of stages. The first, initial contact assessment, may be undertaken by any individual trained to carry it out. This is followed (if required) by an overview assessment which is more rounded and carried out by an appropriate professional. This then may be followed (if required) by a specialist assessment, e.g. a specialist mental health assessment or a comprehensive assessment made by multidisciplinary teams across different agencies. Additionally, assessment (and therefore any ICPs) within older people's mental health services need to consider SAP and the CPA in their content. Whilst current guidance is clear, in that SAP takes priority over CPA for older people with mental health problems (Department of Health 2004), CPA is not discarded. For example, for an older person with severe mental illness, such as schizophrenia, severe functional or organic mental health problems, CPA should be applied whilst assessment of care needs should be based on the four types of assessment set out in SAP. Guidance on the use of CPA in conjunction with SAP suggests, among other things:

- that care pathways into specialist mental health services must be agreed by agencies and understood by professionals, older people, their carers and families
- ensuring that individual older people, and professionals on their behalf, can access specialist mental health services and SAP 24 hours a day, 7 days a week, and 365 days of the year
- ensuring that where it is appropriate for older people to move from CPA to SAP (or vice versa) such transitions are effectively managed with minimum or no disruption to the services that are provided.

With any process, the more agencies and individuals involved, the more difficult it becomes to manage, particularly in terms of ensuring people can access the services they require. Involving people from different professional backgrounds highlights the need to create a care process where all opinions are respected. It is the author's view that ICPs help to manage this complexity if the process mapping phase has been followed and used to design solutions to any problems identified. At this stage, completed process maps (as shown in Figure 13.2) are converted into care pathway documentation. An example of completed care pathway documentation is shown in the Appendix. By using the process maps to 'break' care delivery into manageable stages, services have gained defined criteria for entrance to the care pathway and the assessments to be undertaken, and by whom. A number of assessment tools, guidelines and protocols are also included, with the intention of supporting clinical judgment rather than replacing it. The points within the pathway where key decisions will be made are clearly indicated, together with milestones to monitor performance. Added are prompts for information to be provided to the service user and carers. Obviously, prior to implementation, professionals need to be trained with regard to the content and any new practice in the care pathway document.

IMPLEMENTATION

The ICP pilot stage is a mechanism to test new processes devised, to ensure that these are both robust and help to achieve service targets. In this instance, implementation of the care pathway shown in the Appendix simplifies the assessment process by coordinating the input of different professionals and agencies and ensuring that the new ICP process is consistently applied. It is acknowledged that although other approaches to practice development may seek to simplify the process (in keeping with the intention of the NSF standard), a care pathway also helps to ensure that the new process is introduced in practice. Additionally, the use of variance information as part of the quality improvement cycle means a mechanism exists to improve the process over time. Finally, the inclusion of an assessment component in condition-specific care pathways could help to identify where more comprehensive assessments are required, together with specific interventions and areas of unmet need.

OUTCOMES AND CONCLUSIONS

Implementation of the ICP examples highlighted within this chapter has been found to reduce duplication of documentation and activity. The ICPs have encouraged the coordination of care, in that the professionals are aware of their roles and responsibilities and that there are clear timeframes for their interventions. The development process with the input of service users and carers has offered an overall care pathway that is more service user centred. Examples of evidence for this can be seen in the inclusion of life stories, requirements for carers' assessment and service user and/or carer signatures on care plans. Teams using these ICPs perceive an improvement in standards (although at the time of writing this requires further exploration). Particular reflections have indicated more consistent application of assessment processes post-ICP implementation. Another consequence of pathway development is an improvement in trust between different professionals, agencies, and between professionals, service users and carers. Variance information clearly identifies unmet need which is responded to immediately (when this is possible) and through the quality improvement process.

The experience of using ICPs in older people's mental health services also suggests some key success factors. Firstly, before developing any care pathway it is important to clarify the reasons and motivation for introducing it – 'avoiding change for change's sake'. A formal project plan helps to define expected benefits and ensure development is considered in realistic and manageable stages. It is important to remember that ICPs are rarely a quick fix and developing a pathway that crosses organisational boundaries takes time and the issues raised are invariably complex. It is vital to ensure that a representative sample of all those involved in providing care are part of the ICP development group, and including the perspectives of service users and carers is critical. Pathways need to be owned and agreed by those who will use them. Although there may be a developing trend to use care pathways prescribed by others, in these cases it is equally important to allow stakeholders time for engagement and feedback regarding local processes. Experience has shown that services should not try to put together the pathway document before collecting baseline information and testing it – process mapping is particularly beneficial. Finally, it is necessary to analyse the information generated by the pathway, especially auditing variations and feeding back the results to care teams, as it is this that enables ongoing service improvement.

INTEGRATED CARE PATHWAY FOR OLDER ADULT
ASSESSMENT (INPATIENT CARE)

This integrated care pathway is for individuals admitted to older adult inpatient services. It is intended to guide admission and assessment ensuring that a service user's journey is negotiated, managed and agreed. As inpatient care is implicitly a request for urgent/intensive intervention there needs to be clarity regarding inputs and interventions required and how they will be delivered. It is essential that the expectations of the individual service user and carers are addressed as part of the overall care plan.

Overall objectives of this care pathway are to :
- Initiate a therapeutic relationship and provide prompt expert assessment of individual needs
- Ensure effective care planning, co-ordinated care and risk management; user and carer involvement and communication
- Provide effective, evidence based interventions to help recovery
- Establish effective liaison and ensure that appropriate and necessary treatments and services are offered.

Sources which inform the content of this pathway are :
Department of Health (2001). National Service Framework for Older People
Department of Health; London Audit Commission (2002). Forget-me-not 2002; Audit Commission Update. Audit Commission; London
Department of Health (2003). Discharge from Hospital: pathway, process & practice. Department of Health; London
Standing Nursing & Midwifery Advisory Committee (2001). Caring for Older people a Nursing Priority: Integrating knowledge Practice & Values. Department of Health; London

Instructions for use: When using this document please ensure that you date, time and sign where indicated. It is important to remember that the aim of the Integrated Care Pathway (ICP) is to ensure the most appropriate care is given at the correct time. If an activity outlined in the ICP has not , for whatever reason, been completed then this must be shown as a variance.The variance record sheet at the end of the pathway should then be completed. If further action needs to be taken, e.g. the intervention needs to be repeated, then use the blank spaces in the appropriate time frame of the ICP to record this. These blank spaces can also be used to add interventions which are deemed appropriate for that person but are not already in the ICP. These additions should also be recorded as a variance. To view an example of a completed ICP please read the ICP file which is in your ward/area. It remains each professional's responsibility to ensure that practice is safe. This ICP is not a replacement for experienced clinical judgement and inter-disciplinary discussions. If you require further information please contact your Care Pathway Lead.

LIST OF ABBREVIATIONS:
ICP – Integrated Care Pathway   CPN – Community Psychiatric Nurse GP – General Practitioner   MHA – Mental Health Act   OT – Occupational Therapy   LFTs – Liver Function Tests   EDT – Emergency Duty Team CMHT – Community Mental Health Team   U&Es – Urea & Electrolytes   BP – Blood Pressure   TPR – Temperature, pulse, respiration   FBC – Full Blood Count   HB – Haemoglobin   ESR – Erythrocyte Sedimentation Rate   EEG – Electroencephalogram   ECG – Electrocardiogram   ID – Identification MSE – Mental State Examination   ECT– Electroconvulsive Therapy   CPA – Care Programme Approach AMA – Against Medical Advice   DOB – Date of Birth   MHA – Mental Health Act FACE – Functional Assessment of the Care Environment   NHS – National Health Service SOSCIS – Social Services Care Information System DNAR – Decisions relating to Cardiopulmonary Resuscitation   MADRAS – Montgomery Asberg Depression Rating Scale   MADRAS-S – Montgomery Asberg Depression Rating Scale – Self Rating CSDD – Cornell Scale for Depression in Dementia BSA – Brief Scale for Anxiety   BSI – Beck Scale for Suicidal Ideation BHS – Beck Hopelessness Scale   NPI – Neuropsychiatric Inventory E-BEHAVE-AD – Empirical Behave-ad FrSBe – Frontal Systems Behavioural Scale   MMSE – Mini Mental State Examination   3M's – Modified Mini Mental State Examination   CDIS – Clock Drawing Interpretation Scale   CAMCOG – Cambridge Cognitive Examination SIB – Severe Impairment Battery CDR – Clinical Dementia Rating Scale   FAST – Functional Assessment Staging

PART 1 – PERSONAL INFORMATION

This information is collected to facilitate the care process and completion remains at the discretion of the admitting professional.

Surname:	Forename(s):	Mental Health Act Status:	CPA Status:	Date Applied:
NHS No.	Also known as:	Section 117 (yes/no)	Source of Referral:	
D.O.B	Gender:	Start date (if known)	Method of Referral:	

Address (permanent)	Relationship Status: (e.g. married, single, divorced, partner etc) Religion: National Insurance No:	Employment Status:	Occupation:		
		Unit Number:	Ethnic Group: Circle as appropriate		
			A	White – British	
			B	White – Irish	
		Benefits:	C	White – Any other white background	
			D	Mixed – White & Black Caribbean	
			E	Mixed – White & Black African	
		No of Dependent Children:	F	Mixed – White & Asian	
			G	Mixed – any other mixed background	
Post Code: Tel No(s):					
Address (temporary)	Consultant:	Initial HoNOS Score:	H	Asian or Asian British – Indian	
			J	Asian or Asian British – Pakistani	
			K	Asian or Asian British – Bangladeshi	
			L	Asian or Asian British – Any other Asian background	
			M	Black or Black British – Caribbean	
	Division:	Preferred Language:	N	Black or Black British – African	
			P	Black or Black British – Any other background	
			R	Other Ethnic Groups – Chinese	
Post Code: Tel No(s):			S	Other Ethnic Groups – Any other ethnic group	
Date of this Admission:		Time of Admission:	Ward:		

Appendix 13.1 (*Continued*)

Next of Kin:		Main Carer:	
Relationship:		Relationship (if any):	
Address:		Address:	
Tel No:		Tel No:	

Appraisal of Carer Need Undertaken: (Yes/No/Declined) Date of Appraisal:	Allergies:	Care Plan and Review Date given? (Yes/No/Declined)	Young Carer (Yes/No)

Nearest Relative: (if different from above) Address: Tel No:	GP: Address: Tel No:

Named Nurse: (for in-patients only)	CPA Care Co-ordinator:

1. OTHER PARTIES INVOLVED

Name:	Under 18:	Over 64:	Relationship: (state if carer)	Contact Number/Address:

Please record any special needs that arise from cultural or religious practices:

Appendix 13.1   (Continued)

2. PHYSICAL DESCRIPTION

Height:	Build:	Weight:
Hair Colour (state if dyed/bleached):	Length (Include facial hair):	Eye Colour:
Distinguishing Features:	Physical Disabilities:	

PART 2 – IMMEDIATE RECEPTION & CARE

3. PRACTICE GUIDE

A It is expected that these activities have been completed unless they are recorded as a variance

Code	Activity completed immediately by Admitting Nurse
1.1	Introduce the service user, family & carers to staff, show around the ward and bed space/room
1.2	The Service User is agreeable to admission
1.3	Inform Medical Officer of arrival and agree level of urgency for medical admission
1.4	Determine immediate risk and observation level General ☐ Increased ☐ Maximum ☐
1.5	Offer arrangements to secure property/valuables
1.6	Details recorded on: FireBoard, BedBoard, 24hr Report
1.7	Gather pre-admission information from referral sources and health records
1.8	Sensitively listen to the perspectives and concerns of service user and carers; offer supportive interventions. Discuss anxieties and concerns offering reassurance.
Individualised Interventions (activities offered and not described above)	

Nursing Admission Assessment Completed by:

(name, date, time) _____

4. VARIANCE RECORDING

Only complete when recommended & individualised interventions do not occur as suggested

Code	Date, Time & Sign		Code	Date, Time & Sign

Appendix 13.1   *(Continued)*

PART 3 – NARRATIVE NURSING ADMISSION ASSESSMENT

5. PRESENTING CRISIS

Complete within 3hrs of admission

Reason for Admission	Previous Psychiatric History & Response to Care : (i.e. current/past treatment, hospital admissions, MHA, substance misuse, personal & forensic history)

Mental Health: mood & ideation, anxiety, phobias and panics, somatic preoccupations, lowering energy, drive or interest, sleep disturbance, delusions, hallucinations

Mood & Indication of Depression: (affect, hopelessness, anxiety, guilt, diurnal variation, weight loss, emotional reactivity, low self esteem, loss of interest, energy, concentration)

* Complete Risk Assessment where there is indication of harm to self, others or self neglect

Cognitive & Psychological Wellbeing: memory, attention/ concentration, understanding, communication	Behaviour: wandering, aggressive behaviour, suspicious or accusatory behaviour, sociality, alcohol or substance misuse, over-activity, odd, inappropriate or unacceptable behaviour

Appendix 13.1   *(Continued)*

Activities of Daily Living & Physical Wellbeing: mobility, disability, injury, comorbidity factors, sensory impairment, motor skills, pain, continence, diet

Capacity & Consent:

Social Circumstances: Household Management, Finances, Relationships, Family

Information from previous assessments: (including date completed and by whom, any changes which indicate need for reassessment)

Nursing Admission Assessment Completed by: (name, date, time) _____

PART 4 – ADMISSION COMPLETED & 72 HOUR MANAGEMENT PLAN

6. COMPLETED ADMISSION

	Activity within 5hrs by Admitting Nurse
2.1	**Ward information leaflet offered to the service user and carer** (when the format cannot be understood consider individualised interventions)
2.2	**Refer to Social Work/EDT where urgent situation arises** (i.e. MHA, housing, finance)
2.3	**For detained patients the senior nurse on duty accepts section papers**
2.4	**Help service user to/or inform relatives & carers of admission (with consent)**
2.5	**Establish from the service user, family or carers any immediate needs**

7. 72 HOUR PLAN

The aim of this plan is to ensure that individuals are offered orientation, guidance, information, engagement & reassurance – informed by the vulnerability, capacity and accessibility of the service user. The involvement of the service user (carers and family if possible) is essential and this plan can be supplemented by individualised care plans. **The purpose of the admission has been agreed with the service user as:**

Specific Objectives are to: assess health & wellbeing, provide a safe environment, facilitate health promoting interventions and promote therapeutic relationships.

Appendix 13.1   *(Continued)*

2.6 Obtain consent for and carry out personal search as indicated by risk Yes ☐ N/A ☐ Refused ☐ discuss with MO	**Activities offered by the Named Nurse or Team** **3.1** Level of Observation General ☐ Increased ☐ Maximum ☐
2.7 Obtain consent for disposal of medication/sharp objects Yes ☐ N/A ☐ Refused ☐ discuss with MO	**3.2** Named nurse facilitates individual sessions to develop the therapeutic relationship, assess needs and offer psychological interventions
2.8 Allocate Named Nurse _____ (name) and explain their role and the care planning process	**3.3** Any cultural and spiritual influences upon care are considered and planned for
Activity completed within 5hrs by Medical Officer	**3.4** The nursing team provide orientation, guidance, information, engagement and reassurance
2.9 Assessment of Capacity, Consent, mental, DNAR and Physical State	**3.5** Any changes in physical and mental health, behaviour, mood, capacity, legal status, risk and functioning are documented and result in a review of care/treatment
2.10 Review prescribing & initial plan and explain case review process	**3.6** Support/information is offered to carers and families as appropriate
2.11 Investigations Requested HB ☐ ESR ☐ FBC ☐ U&Es ☐ LFTs ☐ ECG ☐ Other (please state)	**3.7** Where other agencies have been involved in care they are aware of admission
2.12 Observation Level General ☐ Increased ☐ Maximum ☐	**3.9** Referral/Information to Physiotherapy ☐ OT ☐ Social Worker ☐ CPN ☐ Other ☐
Activity completed within 24hrs by Nursing Team	**3.10** Blood samples collected
2.13 Inform Care Coordinator of admission and date of first case review	**Activities by the Ward Administration/Support**
2.14 Care Plan commenced; and wishes and preferences about care established	**3.11** Admission recorded & benefits situation assessed
2.15 Tissue Viability Assessment completed	**3.12** Medical Certificate or BR409 completed and sent to benefits agency
2.16 Moving & Handling Assessment completed	**Activities by Own Medical Team**
2.17 Fall Pathway commenced	**3.13** Review circumstances of admission, Mental Health Act Status and Medication
2.18 TPR:_____ BP:_____ Urinalysis:_____	**3.14** History taken (past psychiatric, family & medical history, personality, social circumstances, medication, self-care & performance)
2.19 Is there need for an interpreter? Yes ☐ No ☐	**3.15** MSE, formulation and management plan recorded
2.20 Plans are in place to address any issues arising from the completed assessments	**3.16** Review physical state & blood result; any abnormalities are recorded
	3.17 Support/information offered to carers and families as appropriate
	3.18 Consider mental state, consent to treatment, functioning, diagnosis and observation level
Activities Coordinated by: (name, date, time) 1. 2.	**Activities Coordinated by:** (name, date, time) 1. 2.

8. VARIANCE RECORDING

Complete when recommended activities do not occur as planned

Code	Date, Time & Sign		Code	Date, Time & Sign

Appendix 13.1   *(Continued)*

CARE PLAN			
Summary of all actions and plans agreed under the Care Programme Approach			
NAME:	D.O.B:	NHS No:	CPA LEVEL Standard ☐ Enhanced ☐

IDENTIFIED NEED	PLANNED OUTCOMES	AGREED ACTION (INCLUDING FREQUENCY)	PERSON/SERVICE RESPONSIBLE & CONTACT DETAILS	DATE NEED MET

Signature of Care Coordinator/Co-worker/Named Nurse: Signature of Service User

Appendix 13.1   *(Continued)*

PART 5 – COMPLETED ASSESSMENTS BY DAY 10

9. COMPLETED ASSESSMENTS

Type of Assessment (√ as completed) (see abbreviation list on page 2 as needed)							
MMSE	☐	MADRS	☐	CDR	☐	Simons	☐
RDRS-2	☐	MADRS-S	☐	FrSBe	☐	SIB	☐
BSS	☐	3MS	☐	BSA	☐	Waterlow	☐
BHS	☐	CAMCOG	☐	NPI	☐	Moving & Handling	☐
CSDD	☐	CDT	☐	Clifton Assessment	☐	Falls	☐
FAST	☐	Risk	☐	Nutritional	☐	Carers	☐

10. OUTCOME OF ASSESSMENTS

Score or indication from assessments:

Problem type:

Intervention

Need for further assessment:

Need for referral:

Completed by (name, date, time) _____

Appendix 13.1   (*Continued*)

It is expected that these activities have been completed unless they are recorded as a variance

Code	Activity completed by Day 10 by Named Nurse
3.20	Assessments have been completed and outcome is recorded above
3.21	The outcome can be cross referenced with the care plan which is in place
3.22	The outcome of the assessments has been discussed at case review
3.23	Appropriate information leaflets have been offered to the Service User & Carer/s
3.24	Delayed Discharge Criteria completed to Part B and faxed

12. VARIANCE RECORDING

Only complete when recommended and individualised interventions do not occur as planned

Code	Date, Time & Sign		Code	Date, Time & Sign

PART 6 - LIFE STORY INFORMATION SHEET

13. LIFE STORY

Personal Attributes: strengths, abilities, personality
Family Details: husband, wife, children, great-grandchildren, visiting
Significant Life Events: significant achievements/events, unpleasant events, marriage, birthdays, anniversaries
Formative Years: birth place, early years, brothers, sisters, school. college, awards or certificates, special places, mother, father
Occupational History: main occupation, work, jobs, main duties & responsibilities, working conditions, achievements at work
Hobbies & Interests: hobbies, interests, sports in the past and now, pastimes and leisure pursuits currently enjoyed, holidays, trips, music, clubs & organisations, songs, books, television, radio, newspaper, church, poetry, sculpture, pets

Appendix 13.1   *(Continued)*

Likes, Dislikes and Fears:
Food & Drinks

Do you need/use glasses or hearing aid?

What type of clothes do you like to wear (colours of clothes)?

Do you have a favourite place to visit, or go for walks?

How do you like to wear your hair?

Do you like to wear a beard or moustache?

How do you like to shave?

What time do you like to go to bed and get up in the morning? How many hours sleep do you prefer to have?

Do you have any fears or phobias?

Are there any likes and dislikes you would like us to know?

Life Story Completed by: (name, date, time) _____

Appendix 13.1   (*Continued*)

INTEGRATED CARE PATHWAY FOR
OLDER ADULT
ASSESSMENT (INPATIENT CARE)

When the pathway is completed please send a
copy of this sheet to:

Variance Record Sheet from _____

Date	Activity Code	Variance Code	Action to be Taken (If you need to repeat an intervention then fill in the blank rows in the appropriate time frame)	Sign

Appendix 13.1   (*Continued*)

VARIATION SOURCE CODES		
User/carer codes	**System codes**	**Other agencies**
1.1 User unavailable	2.1 Date and time of intervention changed	3.1 Accommodation not available
1.2 Carer unavailable	2.2 Awaiting consultation from others	3.2 Community support not available
1.3 User refused	2.3 Staff/Service unavailable	3.3 Day service not available
1.4 Carer refused	2.4 Lack of time	3.4 Funding/benefits not available
1.5 Intervention inappropriate	2.5 Intervention postponed/cancelled	3.5 Transport not available
1.6 Deterioration of mental state:	2.6 Information results not available	3.6 Other (please state)
Intervention inappropriate	2.7 Dept closed/room not available	
1.7 Improvement of mental state:	2.8 Appointment not available/delayed	
Intervention inappropriate	2.9 Other (please state)	
1.8 User refused due to poor motivation		
1.9 Intervention repeated due to lack of		
understanding or skills		
1.10 Other (please state)		

Appendix 13.1   (*Continued*)

REFERENCES

Bullivant J 1997 Introduction to benchmarking for continuous improvement in health and local government. Benchmarking Reference Centre, Wrexham

Department of Health 1999 Effective care coordination in mental health services – modernising the Care Programme Approach. Department of Health, London

Department of Health 2001 National service framework for older people. Department of Health, London

Department of Health 2004 Single assessment process for older people: assessment scales. Department of Health, London

Middleton S, Roberts A 2000 Integrated care pathways: a practical approach to implementation. Butterworth-Heinemann, Oxford

Morse JM 1997 Preventing patient falls. Sage, London

White T 2004 Are you falling down on the prevention of falls? Changing the delivery of care through the development and implementation of a multidisciplinary assessment tool and care pathway. Journal of Integrated Care Pathways 8:19-26

Using a care pathway for electroconvulsive therapy

Alan Pringle

INTRODUCTION	**IMPLEMENTATION**
BACKGROUND	**OUTCOMES AND CONCLUSIONS**
PATHWAY DEVELOPMENT	**REFERENCES**

INTRODUCTION

Within the field of acute mental health care, one form of treatment that remains controversial, and is often criticised for its variation in standards, is electroconvulsive therapy (known as ECT in the United Kingdom and as either ECT or 'Electroshock' in the United States). This chapter outlines the attempt to address both the maintenance of high standards and the process of involving staff in addressing the controversial nature of the treatment, by developing an integrated care pathway (ICP) for the delivery of ECT at Millbrook, a mental health unit in Mansfield, near Nottingham. This chapter proceeds with an overview of ECT, its history and use. Then follows a brief description of the policy and practice context of acute inpatient care where the care pathway is situated. Details of the development and use of the pathway follow and readers can consider how this is used to focus practice development upon one discrete aspect of practice.

Since its earliest days ECT has been the subject of myth, mystique and misrepresentation, and continues to this day to provoke an often visceral and emotive response in those who come into contact with it. Some papers in the nursing and medical press (Fink 1999, Kho 2002, Kho et al 2003, MacEwan 2002, Petrides et al 1994) have come out strongly in favour of ECT and claim that its effectiveness as a treatment for severe depression overrides the controversy that surrounds it. However, other authors write strongly against its use (Drummond 2000, Stephenson 1994, United Kingdom Advocacy Network 1996), stating that the barbarous nature of the process and the variation in care standards in its delivery render it obsolete and untenable as a treatment. Others (Baldwin 2001, Branfield 1992, Perkins 1999) have attempted to give a more balanced picture and suggest that, if questions around standards and delivery could be addressed, there may be a place for ECT despite the limited ability of clinicians and researchers to give definitive explanations of how the treatment actually works.

This range of contradictory views, along with the somewhat gothic and macabre mental image which many people have of ECT, can lead to staff being anxious about taking part in the procedure (Stephenson 1994) and consequently actively avoiding involvement in the treatment. The inability of extensive research to explain conclusively how ECT actually works and why it works (if it does work) is perhaps the greatest reason for the continued controversy that is often expressed by staff in acute inpatient settings where this treatment is usually delivered.

BACKGROUND

Beardsall et al (2002) outline how in 1933 the Hungarian physician Ladislaus von Meduna, working at the Interacademic Institute of Psychiatric Research in Budapest, began to explore what he felt was the biological antagonism between schizophrenia and epilepsy. He believed that these conditions were mutually exclusive and therefore unable to exist together. Von Meduna's belief that epileptic-style convulsions could drive out schizophrenia and cure the condition led him to seek a method of inducing convulsions that were controllable and reproducible. After testing several substances, including camphor and strychnine, he fixed on Metrazol given as an intramuscular injection to induce seizures. In 1937 von Meduna claimed at a symposium in Switzerland that the process was successful, and could boast of dramatic cures and a discharge rate of 50% in those treated. In time, psychiatry would come to accept that the theory of incompatibility between epilepsy and schizophrenia was unfounded but experimentation with the use of convulsions as a method of treatment continued.

In Italy at this time a neurologist called Ugo Cerletti was also convinced about the benefits of convulsive treatments in affective and psychotic disorders but felt that Metrazol injections as a means of induction were too uncontrollable and dangerous. Cerletti's earlier work on epilepsy had involved using electric shocks to trigger convulsions in animals to attempt to understand the neuropathological consequences of repeated grand mal seizures. He then worked with Bini and Kalinowski to develop a machine that could deliver similar electric shocks to humans. The apparatus was designed and the controversial treatment of electro-convulsive therapy began. Soon after its initial introduction, injections of curare and scopolamine were added to the procedure and gradually this 'modified' ECT became known as MECT. This then began to replace Metrazol and insulin-induced shocks to become a treatment of choice in affective disorders in the majority of hospitals and asylums around the world; a place ECT continues to maintain in some countries to this day.

In a time when people who suffer from mental health problems appear to be able to choose from a vast menu of talking therapies, an abundance of medication and a wide range of alternative therapies and approaches, why would anyone agree to attempt to relieve their depressive symptoms by receiving a measured dose of electricity run through their brain instead? This, of course, is a difficult question for staff who work in acute inpatient mental health settings to attempt to answer, as they consider a mass of often conflicting information which provokes perhaps one of the biggest and most emotive controversies in mental health nursing. The reluctance of staff to become involved with, and develop an ownership of, this treatment has contributed to ECT being specifically recognised by the Royal College of Psychiatrists as an area of acute mental health care where standards need to be set, implemented and maintained (Caird et al 2004). Grant (2004) describes how the *Mental health policy implementation guide – adult acute inpatient care provision* (Department of Health 2002) sets out a clear vision of service redesign and care developments to deliver an improvement in the quality of mental health care. This, it may be argued, was in response to mounting criticism of care from amongst others MIND, Rethink and the Sainsbury Centre for Mental Health (1998). This implementation guidance builds upon earlier policy including the National Service Framework for Mental Health (Department of Health 1999) which aims to raise standards and reduce variation and discrepancies in care delivery within trusts and other service providers.

As previously mentioned, ECT is one area where marked variances in standards have been recognised. This was acknowledged by the Royal College of Psychiatrists whose national audit found that many clinics or services were falling short of the standards recommended in their second ECT handbook. Writing in the *British Medical Journal*, Carney & Geddes (2003) described ECT as 'a neglected service with widespread unexplained variations in practice and a low priority with managers'. The Royal College of Psychiatrists subsequently launched an ECT Accreditation Service (ECTAS) with the aim of raising standards (Caird et al 2004). The National Institute of Clinical Excellence (NICE) in their ECT guidelines, published in 2003, state that audits should be carried out to ensure that ECT is used appropriately and that a high standard of care is delivered (National Institute of Clinical Excellence 2003). Furthermore, the Department of Health (2002) suggests that through the construction of national standards and ongoing monitoring of these standards through audit, a culture of good practice can be established and maintained. At Millbrook Mental Health Unit it was felt that one way of developing a culture of good practice around ECT as a treatment was to explore the development of an integrated care pathway.

PATHWAY DEVELOPMENT

So, why develop an integrated care pathway for ECT at Millbrook? Millbrook is a small mental health unit in Mansfield, near Nottingham, with an acute unit comprising of three wards each with 25 beds. Throughout the 1990s ECT at Millbrook had been methodically and systematically managed by one extremely dedicated nurse. This placed a responsibility on this one individual to maintain standards within the department but this inevitably raised potential problems when that nurse was not available for work. As this nurse moved towards retirement, it became apparent that a system was needed that was not heavily reliant upon one person but that helped to develop the skills of a group of staff, whilst not diminishing high standards. It was felt that the answer lay in the development of an ICP for ECT.

An ICP was felt to be a positive direction to take because, according to Riley (1998), an ICP offers a locally agreed multidisciplinary practice, based on guidelines and evidence, for a specific patient/client group. It was suggested by De Luc (2000) that care pathways lead to quality improvement through evidence-based practice and by Hall (2000) that they are a way of meeting local and national agendas in setting and monitoring multi-professional standards of care. An ICP seemed appropriate for ECT as a specific target process because, according to Johnson & Smith (2000), an ICP anticipates all elements of care and treatment from members of the multidisciplinary team and as ECT involves a team (that includes ward staff, recovery staff, doctors and anaesthetists) it was felt that an ICP may help further develop relationships between the members of this team.

A multidisciplinary ECT working group was established to explore developing an ICP. Members were representatives from the ECT department, the unit manager, a consultant psychiatrist, clinical effectiveness officer, practice development nurse and a consultant from the anaesthetic team. The aim of the group was agreed as 'to oversee the development of an ICP specifically designed for use in the coordination and administration of ECT'. This would be used to develop, review and improve the care standards of a variety of clinicians. Care pathways are seen to lend themselves more easily to physical care procedures (Peet & Wakefield 2002), and although the use of ICPs was growing in Britain at this time, and the benefits of ICPs were generally acknowledged, very few existed in mental health. The group initially met bimonthly and began by reviewing the documentation in use at the time, extracting the elements of most use and combining them with essential documents such as the prescription, consent form and anaesthetic assessment forms. The result was the creation of a multidisciplinary document that reflected the client's progression through the treatment, from first suggestion of ECT as a treatment, through the treatment itself, to post-treatment evaluation.

A 'mapping out' of the client's journey followed the review of documentation. This was done stage by stage and followed the variety of routes through treatment a service user might take, either by informed consent or, in certain circumstances, under the provision of the Mental Health Act. Throughout this process, the group brought together their expertise, experience and creativity to the design of the ICP but, perhaps most of all, the multidisciplinary nature of the group gave true ownership to the project. This may sound unimportant until viewed in light of the observation that 48% of responses to a National Pathway Association survey cited clinical ownership as a crucial factor for successful implementation (Riley 1998). Commitment to the project was evident, with regular attendance by different disciplines at the planning meetings. Specific tasks around gathering information,

Box 14.1   PERCEIVED BENEFITS OF USING AN ICP FOR ECT

- Multidisciplinary teamwork and communication
- Coordination of care
- Multidisciplinary documentation
- Access to clinical information
- Delivery of consistent, standardised care
- Identification and reduction of clinical variances
- Auditing of practice against agreed standards
- Training and education of staff.

literature searching and canvassing opinions were delegated to specific group members, and enough time was allowed to complete the tasks well. This helped the group retain its purpose and impetus. Through this process the group identified eight key areas in which it was felt that an ICP could have a major positive impact on standards of care. These were multidisciplinary teamwork and communication, coordination of care, multidisciplinary documentation, access to clinical information, delivery of consistent standardised care, identification and reduction of clinical variances, auditing of practices against agreed standards and training of staff. These are summarised in Box 14.1.

Whether these potential benefits were actually realised would be addressed by an evaluation system built into the process. Hall (2001) suggests that pathways are seen as providing guidelines rather than strict protocols and, as such, a pathway does not aim to create what Jones (2000) calls unthinking care providers. A pathway is not a substitute for professional judgment or individualised interventions (Mullins & Wilson 1994). In this instance, the pathway was created with the express idea of mapping out the ECT care process from start to finish in a way that was concise and easy to follow. In the pathway, each discipline has a clear description of their role and responsibility within the process. This was intended to help clarify each discipline's role without removing the crucial element of clinical judgment. By negotiation, compromise and many drafts, the group finally agreed a product that appeared to be user friendly, clinically sound and included all elements of an individual's care throughout this procedure.

The key activities of different disciplines (doctors, anaesthetists, ward staff and recovery staff) were written into a single document which ran in sequence from identification of the need for ECT and the consent form, through the prescription of treatment, the delivery of treatment, the recovery process and the post-ECT follow-up, to the evaluation of the effectiveness of treatment. There were sections on the pathway to record any reasons why the treatment did not follow the sequence mapped out. The deviations from the planned care (variances) are reported. Each section of text was colour coded so that it was clear at a glance which discipline was responsible for completing which section of the document; and a flow chart using the same colour coding was constructed on the front of each document as a précis and aide memoire about the process. This first flow chart underwent several modifications in light of evaluation and feedback before becoming the one currently in use, which is shown in Figure 14.1.

A review of the current literature on anaesthesia, ECT technique and nursing practice carried out by the various members of the team in their own specialty

Figure 14.1
The current ECT pathway at Millbrook

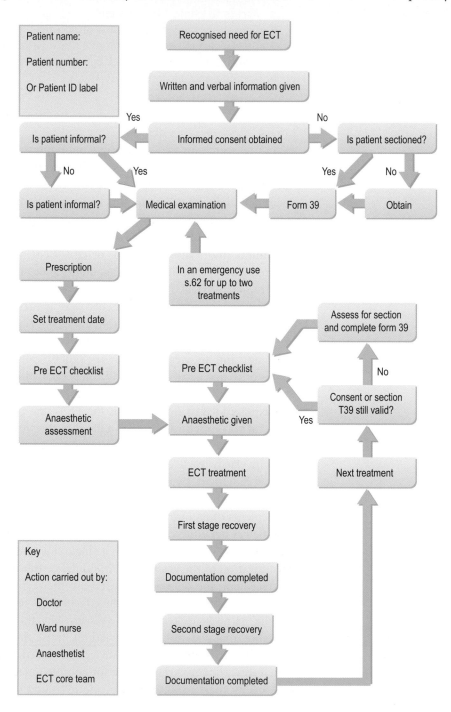

helped underpin the stages of the pathway. This collection of literature was collected into a resource file and was kept in the department for all staff to access.

IMPLEMENTATION

Teaching sessions for the different staff involved in the delivery of care were carried out to introduce them to the pathway; and specific staff from each ward were identified by self-selection to become part of a 'core team' of nursing staff who would be responsible for the delivery of the nursing component of the pathway. The process was clarified by following the flow chart where every area of care was clearly designated to a member of the multidisciplinary team. It was emphasised that if one part of the document was not completed the staff should not progress on to the next part of the document. Following the teaching of staff, the pathway was launched for a 16 week trial period, with a view to an evaluation of its effectiveness after this period. All ECT treatments during this trial time followed the ICP and members of the ICP working group carried out evaluation.

Following the trial of the pathway, the evaluation involved a three-stage process of:

- audit of the pathway documentation
- staff questionnaires and interviews
- semi-structured interviews with the service users who had completed treatment using the pathway (and who wished to be part of the evaluation and discuss their experience of the care).

It was felt that service users would be able to offer a fuller response via face-to-face contact and the use of a semi-structured interview to gather data. This would support clarification and expansion in discussion, which would not be possible with a questionnaire. Gray (2004) suggests that interviews are preferable to questionnaires where the attempt is being made to find about someone's experience of an event. The evaluation of the pilot aimed to gather information about whether the potential benefits of using a pathway that are highlighted in Box 14.1 were seen to be developing. During the 16 week pilot, 15 service users commenced a course of ECT. A course can be as little as two treatments, with the vast majority of courses falling somewhere between six and 12 treatments. Treatment is administered either two or three times a week. During the pilot time at Millbrook the average course of ECT consisted of six treatments with a total of 90 treatments being administered during the pilot period.

Evaluation of ICP documentation

In all, 14 patient records were audited and the pathway documentation had been adopted in all of them, demonstrating that staff had incorporated the pathway into their practice. However, the audit highlighted that there were key sections of the pathway that were either not being completed or being only partially completed.

These areas were:

- administration of anaesthetic – the percentage of oxygen used during the anaesthetic procedure was not always clearly documented
- details of second-stage post-treatment recovery on the ward were not always documented
- review of symptoms and response to treatment were not always completed
- clinical variances were being recorded along the margins of the main pathway document rather than being recorded on the appended variance sheet.

The evaluation of documentation was, however, generally positive and encouraging. Initial findings from audits of notes suggested:

- multidisciplinary teamwork and communication between disciplines had improved
- coordination of care was better
- multidisciplinary documentation was beneficial as all ECT information was together in one place leading to easier access to clinical information
- delivery of care was more consistent.

The audit also highlighted areas of concern around:

- identification and reduction of clinical variances
- training and education of staff.

Staff survey findings

The staff survey regarding use of the ICP was conducted through semi-structured group discussions, interviews and postal questionnaires. All staff involved in ECT were asked to appraise the pathway using a Likert scale, against its aims and objectives and to consider its strengths and weaknesses. The anaesthetists who participated in the evaluation felt they could not objectively appraise changes brought about by the pathway as they worked on a rotational basis and had not been involved in ECT procedures at the unit prior to the pilot. They did however identify weaknesses in the process and provided suggestions to address these. The results of the staff audit reflected some concerns and confusion surrounding the role and responsibility of nursing staff on the wards in the section of the pathway where symptoms and response to treatment should be reviewed. Locally, medical staff had traditionally been responsible for reviewing the client's symptoms and response to ECT. However, prior to this pilot study, both medical and nursing staff had agreed that ward staff were best placed to judge whether ECT had been beneficial to the service user as they spent more time with that person. For the first time, this agreement became 'formalised' with the introduction of the pathway, which caused some concern amongst ward staff. Overall, the staff surveyed expressed the view that the pathway was making progress in achieving its aims and objectives.

Feedback from service users

The views of service users were sought through semi-structured interviews, which were conducted either by the practice development nurse or an experienced healthcare support worker. It is acknowledged that using this approach has a possibility of a biased response, with patients expressing higher levels of satisfaction/positive feedback. Eight clients agreed to participate and they were asked for their views on the information they were given about ECT, the treatment itself and the care and support given by staff.

The majority of service users thought that:

1. they were given enough information about the procedure prior to treatment
2. staff were helpful and reassuring
3. care during the initial recovery period in the clinic was satisfactory
4. ward staff were helpful and reassuring throughout the procedure.

Service users were also asked if there were any aspects of care they would like to change. Whilst no changes were suggested, service users took the opportunity to comment on both positive and negative experiences of undergoing ECT treatment. The positive experiences were the reassurances and explanations given by staff; also, having staff accompany them from the ward to support them prior to, during and after treatment. Negative experiences were the waiting period and anxiety prior to treatment. During the pilot, ECT treatments were carried out in the afternoons. This meant that patients had to maintain their fasting for longer during the day and also that much of the day is spent in a state of anxiety waiting for their treatment. Other negative experiences were wearing the oxygen mask, anxiety generated by people in white coats (anaesthetic staff) and a temporary loss of memory immediately following treatment.

Using the information from evaluation to revise the ICP

Following the ICP evaluation process, the time of ECT sessions was changed and the time needed for fasting was reduced to the minimum time needed. Also in response to the evaluation some areas of the pathway were redesigned, in particular the area given for variance reporting. Campbell et al (1998) suggested using a separate sheet to record all variances from the pathway, as this could be easily removed for audit purposes. This was the system used. It was found, however, that staff had often overlooked the variance sheet and instead used the margins around the page to enter clinical information or variation. By providing a space for variance reporting after each intervention it was felt that staff were more likely to complete variance sections of the pathway. It was suggested that the recording of essential clinical information in a way that was easy to complete and that was legible and succinct, outweighed the ease with which the information could be extracted for the purpose of audit. The importance of regular inspection of variance entries is acknowledged and that shortfalls in standards may never be identified if regular audit is not undertaken.

Addressing variances

Variances are where the care or treatment received differs from the predicted treatment outlined in the pathway. As stated previously, a course of ECT consists of a number of treatments. During the evaluation period any variances from the pathway for each planned treatment for all 14 service users were reviewed by the pathway working group. During the pilot, 18 variances occurred in the 90 planned treatments (20% of treatments). These variances related to seven of the 14 service users studied in the evaluation. The number of variances for these seven service users ranged from one to six. The service user who experienced the greatest number of variances was detained under the Mental Health Act and required compulsory treatment. For the purposes of analysis, the variances were grouped into three broad categories:

- clinical – e.g. inadequate seizure length, adverse reaction to propofol, raised blood pressure
- service user – e.g. fasting protocol prior to treatment not adhered to, agitation in mood during first-stage recovery from treatment
- staff/organisation – e.g. availability of notes.

Of the 18 variances identified, the majority (n = 14) were clinical. The review by the working group concluded that these clinical responses to treatment could not have been predicted, were unavoidable and concurred that the resulting individualised treatment that followed was both necessary and appropriate. These variances were therefore clinically justified and did not indicate that standards of care were not being met. There were three service user related variances, which included the cancellation of a treatment when the fasting protocol was not adhered to and agitation in mood during post-treatment recovery. There was one staff-related variance which concerned the availability of notes when treatment was administered outside the unit at a different location. Reviewing these variances helped the group identify where the process needed to be improved; and changes were made in the observation policy for clients pre-treatment, and in the pathway documentation to ensure that the correct documentation followed the client.

Following evaluation, further training about the pathway was provided for all ward staff and a more in-depth training was provided for those staff who had expressed a desire to become part of the 'core team' who would deliver the treatment in the unit. A training package was subsequently developed which is currently used to train the core team of nursing staff for the ECT clinic. This package is also used to assist in training other members of the multidisciplinary team, for example junior medical staff.

One major change that took place relatively soon after the launch of the pathway was removing ECT from the line management of the Day Therapy Services and reconfiguring it within the acute inpatient structure. The vast majority of clients receiving ECT were from the acute inpatient areas and the new 'core team' of staff providing ECT care were from the inpatient service. To increase further the sense of ownership that the staff had for the pathway, it made perfect sense to move the service under the umbrella of inpatient care. This created the structure under which the ECT team leader works across the three acute wards, with several staff nurses to provide cover for the second-stage recovery process. This appears to have increased the sense of ownership and commitment. The team is the major influence in further development of the pathway and in the instigation of changes that are made at 6 monthly review meetings. They review the workings of the pathway and implement any agreed changes.

The current version of the pathway (shown in Figure 14.1) reflects the changes that have been made to the original structure, noting issues such as ongoing consent during a course of treatment and the completion of specific forms for informal clients and those detained under the Mental Health Act (forms 38 and 39).

OUTCOMES AND CONCLUSIONS

In discussion with the team involved, the strengths of a pathway as a method of care delivery focus primarily around the issues of quality and consistency of care. It is felt that the original aspirations that were held for the pathway have been achieved and are visible:

- multidisciplinary teamwork and communication is better, with each discipline having a clear understanding of their role in the process
- multidisciplinary documentation has been achieved, with each discipline writing directly onto the pathway document
- access to clinical information is better because all information is stored on the pathway document rather than having some in medical notes, some in ECT notes and some in ward nursing notes
- delivery of consistent, standardised care is visible as is seen by recurring, regular audit of the completion rates of the various parts of the pathway
- identification and reduction of clinical variances have been observed as the pathway has become embedded in day-to-day practice
- training and education of staff has been evidenced by the fact that the pathway is an integral part of induction for new nursing staff and new medical staff.

After implementation the pathway was presented at internal trust meetings including the practice development steering group, the clinical effectiveness group and the Trust Board meeting. This ensured that the concept of ICPs could become embedded within the clinical governance agenda of the Trust. Data from the variance reports are disseminated appropriately to ensure that they contribute to further knowledge, development and assurance (McHaffie 2000, Smith & Masterson 1996). Reports of the pathway development were published in the journal *Practice Developments in Health Care* and presented at a European mental health nursing conference. This dissemination was seen as important by staff and derived from pride in the development and a strong sense of ownership.

In conclusion, the Millbrook experience of developing a care pathway for ECT did, in fact, appear to help develop the locally agreed multidisciplinary practice as Riley (1998) suggested. The quality improvement through evidence-based practice proposed by De Luc (2000) and Hall's (2000) way of meeting local and national agendas in setting and monitoring multi-professional standards of care appeared to be the reality. The most important thing to be taken from the

Millbrook experience, however, is the importance of true multidisciplinary working and a genuine sense of ownership in the creation and use of an integrated care pathway. It was that more than anything that helped the pathway to become established as the routine method of care delivery for this specific treatment. As suggested by Johnson & Smith (2000) the ICP did in fact benefit from the multidisciplinary nature of its conception, design, development and implementation. As would be expected, the pathway remains a dynamic document that is constantly under review and developed further by the ECT working group in response to audits, feedback from the staff who use it and the service users who experience care. This is indeed as it should be, with no ICP being the finished article, but merely the current version that is open to further development in light of evidence collected.

REFERENCES

Baldwin H 2001 Shockproof. Nursing Standard 15:21

Beardsall L, Gough J, Pringle A 2002 Developing an ECT integrated care pathway. Practice Development in Healthcare 1(1):21-35

Branfield M 1992 ECT for depression in elderly people. Nursing Standard 6(26):24-27

Caird H, Worrall A, Lelliott P 2004 The electroconvulsive therapy accreditation service. Psychiatric Bulletin 28:257-259

Campbell H, Hotchkiss R, Bradshaw N et al 1998 Integrated care pathways. British Medical Journal 316:133-137

Carney S, Geddes G 2003 Electroconvulsive therapy. Recent recommendations are likely to improve standards and uniformity of use. British Medical Journal 326:1343-1344

De Luc K 2000 Care pathways: an evaluation of their effectiveness. Journal of Advanced Nursing 32(2):485-496

Department of Health 1999 The national service framework for mental health: modern standards and service models. HMSO, London

Department of Health 2002 Mental health policy implementation guide: adult acute inpatient care provision. HMSO, London

Drummond E 2000 The complete guide to psychiatric drugs. John Wiley, New York

Fink M 1999 Electroshock: restoring the mind. Oxford University Press, New York

Grant R 2004 Do integrated care pathways work in acute mental healthcare? A comparative audit based study. Unpublished dissertation, University of Nottingham, Nottingham

Gray DE 2004 Doing research in the real world. Sage, London

Hall J 2000 Establishing an icp within an organic assessment service. Bulletin Old Age Psychiatry 2(1):3-6

Hall J 2001 A qualitative survey of staff responses to an integrated care pathway pilot study in a mental health care setting. Nursing Times Research 6(3):696-705

Johnson S, Smith J 2000 Factors influencing the success of ICP projects. Professional Nurse 15: 776-779

Jones A 2000 Implementation of hospital care pathways for patients with schizophrenia. Journal of Nursing Management 8:215-225

Kho KH 2002 Treatment of rapid cycling bipolar disorder in the acute and maintenance phase with ECT. Journal of ECT 18(3): 159-161

Kho KH, Vreeswick MF, Simpson S 2003 A meta-analysis of electroconvulsive therapy efficacy in depression. Journal of ECT 19(3):139-147

MacEwan T 2002 An audit of seizure duration in electroconvulsive therapy. Psychiatric Bulletin 26(9):337-339

McHaffie H 2000 Ethical issues in research. In: Cormack D (ed) The research process in nursing, 4th edn, pp 51-62. Blackwell Science, Oxford

Mullins E, Wilson J 1994 Medical care paths as part of an integrated organisational strategy. Advisory December 1994, pp 4-6.

National Institute for Clinical Effectiveness 2003 Guidelines on the use of electroconvulsive therapy. NICE, London

Peet M, Wakefield S 2002 Integrated care pathways in mental health: the need for the 'human touch'. Journal of Integrated Care Pathways 6:108-114

Perkins R 1999 Choosing ECT. In: Read J, Reynolds J Speaking our minds: an anthology. Open University Press, Buckingham

Petrides G, Dhossche D, Fink M et al 1994 Continuation ECT, relapse prevention in affective disorder. Convulsive Therapy 10(3):194-198

Riley K 1998 Paving the way. Health Service Journal March 1998, pp 30-31

Sainsbury Centre for Mental Health 1998 Acute problems: a survey of the quality of care in acute psychiatric wards. The Sainsbury Centre for Mental Health, London

Smith P, Masterson A 1996 Promoting the dissemination and implementation of research findings. NT Nurse Researcher 4(4):28-40

Stephenson P 1994 Shock horror Story. No Limits 1(6):11

United Kingdom Advocacy Network 1996 The national experience ECT survey, United Kingdom AN, London

15
An integrated care pathway for crisis triage and assessment

Julie Hall and Jeannette Connelly

CRISIS RESOLUTION AND HOME TREATMENT SERVICES	**THE PATHWAY DEVELOPMENT PROCESS**
ACCESS TO THE PATHWAY	**PROCESS MAPPING AND REDESIGN**
	PILOT, IMPLEMENTATION AND REVIEW
ASSESSMENT AND INTERVENTIONS	**VARIANCE REPORTS AND ANALYSIS**
AN ORGANISATIONAL APPROACH TO CARE PATHWAYS	**MONITORING AND EVALUATION**
THE CASE FOR USING A CARE PATHWAY IN THIS SERVICE	**IMPACTS AND FUTURE DEVELOPMENT**
	REFERENCES

This chapter describes the development and implementation of an integrated care pathway within a Crisis Resolution and Home Treatment (CRHT) service. Discussion begins by outlining the current context of this service setting; the background to home treatment services in the United Kingdom (UK), the characteristics of the team and the interdisciplinary nature of provision. There are brief details about who the service is available to, the interventions offered and how this service integrates with other teams in a whole systems approach to mental health services. The chapter illustrates how the care pathway was developed as part of an organisational approach to service improvement. There are service-specific descriptions of the challenges of development and implementation. Arrangements for monitoring, auditing and variance reporting are described. Details of the specific benefits arising from this pathway are detailed as well as implications for future development.

CRISIS RESOLUTION AND HOME TREATMENT SERVICES

Before providing a review of CRHT services in England, it is appropriate to determine what, in mental health terms, is meant by a crisis. Minghella et al (1998) define a crisis as a time when someone is unable to cope due to either a recent severe deterioration in their mental health or high levels of distress. Parad & Parad (1991) note that crises acutely disturb individuals' abilities to function, and often create major disruption in the lives of their families or friends. Historically, such crises resulted in urgent admission to psychiatric hospitals for treatment, predominantly with medication (Wallcraft 1996). Developments in psychotropic medications in the 1950s (Brimblecombe 2001) and the commencement of outpatient clinics, day hospitals and community psychiatric nursing services (Rose 2001) challenged long-standing attitudes about the need for hospitalisation. Consequently, this resulted in reduced hospital admissions and the closure of mental hospitals (Freeman 1993). The development of a broader knowledge base about crisis intervention by Caplan (1964) and others, in conjunction with the more extensive provision of community-based care, led to the creation of the first community-based crisis intervention and home treatment services (Burns et al 1993, Dean & Gadd 1990, Muijen et al 1992).

Early CRHT teams demonstrated their efficacy in terms of clinical results (Dean et al 1993), reduced inpatient bed occupancy (Whittle & Mitchell 1997) and service user satisfaction (Coleman et al 1998, Kwakwa 1995). Government recognition of those and subsequent CRHT teams was demonstrated in the National Health Service (NHS) Plan (Department of Health 2000), which announced the establishment of 335 crisis resolution services in England by 2004. Hospitalisation in response to crisis for too long had paid little attention to the individual or to the life circumstances that had brought about the crisis (Punukollo 1991). This viewpoint is now embedded into current mental health policy and service design. It is firmly acknowledged in the literature that therapeutic outcomes are positive when individuals can fully engage with their recovery process and are offered appropriate interventions and information in a timely manner. The feasibility of crisis assessments and interventions outside of restrictive settings has been a preoccupation of services for some time.

CRHT teams generally have representation from several different professional groups. According to the Durham mapping database (University of Durham & Department of Health 2004), which lists the services provided by all of England's Mental Health Trusts, in September 2004 every CRHT team had nurses in their teams, 89% had managers and/or administrative support, 73% had social workers, 54% had medical input (from consultant psychiatrists and/or career grade doctors), 38% had social care support and development staffing, 10% had psychologists and 24% of the teams had input from other therapists. This is similar to the findings of Orme (2001), who noted the wide diversity in the staff disciplines represented in the CRHT teams she appraised. Concern has been expressed that the mixing of so many different disciplines within a single team might create conflict due to different professional philosophies. However, this can also be interpreted as the richness of integrated working and demonstrating the need for an integrative service philosophy. The team who developed this care pathway comprised nurses, managers, an administrator, an approved social worker, a consultant psychiatrist and a staff grade doctor. Interdisciplinary differences were a feature that arose within the integrated care pathway development and review process. It is believed that using the pathway has enabled team members to maintain a common focus on clients' assessments and in the planning and delivery of the most appropriate therapeutic interventions.

ACCESS TO THE PATHWAY

Review of the criteria for referral to the CRHT teams around England (University of Durham & Department of Health 2004) indicates a general consensus in the problems that service users experience when they access CRHT services. There is a general view that crisis resolution and home treatment is available for individuals who are suffering from deteriorated mental health. Many of these people will be previously known to the local mental health teams, with care coordinators and existing Care Programme Approach (CPA) care plans. Those care plans may include contingency plans to indicate how similar crises have been managed previously. Some CRHT teams designate one member of their team to take over as a service user's CPA care coordinator for the duration of their crisis (Orme 2001). For the team whose pathway is the focus of this chapter, this does not occur and that role remains within the local Community Mental Health Team (CMHT). The CRHT team manages care using a team approach, rather than one individual worker being responsible for each client's care. The coordination and liaison required for team case management to be effective are facilitated by the integrated care pathway approach. However, where there is no previous care coordinator and these arrangements are required during CRHT then CPA is triggered by the team.

As well as those with previous identified and long-term mental health problems, crisis intervention and home treatment also help individuals who find themselves in a psychiatric or psychological crisis following a major life event (perhaps a loss or bereavement they feel unable to cope with). These referrals originate from the local general hospitals and often involve people not previously known to mental health services. Many CRHT teams try to be available to all individuals who are experiencing crises due to deteriorated mental health or life trauma, but most teams have some exclusion criteria (Orme 2001). For example, many teams do not accept referrals for individuals who are intoxicated due to illicit drugs and/or alcohol at the point of referral or individuals for whom drug or alcohol dependence is their primary problem (Audini et al 1994). The triage process in this CRHT team prompts staff to ask referrers about the drug or alcohol usage of referred individuals, to allow staff to signpost to specialist services where this is needed. The philosophy regarding fair access to services is applied. Crisis resolution is generally restricted to adult mental health services (Sainsbury Centre for Mental Health 2001) and this CRHT team does not accept referrals for people under the age of 16 years; and although opinions vary from team to team, this service accepts referrals for those over 65 years old (Marks et al 1994, Orme 2001, Ratna 1991).

ASSESSMENT AND INTERVENTIONS

Due to the wide scope of the service offered, CRHT teams require crisis workers to be skilled and knowledgeable in mental health assessment. Assessment involves collecting and evaluating the incidence and significance of the service user's problems and needs along with how they are influenced by psychological stressors (Freud 1991), socio-economic factors (Gomm 1996, Sims & Owens 1993) or physical health problems (Snowley 1992). The need to formulate an impression of the individual's risk to themselves and others is essential (Motto et al 1985, Williams 1997). It is essential that the service user is a partner in this process and able to make decisions from as early a stage as possible in the care process. The service user's definition of recovery should be established to underpin all future care arrangements. The involvement and assessment of carers' requirements are integral to this process (as outlined in statutory statements and good practice guidance). Assessment will allow the worker to ascertain the individual's need for home treatment and indicate the type of interventions which will best help recovery. If assessment reveals that home treatment is not appropriate, the team facilitates access to other services; perhaps inpatient admission or access to another agency. The integrated care pathway developed provides a format that enables crisis workers to provide consistently thorough and rigorous assessments to all referred clients.

The interventions provided by the CRHT team can be many and varied. Many people need support and reassurance during their time of crisis, which the CRHT team can provide with home visits or telephone support. Visits may be used to offer advice about anxiety management, confidence-building techniques or methods for improving assertiveness (Powell 2001); or they may be used to help people to improve their problem-solving skills (Spivack et al 1976). Some people may need support to cope safely with suicidal ideas and depressive symptoms (Morgan 1997). Others may need medication to help them overcome the deterioration in their mental health or heightened distress (Davies & Winter 2001, Nagamoto 2001, Vasile 2001). The CRHT team may then have a role in overseeing use of medication, encouraging compliance and monitoring the effects of the medication. CRHT workers often fulfil an important role in informing individuals about their illnesses, treatments and self-help to maintain good mental health in the future. This is not a complete list of the interventions a CRHT team can offer, but it is intended to demonstrate how a CRHT team can help an individual and their family overcome a crisis without needing to be admitted to a psychiatric hospital. The integrated care pathway guides the assessment process to establish areas of need, which can be addressed by the therapeutic alliance, and the interventions offered.

AN ORGANISATIONAL APPROACH TO CARE PATHWAYS

The Trust in which this care pathway is used places importance upon maintaining high-quality integrated health services that are organised around the health needs of individuals. Underpinning this is a care pathway strategy which has the ambition of establishing programmes of care, which span professional boundaries and determine how needs might be met over a period of time (Department of Health 1998). The care pathway described in this chapter was one of the first developed in the Trust and was viewed as integral to the Trust's modernisation processes. The Trust's approach aspires to use integrated care pathway arrangements as a formula for ensuring that care experiences are built around the needs of service users, their families and carers. Implementation seeks to ensure that a journey across services is negotiated, managed and agreed. Specifically, in this case, the pathway is used to determine, plan and coordinate therapeutic and organisational activities for the CRHT service.

The CRHT service has two care pathways available for use: one for crisis triage and assessment (which is the focus of this chapter) and the other for home treatment. Both care pathways:

> *determine locally agreed, multidisciplinary practice based upon guidelines and evidence where available, for a specific patient/client group. It forms all or part of the clinical record, documents the care given and facilitates the evaluation of outcomes for continuous quality improvement.*

> (Riley 1998)

The general aim of the organisational strategy is to improve the experience of receiving services by using care pathways as a tool for monitoring, coordinating and improving standards of care. This approach hopes to secure a culture of practice development and pursuit of improvement which places service users at the centre of care. All care pathways developed and implemented in the Trust:

- Are a consequence of rigorous review of existing practices and involve all stakeholders in development.
- Adopt an integrative philosophy and deliberately use teamworking and shared belief systems from the outset. Collaboration is visible during development, within the pathway content and in subsequent feedback of variance.
- Form all or part of the patient record and describe a pathway of care that articulates expected interventions. The document in conjunction with others satisfies existing standards of record keeping and is multidisciplinary in nature.
- Describe effective interventions targeted to effect the greatest clinical benefit. This incorporates evidence-based practice and clear reference to available clinical guidelines, outcome measures, benchmarks, research and expert opinion.
- Identify through variance analysis: clinical deterioration, variation in care delivery and clinical outcomes. This specific information is used to facilitate clinical decision-making, risk management, individualised interventions and continuous quality improvement.

- Focus upon benefits management – reviewing service availability, 'gate-keeping' arrangements and reducing delays, duplications, hold-ups and deficiencies.

THE CASE FOR USING A CARE PATHWAY IN THIS SERVICE

This care pathway was selected as an early priority for the Trust for several reasons. Generally it is known that target processes suitable for pathway development are:

- high-cost services
- high-volume processes
- high-risk practices, and
- difficult to manage case groups.

However, these criteria have quite limited applicability in a mental health context. Compared with situations in acute care (medicine) CRHT cannot be described as high cost or high volume. However, the nature of the CRHT service and the interventions offered involve high clinical risk and difficult to manage case groups. Most significant is the complex nature of situations and the need to coordinate the interventions of different agencies when service users and their carers first access mental health services. As new mental health services have been developed as part of the mental health modernisation agenda, there has been the need to ensure that new care experiences are built to provide a whole patient journey and that interfaces are managed. Relevant to this pathway, patient journeys may begin and end purely within CRHT or continue with other agencies or mental health services. The CRHT service where this pathway was developed was a new service and interfaces had to be agreed and established. This made the pathway a priority process for development. Alongside this was the need for clear risk assessment and management processes to be built in to routine practice. It was believed that there would be advantages to the process mapping involved in considering the variations in patient journeys through CRHT and seeing how processes vary as a consequence of clinical and individual variations.

Notably successful development of pathways has been seen in:

- areas where there is a high level of interest among professionals
- services which wish to monitor implementation of clinical guidelines
- areas where considerable variations in practice affect patient outcomes, and
- new services.

There was a high level of interest amongst the CRHT team to develop the care pathway, which was spearheaded by the Locality Team Manager and Clinical Team Manager. Also, this area of service has grown in interest locally and nationally. The volume of literature around crisis mental health services has expanded pre and post-pathway development. The National Institute for Clinical Excellence (NICE) published guidelines for treating and managing schizophrenia (National

Institute for Clinical Excellence 2002) during the period when the pathway was being developed, and guidelines for self-harm and eating disorders subsequently followed. Each guideline has implications in terms of monitoring the implementation of evidence-based practice. The development of CRHT services had been cemented in the UK by the mental health policy implementation guidance and subsequent performance indicators (Department of Health 2001). The team that developed the pathway was piloting a model for CRHT before this was developed as a Trust-wide service.

THE PATHWAY DEVELOPMENT PROCESS

Over the last decade, models for care pathway development have evolved and a general pattern was followed in this case. The process began by defining the pathway parameters and continued through the process of authoring and implementation. Contributing to the model used were the works of Campbell et al (1998), Ignatavicius & Hausman (1995), Johnson (1997) and Stephens (1997).

The first stage of the care pathway development process was that of selecting a case type, client group or care process. The team debated whether to have specific care pathways for individual case types or need. However, after considerable discussion, the team agreed to begin by generally mapping journeys through the service and examining how these varied for specific problems or needs; and then indeed what impact this had upon the patient journey. Through this process it was found that, especially in the early part of crisis work carried out by the team, there were core activities that occurred within most patient journey processes. There were, however, significant differences where interventions for specific individual needs were concerned. These differences had to be accounted for within the care pathway. After versions of early process maps were developed it was felt that to develop one care pathway for the whole of the journey through CRHT was not viable. Data collection determined that many service users left the service following short crisis interventions and not all required intensive home treatment offered by the CRHT team. It was felt that to make the care pathway development manageable the processes would be broken down into discernible chunks or elements. The first chunk (or pathway) would begin at the point of referral through crisis intervention (where this is required), to the point that service users leave the CRHT service or access a subsequent pathway for home treatment. This decision involved data collection to determine the needs of the service users and carers accessing the service, the interventions offered, any measurable outcomes and services accessed following immediate crisis care. At this point, it was acknowledged that pathways for specific needs at the point of home treatment would be desirable at a later stage of development by the team. It was decided that a Crisis Triage and Assessment Integrated Care Pathway could be flexible enough to portray the patient journey for most cases in the early process of CRHT. It was agreed that later development could see the boundaries of the pathway suitably extended to incorporate gate-keeping arrangements and transfer arrangements with other services and agencies (indeed, joining together with subsequent pathways).

So, having selected the process to be subject to the integrated care pathway, crisis triage and assessment, the next stage in the process was to establish an authoring team. This involved any stakeholders with an interest in the process. A small group of core members was established, which included health and social care representatives, service users and carers. Co-opted onto the authoring team as required were professionals not available at that time within the CRHT team, and representatives of other services and voluntary agencies. A significant issue for pathway authoring was that not all disciplines which normally exist in a CRHT team were in post. Hence, opinions from these professionals had to commissioned for the development process. Once the authoring team was formed, education into the care pathway development process took place. Authoring team members then were able to raise awareness of development and secure support from others. The care pathway manager took responsibility for leading the process and administration.

An early task of the authoring team was to clarify the timeframe and parameters of the pathway. This determined where the pathway began and ended. Patient journeys can span many services and in their entirety are extremely complex, as mentioned previously. Integral to this is some form of a timeframe. Often in mental health care pathways the timeframe is elusive and phases are used rather than absolute time periods. It was agreed by the authoring team that the first pathway developed by the CRHT would begin on referral to the service and end at the point where the immediate crisis abated or the service user accessed the home treatment interventions offered by the team, or accessed alternative sources of help. Previous mapping indicated that within the crisis triage and assessment process offered by the CRHT there are discernible timeframes which could underpin certain activities and these could be built into the pathway.

PROCESS MAPPING AND REDESIGN

A key activity undertaken by the team during these early stages was to determine the goals and outcomes of the care process. At this stage the views of different stakeholders were extremely valuable. As in many cases, professionals view processes and outcomes from a specific perspective whereas the only stakeholder group to experience the entire process is the services user (and carer). Thus the expression of aims and outcomes from a pluralistic perspective is essential. This moves away from a process dominated exclusively by professional opinion. After much debate and editing the authoring team agreed the following aims and outcomes of the pathway. Overall objectives of the crisis triage and assessment care pathway are to:

- initiate a therapeutic relationship
- provide prompt and expert assessment of individual needs during crisis

- provide effective, evidence-based interventions to reduce and resolve crisis
- establish effective liaison and ensure that appropriate and necessary treatments are planned.

The task of reaching this consensus must not be underestimated. This involves acknowledging the parameters of the pathway as CRHT teams offer much more than crisis triage and assessment (i.e. home treatment). But also there were huge and inevitable debates around the sociological understanding of the process and use of terms such as triage and its suitability in this context.

The next stage was to process map the patient journey from all perspectives. This involved all contributors mind-mapping the major steps and activities throughout the timeframe. This produced high-level process maps and more detailed maps of activity (examples can be seen in Figures 15.1 and 15.2). It was quite clear from this exercise that even short processes involve many steps and individual activities. At some points contributors were able to include approximate time periods and parallel processes. The mapping made known loops, complexities, roles and relationships. Different stakeholders mapped their experiences and inputs but were also asked to articulate improvements to the process. Previous medical records were used to establish practice patterns that may have been overlooked. One service user offered extracts from a personal journal to describe needs, activities, timing and experiences. Interestingly, this activity did establish that although the service was newly developed there were already considerable variations in practice and views of the service being offered.

Once the early maps had been drawn, then began the process of redesign. First, this involved a rigorous scrutiny of current practices from different perspectives. The variations in practice and standards were viewed critically as were

Figure 15.1
The crisis triage and assessment high-level process map

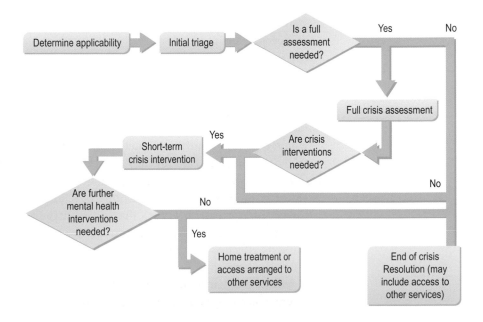

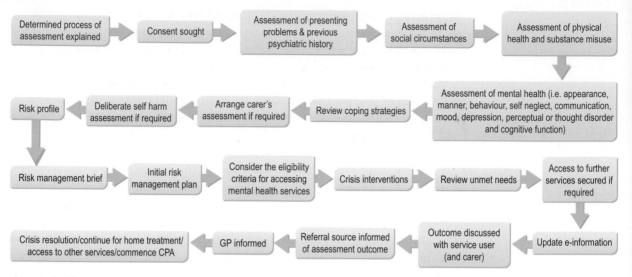

Figure 15.2
Crisis assessment extract of a lower-level process map

the potential of these activities in meeting the outcomes of the pathway. Also, important discussions followed about what this process feels like. All the steps in the map were reviewed for appropriateness, value and timeliness. Each stakeholder group was able to consider their roles within the map and determine duplications, delays, and added value. The authoring team considered problems and issues at each step. Some activities without value were removed from the process at this stage. Other steps were re-ordered to make processes clearer and more efficient. Some activities, for example, administration of GP (general practitioner) letters, were changed from the role of clinical staff to administrative staff. Examples of specific steps added related to consent, education for service users and carers, access to other services and interagency communication. Contributing to redesign was the comparison of activities with established clinical guidelines and benchmarks from other organisations. A review of the literature, guidelines and national recommendations which influenced the expected integrated care pathway identified key areas for pathway development. A wealth of literature was reviewed with regard to its contribution to the care pathway content and later made available to those using the pathway. Key sources of evidence used were: Churchill et al (2001), Cormac et al (2003), Department of Health (2001), Gould et al (1997), House et al (1998), National Institute of Clinical Excellence (2002, 2004), Royal College of Psychiatrists (1994), the Sainsbury Centre for Mental Health (2001).

The aim of this stage of the process was to discern the evidence-based interventions effective for those experiencing a mental heath crisis; and then, consequently, where appropriate, to integrate these within a redesigned process which is built around the experience of receiving care. There followed an analysis of training needs, any requirements to extend roles and issues around matching capacity to demand. The aim was to make the process into a sustainable, feasible vision based upon best practice. Subsequently, the redesigned process map content was redefined then moulded into the corporate care pathway template, variance analysis system and prevailing clinical documentation.

PILOT, IMPLEMENTATION AND REVIEW

Following training of the team in the use of the pathway, the first version of the pathway was piloted in February 2003 for a period of 2 months. During this time the pathway was offered for consultation within the Trust and to others outside the Trust with a known profile in CRHT. The pathway content was validated through the Trust's clinical governance processes and agreed for use by the Trust. One significant issue arising from the pilot was that the pathway was not required for a number of people who only contacted the service by telephone and for a variety of reasons were not seen or assessed by the team. Thus it was agreed that an initial triage document would be used as an appendix to the pathway. This document spans two sides of paper and includes contact details, reasons for contacting the CRHT service and the outcome of the triage or later assessment after the pathway is used. The primary use of the second page of the two-page triage sheet is to record the outcome of triage and/or crisis interventions. Following revisions the pathway was reissued ready for use.

The two-page triage document is shown in Appendix 15.1 and the current version of the pathway in use is shown in Appendix 15.2. In the 20 months that the pathway has been in use, it has been subject to revision on three occasions and is now in its fourth version. Revisions have been due to changes in the evidence base and organisational arrangements. The pathway is now used by three teams. Each team has a care pathway champion who oversees its use within the CRHT team. Any changes to the version or arrangements are recorded on the care pathway implementation plan to provide an open audit trail. The pathway content is subject to at minimum an annual review. This review is essential to ensure that the pathway is revised and upgraded according to emerging evidence, variance analysis and organisational developments.

It has been acknowledged that there is a need to monitor how the care pathway is used within teams and the level of completion. The use of the care pathway has been audited twice since its implementation to assure the Trust regarding levels of completion. An audit tool such as that shown in Figure 15.3 is used to define a level of compliance. The audit tool essentially turns each place on the pathway into an audit point. Therefore the audit results identify the parts of the pathway completed (or not).

Figure 15.4 shows the findings of an audit of usage and completion of 20 care pathways randomly selected in May 2003, just a few months after the care pathway was fully implemented. At that time the pathway was not dissimilar from its current version. In part 2 the rate of compliance for completion measured between

<table>
<tr><td>CRISIS RESOLUTION & HOME TREATMENT</td></tr>
</table>

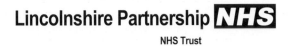

Lincolnshire Partnership **NHS**

NHS Trust

INITIAL TRIAGE

1. PERSONAL INFORMATION

Last name:	First name(s):
Maiden Name:	Date of Birth: / / (DD / MM / YR)
Address:	Marital Status:
Postcode	
Telephone:	Spoken Language:
Male/Female: (circle as appropriate)	Ethnic Origin:
Next of Kin: (name, address, telephone)	
GP: (name, address, telephone)	

CPA level: (circle as appropriate) None/Standard/Enhanced	Psychiatrist:	Care Coordinator:

Appendix 15.1
The two-page triage document

2. REFERRAL INFORMATION

Date and Time:	Referral Source:	CRHT No:
Mode: phone/F2F/other (circle as appropriate)	Home Treatment	Crisis Referral

Reason for Contact:

3. TRIAGE RESPONSE

Triage Category: 1. Emergency   2. Urgent/Acute   3. Non-Urgent   4. Triage Coordinator Response

5. Other Agency Referral   6. Inconclusive Contact   7. Inappropriate Referral (circle as appropriate)

Actions Required: 1. Return Phone Call   2. F2F Assessment Onsite/Off-site   3. D/W Care Coordinator

4. D/W Psychiatrist   5. MHA   6. No further action (circle as appropriate)

Assessed: Yes/No	Alert Form: Yes/No
Triage by: (signed)	Date:

Appendix 15.1   *(Continued)*

4. TRIAGE SUMMARY

Presenting Circumstances:

Formulation & Needs:

Drug/Alcohol Use:

Medication:

Other Agencies Involved:

5. TRIAGE OUTCOME

Crisis & Risk Management Plan/Outcome (inc referral/signposting, or why no services are offered)

Contact details entered onto the electronic information system	Yes/No
Triage information faxed/telephoned to GP	
Crisis team member assigned **Name**	Yes/No
Outcome shared with service user and carer as appropriate	Yes/No
Triage Response by: (name, date & time)	Yes/No

Appendix 15.1   *(Continued)*

INTEGRATED CARE PATHWAY FOR CRISIS TRIAGE & ASSESSMENT

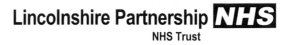

This Integrated Care Pathway is for individuals referred to the Crisis Resolution Home Treatment Service. It is intended to guide crisis assessment. Wherever possible the interventions are based upon evidence and best practice.

Overall Objectives of this care pathway are to

- Initiate a therapeutic relationship
- Provide prompt and expert assessment of individual needs during crisis
- Provide effective, evidence based interventions to reduce and resolve crisis
- Establish effective liaison and ensure that appropriate and necessary treatments are planned.

1. PERSONAL DETAILS

Name, Date of Birth & Address:	Service Location:
	Pathway Start Date:
	Pathway End Date:

Sources and evidence which inform the content of this pathway are:
DEPARTMENT OF HEALTH (2001). Mental Health Policy Implementation Guide. Department of Health; London
HOUSE A., OWENS D., & PATCHETT L. (1998). Effective Health Care – Deliberate Self Harm. NHS Centre for Dissemination and Reviews; University of York
ROYAL COLLEGE OF PSYCHIATRISTS (1994). The General Hospital Management of Adult Deliberate Self-Harm. Royal College of Psychiatrists; London
THE SAINSBURY CENTRE FOR MENTAL HEALTH (2001). Mental Health Topics; Crisis Resolution. The Sainsbury Centre; London

---

Instructions for use:
Before writing in this Integrated Care Pathway, please ensure you have signed the signature sheet (overleaf). When using this document please ensure that you date, time and sign against each activity when it has been completed. It is important to remember that the aim of the Integrated Care Pathway (ICP) is to ensure the most appropriate care is given at the correct time.

If an activity outlined in the ICP has not, for whatever reason, been completed then this must be shown as a Variance. A 'V' should therefore be placed in the box next to the intervention. The variance record sheet should then be completed. If further action needs to be taken, e.g. the intervention needs to be repeated, then use the blank spaces in the appropriate time frame of the ICP to record this. These blank spaces can also be used to add interventions which are deemed appropriate for that person but are not already in the ICP. These additions should also be recorded as a variance.

To view an example of a completed ICP please read the ICP file which is in your ward/area. It remains each professional's responsibility to ensure that practice is safe. This ICP is not a replacement for experienced clinical judgement and inter-disciplinary discussions. If you require further information please contact your Clinical Team Leader or Care Pathway Manager.

LIST OF ABBREVIATIONS:
CRHT: Crisis Resolution Home Treatment. D/W: Discussed with. F2F: Face to Face. GP: General Practitioner
ICP: Integrated Care Pathway. MHA: Mental Health Act. HONOS: Health of the Nation Outcome Scales. DSH: Deliberate Self Harm

---

Appendix 15.2
The current version of the pathway in use.

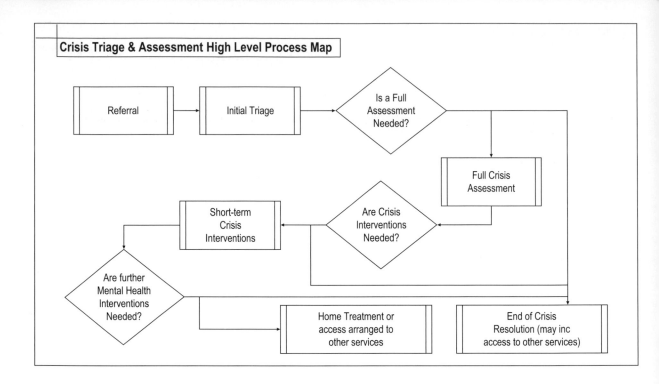

Crisis Triage & Assessment High Level Process Map

2. SIGNATURE SHEET

Would all disciplines please sign below prior to writing in this ICP.

Full Name (print)	Designation	Signature	Initials	Date

Appendix 15.2   *(Continued)*

PART 1 – CRISIS ASSESSMENT

3. PRESENTING CRISIS ASSESSMENT

Complete within 4 hrs of referral (or otherwise as agreed)

Code:	Activity: It is expected that these activities have been completed unless they are recorded as a variance	'V'	Date/Time/Sign:
1.1	**Process of assessment explained and agreement sought**		

Presenting Problems (e.g. mental disorder, self injury, loss)

Previous Psychiatric History: (i.e. current/past treatment, hospital admissions, MHA)

Daytime Occupation, Finances, Spiritual Needs:

Household Management: (accommodation, cooking, shopping)

Physical Illness/Injury/Access/Mobility/Sexual Health: (e.g. head injury, epilepsy, comorbidity factors, family planning)

Registered Disabled: **Yes/No** (circle as appropriate)

Substance Misuse

Social Relationships, Family/Dependants:

Personal and/or Forensic History: (i.e. childhood development)

Information provided by: patient, family/carer, other (circle as appropriate)

Appendix 15.2   *(Continued)*

4. MENTAL HEALTH ASSESSMENT

Appearance, Manner and Behaviour: (self care, eye contact, agitation, hostility)

Self Neglect: (physical, social, environment, bathing, toileting, managing medication)

Communication; Speech, Content: (flow, content, amount)

Mood: (affect, hopelessness, anxiety, guilt)

Indication of Depression: (diurnal variation, weight loss, emotional reactivity, low self esteem, loss of interest, energy, concentration)

Evidence of Perceptual/Thought Disorder/Insight: (form, content, perception, awareness)

Cognitive Function: (orientation, concentration, cognitive ability, memory)

COPING ABILITIES

Does the person feel able to utilise any mechanisms to cope with crisis situations? (problem solving skills, networks)

<u>Scale 0-10</u> **Coping Abilities**

Is a Carer's Assessment required?   **Yes/No** (delete as required)

Code	Activity: It is expected that this activity has been completed unless it is recorded as a variance	'V'	Date/Time/Sign:
2.1	**Assessment of presenting crisis & mental health completed**		

Appendix 15.2   *(Continued)*

5. DELIBERATE SELF HARM ASSESSMENT

Complete only where indicated

Consider all of the following

1. **Presenting DSH Problem** (ideation, statement of intent, frequency of thoughts, preparation. Act – description of event i.e. method, where took place, did seek help, suicide note, what was the problem/stressor)

2. **Planning element of Intent** (suicide note – access to means, put affairs in order)

3. **Clarification of the reasons why wanting to harm self** (expected outcome)

4. **Specific Risk Factors** (i.e. age, sex, living alone, employment status, family history of self harm, history of substance misuse, recently discharged, mental/physical illness, past DSH, bereavement)

5. **Evaluate the context of any suicidal act/thoughts and meaning to the individual** (what happened in preceding days, did they seek help after the attempt, regret, effects on others, likelihood of being discovered)

6. **Level of Hopelessness** (the belief that things are not going to change, future life plans)

7. **Is self-injury a coping mechanism?** (details e.g. any established patterns, rituals, frequency, eating disorder, is self harm a result of religious belief)

8. **Has there been involvement of specific support services regarding self-injury?**

9. **Extent of social support/protective factors**

10. **Strengths Assessment/Coping Strategies**

Likelihood of further self harm (delete as appropriate) Low / Moderate / High	Potential level of harm (delete as appropriate) Low / Medium / High
Completed by: (Name / designation)	**Date:**

Appendix 15.2   *(Continued)*

PART 2 – SAINSBURY RISK PROFILE & MANAGEMENT BRIEF

6. PERSONAL DETAILS

Complete for all referrals

Name:	Date of Birth:	Source of Information:

This format is part of a comprehensive mental health assessment and care planning process. This is not an exhaustive list of risk factors; it indicates the potential sources of risk, and possible management responses. Accurate prediction of risk is difficult, as initial assessment may be based on incomplete/inaccurate information. This assessment offers a guide to further discussion and investigation, and an initial management plan. If completed by one person, this assessment should be quickly discussed with Medical Officers and multi-disciplinary team (inc. users and carers, where appropriate).

7. RISK INDICATORS

($\sqrt{}$) Tick only the indicators that apply

Suicide	Yes	No	Don't Know		Yes	No	Don't Know
Previous attempts on their life				Expressing high levels of distress			
Previous use of violent methods				Helplessness or hopelessness			
Misuse of drugs and/or alcohol				Family history of suicide			
Major psychiatric diagnoses				Separated/widowed/divorced			
Expressing suicidal intent				Unemployed/retired			
Considered/planned intent				Recent significant life events			
Believe no control over life				Major physical illness/disability			
Other (please specify)			Comments:				

Neglect	Yes	No	Don't Know		Yes	No	Don't Know
Previous history of neglect				Lack of positive social contacts			
Failing to drink properly				Unable to shop for self			
Failing to eat properly				Insufficient/inappropriate clothing			
Difficulty managing physical health				Difficulty maintaining hygiene			
Living in inadequate accommodation				Experiencing financial difficulties			
Lacking basic amenities (water/heat/light)				Difficulty communicating needs			
Pressure of eviction/repossession				Denies problems perceived by others			
Other (please specify)			Comments:				

Appendix 15.2   *(Continued)*

Aggression/Violence	Yes	No	Don't Know		Yes	No	Don't Know
Previous incidents of violence				Paranoid delusions about others			
Previous use of weapons				Helplessness or violent command hallucinations			
Misuse of drugs and/or alcohol				Signs of anger and frustration			
Male gender, under 35 yrs/age				Sexually inappropriate behaviour			
Known personal trigger factors				Preoccupation with violent fantasy			
Expressing intent to harm others				Admissions to secure settings			
Previous dangerous impulsive acts				Denial of previous dangerous acts			
Other (please specify)			Comments:				

Other	Yes	No	Don't Know		Yes	No	Don't Know
Self-injury (e.g. cutting, burning)				Exploitation by others (e.g. financial)			
Other self-harm (e.g. eating disorders)				Exploitation of others			
Stated abuse by others (e.g. physical, sexual)				Culturally isolated situation			
Abuse of others				Non-violent sexual offence (e.g. exposure)			
Harassment by others (e.g. racial, physical)				Arson (deliberate fire-setting only)			
Harassment of others				Accidental fire risk			
Risks to child(ren)				Other damage to property			
Failure to attend appointments				Unplanned disengagement with services			
Other (please specify)			Comments:				

Summary/Plan: (inc. those informed)

Continue with detailed risk profile and management brief?		Yes / No	(delete as appropriate)

Code	Activity : It is expected that this activity has been completed unless it is recorded as a variance	'V'	Date/Time/Sign:
2.2	**Risk Profile completed**		

Appendix 15.2   (Continued)

DETAILED RISK PROFILE & MANAGEMENT BRIEF

8. RISK FACTORS

Complete only as required

Situational Context of Risk Factors: (including for example – arousal in official settings, risks in community locations, friends/neighbours/carers, need for two workers, race or gender considerations, etc.)

Historical and/or Current Context of Factors:

Summary of 'Positive' Resources and Potentials:

9. SUMMARY OF RISK ASSESSMENT

Involvement of Service User and/or Carers In Assessment:

Primary Risks Identified:

Other Risks Identified: (inc. for example factors, context, gut reactions/intuition)

INITIAL RISK MANAGEMENT PLAN

SHORT- TERM CRISIS MANAGEMENT OPTIONS			
Precautions:	To be discussed with	Information needed:	Actions & Responsibilities for Actions:
Complete By:	Date:	Time:	Review Date:
LONG-TERM RISK MANAGEMENT OPTIONS			
Precautions:	To be discussed with	Information needed:	Actions & Responsibilities for Actions:
Complete By:	Date:	Time:	Review Date:
POSITIVE RISK OPTIONS (and support needed)			

Appendix 15.2   *(Continued)*

10. RISK MANAGEMENT CONSIDERATIONS

(including for example – who, what, how, when, expected outcome, positive potentials, etc.)

Care Programme Approach registration (√ tick all relevant areas)	Y	N			
CPA			Level (delete as appropriate)	Standard	Enhance
Section 117					
Other Section			State which		
Supervised discharge					
Role of client and/or carer in plan	Y	N		Yes	No
Client involved			Carer involved		
Client agreed to plan			Carer agreed to plan		

Comments:

Opportunities for Risk Prevention: (including risk mitigating/protective factors)

Responsibilities for future actions: (not stated in the management options)

Date of Next Review:	Plan:
Completed by: (for collective responsibility)	**Date:**

Adapted from: MORGAN S (2000) Clinical Risk Management – A Clinical Tool and Practitioner Manual. The Sainsbury Centre for Mental Health London

Appendix 15.2   *(Continued)*

PART 3 – ASSESSMENT OUTCOME

12. CRHT RESPONSE
Completed following Crisis Assessment

Are the Eligibility Criteria for accessing mental health services met?			Yes / No	
Code	**Activity** It is expected that these activities have been completed unless they are recorded as a variance	'V'	Date/Time/Sign	
3.1	**Interventions offered during crisis** (or how needs will be met for those who do not meet the criteria for accessing mental health services) **and the Crisis Plan/Outcome** (inc CPA, referral/signposting, or why no services are offered) **are recorded on the triage document**			
3.2	**Access to other services secured** (as above plan)			
3.3	**Referral source informed of the outcome**			
3.4	**Contact details entered onto the electronic information system**			
3.5	**Information faxed/telephoned to GP**			
3.6	**Outcome shared with service user and carer**			
3.7	**Continue with further care in this team**			
3.8	**HONOS**			

Appendix 15.2   *(Continued)*

	VARIANCE REPORT: INTEGRATED CARE PATHWAY FOR CRISIS TRIAGE & ASSESSMENT	When the pathway is completed please send a copy of this sheet to: LPT Trust Audit Department, Rauceby, Sleaford, Lincs. NG34 8PP

Variance Record Sheet from _____

Date	Activity Code	Variance Code	Action to be Taken or Details of added intervention	Sign

VARIATION SOURCE CODES

User/carer codes
1.1 User unavailable
1.2 Carer unavailable
1.3 User refused
1.4 Carer refused
1.5 Intervention inappropriate
1.6 Deterioration of mental state:
        intervention inappropriate
1.7 Improvement of mental state:
        intervention inappropriate
1.8 User refused due to poor motivation
1.9 Intervention repeated due to lack of
        understanding or skills
1.10 Other (please state)

System codes
2.1 Date and time of intervention changed
2.2 Awaiting consultation from others
2.3 Staff unavailable
2.4 Lack of time
2.5 Intervention postponed/cancelled
2.6 Information results not available
2.7 Dept closed /room not available
2.8 Appointment not available/delayed
2.9 Other (please state)

Other agencies
3.1 Accommodation not available
3.2 Community support not available
3.3 Day services not available
3.4 Funding/benefits not available
3.5 Transport not available
3.6 Other (please state)

Appendix 15.2   *(Continued)*

95 and 97.5%. The average compliance across parts 1 and 2 (total of 11 activity codes) was 95.45%.

The pathway up until that time had been used for 116 referrals. Completion rates were extremely high (which may be viewed sceptically by some). Indeed, the compliance rate for this pathway vastly exceeds rates for all other pathways used in the Trust, where compliance rates typically range from 58 to 76%. There are a number of factors which may explain the high completion rate. Firstly, the pathway

Figure 15.3
Audit of usage and
compliance tool

		AUDIT OF USAGE & COMPLETION CRISIS TRIAGE & ASSESSMENT CARE PATHWAY		
			COMPLETED	
	OTHER			
	Personal Details			
	Signature Sheet (check signatures correspond with those throughout the care plan)			
	Variance Record Sheet			

Code	Activity:	COMPLETED	
	PART 1		
1.1	Process of assessment explained and agreement sought		
	Is a carer's assessment required (yes/no)		
2.1	Assessment of presenting crisis & mental health completed		
	Deliberate Self Harm Assessment - Likelihood of further self harm		
	Deliberate Self Harm Assessment - Potential level of harm		
	Deliberate Self Harm Assessment - Completed by		
	PART 2		
	Sainsbury Risk Profile attempted		
	Continue with Detailed Risk Profile and Management Brief (yes/no)		
2.2	Risk Profile completed		
	Initial Risk Management Plan		
	CPA sections		
	CPA - Completed by		
	PART 3		
	Are the Eligibility Criteria for accessing mental health services met (yes/no)		
3.1	Interventions offered during crisis (or how needs will be met for those who do not meet the criteria for accessing mental health services) and the Crisis Plan/Outcome (inc CPA, referral/signposting, or why no services are offered) are recorded on the triage document		
3.2	Access to other services secured (as above plan)		
3.3	Referral source informed of the outcome		
3.4	Contact details entered onto the electronic information system		
3.5	Information faxed/telephoned to GP		
3.6	Outcome shared with service user and carer		
3.7	Continue with further care in this team		
3.8	HONOS		

is relatively short. Also, the pathway is not subject to many handovers between professionals – which can influence compliance rates to their detriment. A further influential factor was the enthusiasm of the team in developing the pathway and their involvement in the development process; which greatly affected ownership. Leadership at the team level was a further contributing factor. To examine whether the compliance rates remained high, a repeat audit was completed in September 2004, using the tool shown in Figure 15.3; the results can be seen in Figure 15.5.

Audit results still continue to show a high average completion rate (83.6%) which 18 months after development still far exceeds the rates found for traditional forms of record keeping.

Figure 15.4
Compliance audit results
May 2003

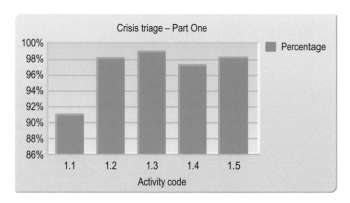

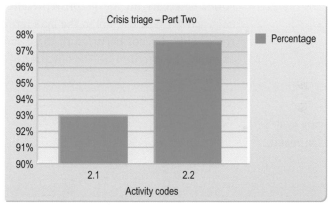

Figure 15.5
Compliance audit results
September 2003

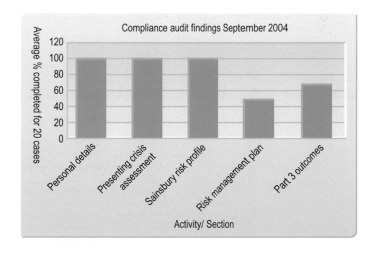

VARIANCE REPORTS AND ANALYSIS

From the outset, it was planned that variance reports for the pathway would be produced quarterly. The variance record sheets on the final page of the pathway are sent to the audit department and collated in a simple database. At quarterly intervals, the variances are converted to a graphical form. The relationship between the activity codes and variance codes is analysed and a short narrative summary is offered. An extract from such a report is shown in Figure 15.6.

This graph shows the incidence of variances for nine activities plotted along the x-axis. The activities can be cross-referenced to Table 15.1 by their activity codes. The bars on the graph represent the number of variances reported for each activity. The colours in the bars represent the variance code (the reason why the activity did not occur), and these can be cross-referenced to Table 15.2. For example, the activity 1.6 – the outcome of the assessment is shared with the service

Figure 15.6
Extracts from an early quarter variance report

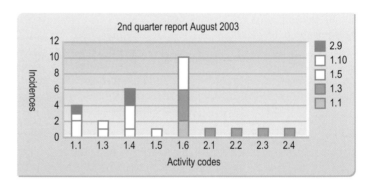

Table 15.1
Activity codes (shown on the x-axis in Figure 15.6)

Code	Activity
1.1	Access to other services secured (as plan) Yes/No/NA
1.3	Contact details entered onto the electronic information system
1.4	Triage information faxed/telephoned to GP
1.5	Crisis team member assigned: Yes/No/NA
1.6	Outcome shared with service user and carer as appropriate
2.1	Process of assessment explained and agreement sought
2.2	Assessment of presenting crisis, mental health and coping
2.3	Crisis risk assessment and first contact risk profile
2.4	HONOS Health of the Nation Outcome Scales
2.5	Assessment outcome is recorded in the triage response (tab 7)

Table 15.2
Variation source codes
(shown in Figure 15.6)

Code	User/carer codes
1.1	User unavailable
1.3	User refused
1.5	Intervention inappropriate
1.10	Other (please state)
	System codes
2.9	Other (please state)

user and carer – was recorded as a variance on 10 occasions. According to the variance source codes, in two cases this could not occur as the service user was not available.

Summary of the variance analysis (as shown in Figure 15.6)

- Information from the exception reporting suggests that variances remain low.
- The most significant variances reported refer to:

1. *Access to other services (activity 1.1)* This variance is consistent with the last report, although the variance sources differ in this case. Reports of this variance generally indicate that this is, in some cases, an inappropriate intervention. Therefore this is suitably reported as a variance determined by individual need and circumstances. This does indicate some development following the last variance report in terms of system influences upon the process of care.
2. *Details of referral entered onto the electronic information system (activity 1.3)* This did not occur in two cases. Reports suggest that details required to complete this activity were not available.
3. *Information faxed to the GP (activity 1.4)* This activity was recorded as a variance for a wide range of reasons. For example, the service user had no GP, these details had not been disclosed, this activity was being completed by another service or the intervention was considered as inappropriate at that time.
4. *Outcome of the assessment shared with the service user and carer as appropriate (activity 1.6)* This activity accounted for the most number of variances (reported in 10 cases). The most frequently cited reason for this variance was referral to other services/agencies (although this would not exclude the need for this activity).

Quarterly variance analysis reports are presented to identified members of the multidisciplinary team and organisation. This information is considered in the ongoing review of clinical activity and care processes. The CRHT teams are expected to develop action plans and consider reviewing the pathway to address

Figure 15.7
Variance chart for July
2004

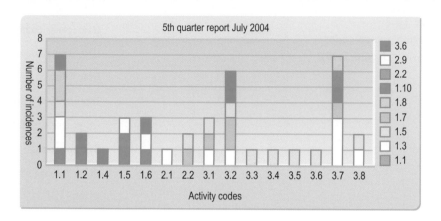

adverse variances. This process relies upon a variance tracking system. Recording variances involves identifying what the variance is, the cause of the variance and any action plan needed to address the variance. The reasons why practice digresses from the integrated care pathway can be examined to identify variation in professional standards or if the process is failing to meet the stated outcomes. This information is used for both day-to-day clinical management and continuous quality improvement. Over a period of time these data can be examined to establish trends, develop action plans and improve practice. For example, considering the findings of a later variance report (Figure 15.7), there is a clear pattern in subsequent reports related to activity 1.1.

The roles and responsibilities of those involved in development and implementation are summarised in Box 15.1.

MONITORING AND EVALUATION

This care pathway has its own implementation plan which documents changes in practice arising from changes to the pathway content and the actions plans arising from variance reports. Action plans from past variance reports have included taking action to address a number of quality problems, for example:

- To recruit a medical staff grade for the crisis team; an advert due to be sent out for staff grade.
- Working on backlogs to access other services, and ways of improving this have been discussed with team managers.
- To improve the triage procedure. Training has been arranged for all crisis team members to address inconsistencies in the screening process.
- The outcome of the assessment is not being shared – this will be highlighted with the team at staff meetings, and added checks will be completed to ensure that assessments are appropriately shared.

Box 15.1   ROLES AND RESPONSIBILITIES

Care Pathway Manager
- Lead implementation of the care pathway strategy
- Maintain a database of care pathways in use
- Identify target processes in conjunction with clinical staff and organisational priorities
- Facilitate the development process
- Provide education, training and support during implementation
- Monitor and audit care pathway implementation/use
- Ensure that variance analysis data are disseminated
- Pursue appropriate opportunities for evaluation
- Review the care pathway strategy in accordance with organisational and health policy developments.

Clinical Governance Committee
- Provide organisational validation of care pathway content
- Support a culture of multidisciplinary care pathways within the organisation
- Use variance analysis data to inform governance processes, systematic evaluation and improvement.

Authoring Teams
- Participate in the development process as identified in the model
- Support implementation, audit and evaluation as required.

Local Champions
- Participate in care pathway development
- Provide 'on the ground' support and monitoring during implementation.

Divisional Staff
- Identify target processes
- Support development, implementation, audit and evaluation
- Use variance data to inform service development, improve efficiency, outcomes and reduce variation in practice.

Clinical Audit Support
- Maintain the variance databases
- Administer quarterly variance reports.

Following full implementation there has been one planned annual review by the authoring team and this will be repeated. The pathway will be revised and upgraded and it is intended that any opportunities to evaluate its impact are integral to the implementation plan. The effects of the pathway upon the delivery of the service are being viewed through a number of mechanisms. Perspectives offered by the team suggest that the pathway:

- enables the team to work with a client through an expected process
- guides activities

- aids decision-making
- encourages the team to communicate effectively (within their own team)
- improves standards of communication with other services
- allows monitoring at each stage
- describes good practice and expected standards
- documents the process in an accessible format
- informs others without the need for additional notes or explanations to be added.

The view offered is that utilising an integrated care pathway has enhanced the team's ability to deliver crisis resolution and home treatment care to a consistently high standard and may be recommended to other teams.

IMPACTS AND FUTURE DEVELOPMENT

The CRHT have in use a pathway that exists as all or part of the clinical documentation and any deviation from the plan is documented as a variance. This information is used for day-to-day monitoring and periodic analysis for quality improvement. The pathway documents the anticipated evidence-based multidisciplinary care (including interventions, activities, assessments etc.) required to achieve agreed outcomes for the early stages of CRHT. Benefits of the pathway reported in the Trust are summarised as:

- development of care processes that involve all stakeholders
- changes in practice and implementation of evidence
- standardised processes across the organisation
- process and systems coordination which 'fits' specific patient journeys
- increased ownership and professionalisation for those who use pathways
- less duplication and fewer errors due to improved communication and role clarification
- improved access to clinical information and evidence
- audit and identification of variance for risk management and continuous quality improvement.

The pathway has been implemented with a high degree of completion and is now in use by three CRHT teams. Within the Trust the pathway has clarified the philosophy of pathways to other stakeholders pursuing similar development. The CRHT pathway has confirmed how an organisation can use the care pathway process to implement new practices supported by evidence for specific services and service users. The involvement of all stakeholders within the development process has been critical to success.

This care pathway has been modelled specifically for its purpose, and current electronic Patient Administration Systems and electronic Care Programme Approach systems (with rare exceptions) are not dynamic enough to support care pathway activity such as this. It is clear that for development to flourish in the current informatics climate there needs to be sustained enthusiasm by all stakeholders and influence upon the emerging informatics infrastructure. Whilst the current version of the pathway meets the general criteria for care pathways documented in the literature, a great deal of development is required to model and support such processes electronically. There are growing indications that some service providers are grasping the challenges for the future development of process such as the one documented in this chapter.

Acknowledgements

The contribution of South West Lincolnshire's Crisis Resolution and Home Treatment team (part of Lincolnshire Partnership NHS Trust) and the Lincolnshire Partnership Trust Audit Department is gratefully acknowledged. The risk assessment within the care pathway document was reproduced by kind permission of Steve Morgan, Independent Consultant, Practice Based Evidence, c/o Top Flat, 87 Charlton Road, Blackheath, London SE3 8TH, UK.

REFERENCES

Audini B, Marks I M, Lawrence R E et al 1994 Home-based versus out-patient/in-patient care for people with serious mental illness. Phase II of a controlled study. British Journal of Psychiatry 165:204-210

Brimblecombe N 2001 Community care and the development of intensive home treatment services. In: Brimblecombe N (ed.) Acute mental health care in the community: intensive home treatment. Whurr Publishers Ltd, Chichester, p 5-28

Burns T, Beadsmore A, Bhat A V et al 1993 A controlled trial of home-based acute psychiatric services I: clinical and social outcome. British Journal of Psychiatry 163:49-54

Campbell H, Hotchkiss R, Bradshaw N et al 1998 Integrated care pathways. British Medical Journal 316:113-137

Caplan G 1964 Principles of preventive psychiatry. Basic Books, New York

Churchill R, Hunot V, Corney R et al 2001 A systematic review of controlled trials of the effectiveness and cost-effectiveness of brief psychological treatments for depression. The National Coordinating Centre for Health Technology Assessment (NCCHTA) 2001:173

Coleman M, Donnelly P, Davies A et al 1998 Evaluating intensive support in community mental health care. Mental Health Nursing 18(5):8-11

Cormac I, Jones C, Campbell C, et al 2003 Cognitive behaviour therapy for schizophrenia (Cochrane Review). In: The Cochrane Library, Issue 2, 2003. Update Software, Oxford

Davies R D, Winter L 2001 Antianxiety agents. In: Jacobson J L, Jacobson A M (eds) Psychiatric secrets, 2nd edn. Hanley & Belfus, Inc., Philadelphia, p 268-271

Dean C, Gadd E M 1990 Home treatment for acute psychiatric illness. British Medical Journal 301:1021-1023

Dean C, Phillips J, Gadd E M et al 1993 Comparison of community based service with hospital based service for people with acute, severe psychiatric illness. British Medical Journal 307:473-476

Department of Health 1998 The new NHS – modern and dependable. HMSO, London

Department of Health 2000 The NHS plan. Department of Health, London

Department of Health 2001 The mental health policy implementation guide. HMSO, London

Freeman H 1993 The history of British community psychiatry. In: Dean C, Freeman H (eds) Community mental health care: international perspectives on making it happen. The Royal College of Psychiatrists, London

Freud S 1991 Volume 1: Introductory lectures on psychoanalysis. Penguin Books, London

Gomm R 1996 Mental health and inequality. In: Heller T, Reynolds J, Gomm R et al (eds) Mental health matters. A reader. Macmillan Press Ltd, Basingstoke

Gould R A, Otto M W, Pollack M H et al 1997 Cognitive behavioural and pharmacological treatment of generalized anxiety disorder: a preliminary meta-analysis. Behaviour Therapy 28: 285-305

House A, Owens D, Patchett L 1998 Effective health care – deliberate self harm. NHS Centre for Dissemination and Reviews; University of York

Ignatavicius D, Hausman K 1995 Clinical pathways for collaborative practice. Saunders, London

Johnson S 1999 Pathways of care. Blackwell Science, London

Kwakwa J 1995 Alternatives to hospital-based mental health care. Nursing Times 91(23):38-39

Marks I M, Connolly J, Muijen M et al 1994 Home-based care for people with serious mental illness. British Journal of Psychiatry 165:179-194

Merson S 1990 The early intervention service: the first 18 months of an Inner London demonstration project. Psychiatric Bulletin 14:267-269

Minghella E, Ford R, Freeman T et al 1998 Open all hours. 24-hour response for people with mental health emergencies. Sainsbury Centre for Mental Health, London

Morgan G 1997 Management of suicide risk. Psychiatric Bulletin 21:214-216

Motto J A, Heilbron D C, Uster R P 1985 Development of a clinical instrument to estimate suicide risk. American Journal of Psychiatry 142(6):680-686

Muijen M, Marks I, Connolly J et al 1992 Home based care and standard hospital care for patients with severe mental illness: a randomised controlled trial. British Medical Journal 304:749-754

Nagamoto T 2001 Antipsychotic medications. In: Jacobson J L, Jacobson A M (eds) Psychiatric secrets, 2nd edn. Hanley & Belfus, Inc., Philadelphia, p 252-259

National Institute of Clinical Excellence (NICE) 2002 Schizophrenia – core interventions in the treatment and management of schizophrenia in primary and secondary care. NICE, London

National Institute of Clinical Excellence (NICE) 2004 Self harm – the short-term physical and psychological management and secondary prevention of self-harm in primary and secondary care. NICE, London

Orme S 2001 Intensive home treatment services: the current position in the UK. In: Brimblecombe N (ed.) Acute mental health care in the community: intensive home treatment. Whurr Publishers Ltd, Chichester, p 29-53

Parad H J, Parad L G 1991 Crisis intervention: yesterday, today and tomorrow. In: Punukollu N R (ed.) Recent advances in crisis intervention, vol 1. International Institute of Crisis Intervention and Community Psychiatry Publications, Huddersfield, p 3-23

Powell T 2001 The mental health handbook (revised edition). Speechmark Publishing Ltd, Bicester

Punukollu N R 1991 Crisis intervention in practice – an international perspective. In: Punukollu N R (ed.) Recent advances in crisis intervention, vol 1. International Institute of Crisis Intervention and Community Psychiatry Publications, Huddersfield, p 25-36

Ratna L 1991 Crisis resolution where it is contraindicated. In: Punukollu N R (ed.) Recent advances in crisis intervention, vol 1. International Institute of Crisis Intervention and Community Psychiatry Publications, Huddersfield, p 59-65

Riley K 1998 Paving the way. Health Service Journal 108:30-31

Rose N 2001 Historical changes in mental health practice. In: Thornicroft G, Szmukler G (eds) Textbook of community psychiatry. Oxford University Press, Oxford

Royal College of Psychiatrists 1994 The general hospital management of adult deliberate self-harm. Royal College of Psychiatrists, London

Sainsbury Centre for Mental Health 2001 Mental health topics: crisis resolution. The Sainsbury Centre, London

Sims A, Owens D 1993 Psychiatry (6th edn). Baillière Tindall, London

Snowley G 1992 Stress, pain and the individual. In: (Kenworthy N, Snowley G, Gilling C (eds) Common foundation studies in nursing. Churchill Livingstone, Edinburgh

Spivack G, Platt J J, Shure M B 1976 The problem-solving approach to adjustment. Jossey-Bass Publishers, San Francisco

Stephens R 1997 Setting up pathways in mental health. In: Wilson J Integrated care management – the path to success, ch 9. Butterworth Heinemann, Oxford

University of Durham & Department of Health 2004 Durham mapping adult mental health service mapping: crisis resolution teams. Online. Available at: http://www.dur.ac.uk/service.mapping/amh/index.php 18 September 2004

Vasile R G 2001 Medical treatment of depression. In: Jacobson J L, Jacobson A M (eds) Psychiatric secrets (2nd edn). Hanley & Belfus, Inc., Philadelphia, p 241-252

Wallcraft J 1996 Some models of asylum and help in times of crisis. In: Tomlinson D, Carrier J (eds) Asylum in the community. Routledge, London

Whittle P, Mitchell S 1997 Community alternatives project: an evaluation of a community-based acute psychiatric team providing alternatives to admission. Journal of Mental Health 6(4):417-427.

Williams M 1997 Cry of pain: understanding suicide and self-harm. Penguin, London

INDEX